Fitness and Exercise

SOURCEBOOK

Fifth Edition

Health Reference Series

Fifth Edition

Fitness and Exercise
SOURCEBOOK

*Basic Consumer Health Information about the Benefits of
Physical Fitness, including Strength, Endurance, Longevity,
Weight Loss, Bone Health, and Stress Management, with
Exercise Guidelines for People of All Ages and Tips for
Maintaining Motivation, Measuring Exercise Intensity,
Preventing Injuries, and Exercising with a Health Condition*

*Along with Information on Exercise Equipment, Fitness
Tourism, and Wearable Technology, a Glossary of
Related Terms, and a Directory of Resources for
Additional Help and Information*

OMNIGRAPHICS

615 Griswold, Ste. 901, Detroit, MI 48226

Bibliographic Note

Because this page cannot legibly accommodate all the copyright notices, the Bibliographic Note portion of the Preface constitutes an extension of the copyright notice.

* * *

Health Reference Series
Keith Jones, *Managing Editor*
***

OMNIGRAPHICS
A PART OF RELEVANT INFORMATION
***

Copyright © 2017 Omnigraphics
ISBN 978-0-7808-1534-6
E-ISBN 978-0-7808-1535-3

Library of Congress Cataloging-in-Publication Data

Names: Omnigraphics, Inc., issuing body.

Title: Fitness and exercise sourcebook : basic consumer health information about the benefits of physical fitness, including strength, endurance, longevity, weight loss, bone health, and stress management, with exercise guidelines for people of all ages and tips for maintaining motivation, measuring exercise intensity, preventing injuries, and exercising with a health condition; along with information on different types of exercises and exercise equipment, a glossary of related terms, and a directory of resources for additional help and information.

Description: Fifth Edition. | Detroit, MI : Omnigraphics, [2016] | Series: Health Reference Series | Includes bibliographical references and index.

Identifiers: LCCN 2016037386 (print) | LCCN 2016038302 (ebook) | ISBN 9780780815346 (hardcover : acid-free paper) | ISBN 9780780815353 (eBook)

Subjects: LCSH: Physical fitness--Handbooks, manuals, etc. | Exercise--Handbooks, manuals, etc.

Classification: LCC GV436 .F53 2016 (print) | LCC GV436 (ebook) | DDC 613.7--dc23

LC record available at https://lccn.loc.gov/2016037386

5/17

Table of Contents

v

Part III: Start Moving

Part V: Fitness Safety

Part VII: Health and Wellness Trends

Part VIII: Additional Help and Information

Preface

About This Book

Regular physical activity provides numerous health benefits, including a reduced risk of diabetes, osteoporosis, obesity, some cancers, and heart disease, as well as increased mental well-being, longevity, and life satisfaction. Yet, despite the many obvious health benefits of physical activity, only 1 in 5 adults (21%) meet the physical activity guidelines established by the U.S. Department of Health and Human Services, and less than 3 in 10 high school students get at least 60 minutes of physical activity every day.

Fitness and Exercise Sourcebook, Fifth Edition, provides updated information about the health benefits of physical activity. It discusses the guidelines for physical activity in people of all ages and diverse fitness levels—including those with disabilities, chronic diseases, and other challenges. It offers suggestions for incorporating fitness into everyday activities. Ways to maintain motivation and set fitness goals are described, and different types of physical activity—including aerobic, strength, balance, and mind-body—are detailed. Information on safety concerns, nutrition and hydration, equipment needs, and wearable technology is included, and an end section offers a glossary of related terms and a directory of organizations that provide information about physical fitness and exercise.

How to Use This Book

This book is divided into parts and chapters. Parts focus on broad areas of interest. Chapters are devoted to single topics within a part.

Part I: The Health Benefits of Physical Activity details the physical and mental benefits of physical activity, including disease prevention, increased mental health, and a healthy weight. It also discusses the genetic correlation and health burden of physical inactivity.

Part II: Guidelines for Lifelong Physical Fitness offers readers specific fitness suggestions, age-appropriate guidelines, and tips for promoting physical activity among children, teenagers, adults, and the elderly.

Part III: Start Moving explores practical suggestions for adding activity to everyday life and for beginning an exercise program. It explains how to create a fitness plan, overcome barriers to exercise, find a fitness club or workout partners, and measure and track exercise intensity and calorie expenditure. It also provides tips on things to consider when joining a gym or buying exercise equipment for home.

Part IV: Exercise Basics includes facts about specific forms of exercise, from basics—such as aerobic activity and strength training—to individual activities—such as walking, cross training, biking, running, kickboxing, aquatic exercise, and bicycling. Mind-body exercises, such as yoga, Tai Chi, and Pilates, are also discussed.

Part V: Fitness Safety offers suggestions about how to be safe during physical activity through warming up, avoiding common mistakes, choosing safe and comfortable equipment, eating and hydrating properly, and preventing sports injuries. It also discusses the risks of over-training and compulsive exercise and offers tips for exercising safely out of doors.

Part VI: Physical Fitness for People with Health Conditions describes specific steps to physical fitness for people with disabilities, people who are overweight, and people with other health challenges, such as heart disease, bone disorders, breathing difficulties, diabetes, or cancer.

Part VII Health and Wellness Trends discusses recent developments in health and fitness including online training, wellness tourism, and wearable technology.

Part VIII: Additional Help and Information includes a glossary of important terms and a directory of organizations able to provide information on physical fitness and exercise topics.

Bibliographic Note

This volume contains documents and excerpts from publications issued by the following U.S. government agencies:

Agency for Healthcare Research and Quality (AHRQ); Centers for Disease Control and Prevention (CDC); Division of Commissioned Corps Personnel and Readiness (DCCPR); Federal Occupational Health (FOH); Federal Trade Commission (FTC); National Cancer Institute (NCI); National Center for Complementary and Integrative Health (NCCIH); National Heart, Lung, and Blood Institute (NHLBI); National Institute of Arthritis and Musculoskeletal and Skin Diseases (NIAMS); National Institute of Diabetes and Digestive and Kidney Diseases (NIDDK); National Institute on Aging (NIA); National Institutes of Health (NIH); NIHSeniorHealth; Office of Disease Prevention and Health Promotion (ODPHP); Office of Disease Prevention and Health Promotion (ODPHP); Office of Disease Prevention and Health Promotion (ODPHP); Office on Women's Health (OWH); Office on Women's Health(OWH); U.S. Department of Agriculture (USDA); U.S. Department of Health and Human Services (HHS); U.S. Department of Veterans Affairs (VA); U.S. Environmental Protection Agency (EPA); and WhiteHouse.gov.

In addition, this volume contains copyrighted documents from the following organization: The Nemours Foundation

It may also contain original material produced by Omnigraphics and reviewed by medical consultants.

About the Health Reference Series

The *Health Reference Series* is designed to provide basic medical information for patients, families, caregivers, and the general public. Each volume takes a particular topic and provides comprehensive coverage. This is especially important for people who may be dealing with a newly diagnosed disease or a chronic disorder in themselves or in a family member. People looking for preventive guidance, information about disease warning signs, medical statistics, and risk factors for health problems will also find answers to their questions in the *Health Reference Series*. The *Series*, however, is not intended to serve as a tool for diagnosing illness, in prescribing treatments, or as a substitute for the physician/patient relationship. All people concerned about medical symptoms or the possibility of disease are encouraged to seek professional care from an appropriate health care provider.

A Note about Spelling and Style

Health Reference Series editors use *Stedman's Medical Dictionary* as an authority for questions related to the spelling of medical terms and the *Chicago Manual of Style* for questions related to grammatical structures, punctuation, and other editorial concerns. Consistent adherence is not always possible, however, because the individual volumes within the *Series* include many documents from a wide variety of different producers, and the editor's primary goal is to present material from each source as accurately as is possible. This sometimes means that information in different chapters or sections may follow other guidelines and alternate spelling authorities.

Medical Review

Omnigraphics contracts with a team of qualified, senior medical professionals who serve as medical consultants for the *Health Reference Series*. As necessary, medical consultants review reprinted and originally written material for currency and accuracy. Citations including the phrase, "Reviewed (month, year)" indicate material reviewed by this team. Medical consultation services are provided to the *Health Reference Series* editors by:

Dr. Senthil Selvan, MBBS, DCH, MD
Dr. K. Sivanandham, MBBS, DCH, MS (Research), PhD

Our Advisory Board

We would like to thank the following board members for providing initial guidance on the development of this series:

- Dr. Lynda Baker, Associate Professor of Library and Information Science, Wayne State University, Detroit, MI

- Nancy Bulgarelli, William Beaumont Hospital Library, Royal Oak, MI

- Karen Imarisio, Bloomfield Township Public Library, Bloomfield Township, MI

- Karen Morgan, Mardigian Library, University of Michigan-Dearborn, Dearborn, MI

- Rosemary Orlando, St. Clair Shores Public Library, St. Clair Shores, MI

Health Reference Series *Update Policy*

The inaugural book in the *Health Reference Series* was the first edition of *Cancer Sourcebook* published in 1989. Since then, the *Series* has been enthusiastically received by librarians and in the medical community. In order to maintain the standard of providing high-quality health information for the layperson the editorial staff at Omnigraphics felt it was necessary to implement a policy of updating volumes when warranted.

Medical researchers have been making tremendous strides, and it is the purpose of the *Health Reference Series* to stay current with the most recent advances. Each decision to update a volume is made on an individual basis. Some of the considerations include how much new information is available and the feedback we receive from people who use the books. If there is a topic you would like to see added to the update list, or an area of medical concern you feel has not been adequately addressed, please write to:

Managing Editor
Health Reference Series
Omnigraphics
615 Griswold, Ste. 901
Detroit, MI 48226

Part One

The Health Benefits of Physical Activity

Chapter 1

Physical Activity Has Many Health Benefits

Chapter Contents

Section 1.1

An Overview of Physical Activity

This section includes text excerpted from "Physical Activity," ChooseMyPlate.gov, U.S. Department of Agriculture (USDA), June 10, 2015.

What Is Physical Activity?

Physical activity simply means movement of the body that uses energy. Walking, gardening, briskly pushing a baby stroller, climbing the stairs, playing soccer, or dancing the night away are all good examples of being active. For health benefits, physical activity should be moderate or vigorous intensity.

Moderate physical acitivities include:

- Walking briskly (about 3½ miles per hour)

- Bicycling (less than 10 miles per hour)

- General gardening (raking, trimming shrubs)

- Dancing

- Golf (walking and carrying clubs)

- Water aerobics

- Canoeing

- Tennis (doubles)

Vigorous physical activities include:

- Running/jogging (5 miles per hour)

- Walking very fast (4½ miles per hour)

- Bicycling (more than 10 miles per hour)

- Heavy yard work, such as chopping wood

- Swimming (freestyle laps)

- Aerobics

- Basketball (competitive)

- Tennis (singles)

You can choose moderate or vigorous intensity activities, or a mix of both each week. Activities can be considered vigorous, moderate, or light in intensity. This depends on the extent to which they make you breathe harder and your heart beat faster.

Only moderate and vigorous intensity activities count toward meeting your physical activity needs. With vigorous activities, you get similar health benefits in half the time it takes you with moderate ones. You can replace some or all of your moderate activity with vigorous activity. Although you are moving, light intensity activities do not increase your heart rate, so you should not count these towards meeting the physical activity recommendations. These activities include walking at a casual pace, such as while grocery shopping, and doing light household chores.

Why Is Physical Activity Important?

Regular physical activity can produce long term health benefits. People of all ages, shapes, sizes, and abilities can benefit from being physically active. The more physical activity you do, the greater the health benefits.

Being physically active can help you:

- Increase your chances of living longer

- Feel better about yourself

- Decrease your chances of becoming depressed

- Sleep well at night

- Move around more easily

- Have stronger muscles and bones

- Stay at or get to a healthy weight

- Be with friends or meet new people

- Enjoy yourself and have fun

When you are not physically active, you are more likely to:

- Get heart disease

- Get type 2 diabetes

- Have high blood pressure
- Have high blood cholesterol
- Have a stroke

Physical activity and nutrition work together for better health. Being active increases the amount of calories burned. As people age their metabolism slows, so maintaining energy balance requires moving more and eating less.

Some types of physical activity are especially beneficial:

- Aerobic activities make you breathe harder and make your heart beat faster. Aerobic activities can be moderate or vigorous in their intensity. Vigorous activities take more effort than moderate ones. For **moderate activities,** you can talk while you do them, but you can't sing. For **vigorous activities,** you can only say a few words without stopping to catch your breath.

- Muscle-strengthening activities make your muscles stronger. These include activities like push-ups and lifting weights. It is important to work all the different parts of the body–your legs, hips, back, chest, stomach, shoulders, and arms.

- Bone-strengthening activities make your bones stronger. Bone strengthening activities, like jumping, are especially important for children and adolescents. These activities produce a force on the bones that promotes bone growth and strength.

- Balance and stretching activities enhance physical stability and flexibility, which reduces risk of injuries. Examples are gentle stretching, dancing, yoga, martial arts, and Tai chi.

How Much Physical Activity Is Needed?

Physical activity is important for everyone, but how much you need depends on your age.

Adults (18–64 Years)

Adults should do at least 2 hours and 30 minutes each week of aerobic physical activity at a moderate level or 1 hour and 15 minutes each week of aerobic physical activity at a vigorous level. Being active 5 or more hours each week can provide even more health benefits. Spreading aerobic activity out over at least 3 days a week is best. Also, each activity should be done for at least 10 minutes at a time.

Adults should also do strengthening activities, like push-ups, sit-ups and lifting weights, at least 2 days a week.

Children and Adolescents (6–17 Years)

Children and adolescents should do 60 minutes or more of physical activity each day. Most of the 60 minutes should be either moderate- or vigorous intensity aerobic physical activity, and should include vigorous-intensity physical activity at least 3 days a week. As part of their 60 or more minutes of daily physical activity, children and adolescents should include muscle-strengthening activities, like climbing, at least 3 days a week and bone-strengthening activities, like jumping, at least 3 days a week. Children and adolescents are often active in short bursts of time rather than for sustained periods of time, and these short bursts can add up to meet physical activity needs. Physical activities for children and adolescents should be developmentally appropriate, fun, and offer variety.

Young Children (2–5 Years)

There is not a specific recommendation for the number of minutes young children should be active each day. Children ages 2–5 years should play actively several times each day. Their activity may happen in short bursts of time and not be all at once. Physical activities for young children should be developmentally appropriate, fun, and offer variety.

Physical activity is generally safe for everyone. The health benefits you gain from being active are far greater than the chances of getting hurt. Here are some things you can do to stay safe while you are active:

- If you haven't been active in a while, start slowly and build up.
- Learn about the types and amounts of activity that are right for you.
- Choose activities that are appropriate for your fitness level.
- Build up the time you spend before switching to activities that take more effort.
- Use the right safety gear and sports equipment.
- Choose a safe place to do your activity.
- See a healthcare provider if you have a health problem.

Section 1.2

Benefits of Physical Activity

This section includes text excerpted from "Physical Activity and Health," Centers for Disease Control and Prevention (CDC), June 4, 2015.

Control Your Weight

Looking to get to or stay at a healthy weight? Both diet and physical activity play a critical role in controlling your weight. You gain weight when the calories you burn, including those burned during physical activity, are less than the calories you eat or drink. When it comes to weight management, people vary greatly in how much physical activity they need. You may need to be more active than others to achieve or maintain a healthy weight.

To maintain your weight: Work your way up to 150 minutes of moderate-intensity aerobic activity, 75 minutes of vigorous-intensity aerobic activity, or an equivalent mix of the two each week. Strong scientific evidence shows that physical activity can help you maintain your weight over time. However, the exact amount of physical activity needed to do this is not clear since it varies greatly from person to person. It's possible that you may need to do more than the equivalent of 150 minutes of moderate-intensity activity a week to maintain your weight.

To lose weight and keep it off: You will need a high amount of physical activity unless you also adjust your diet and reduce the amount of calories you're eating and drinking. Getting to and staying at a healthy weight requires both regular physical activity and a healthy eating plan. The Centers for Disease Control and Prevention (CDC) has some great tools and information about nutrition, physical activity and weight loss.

Reduce Your Risk of Cardiovascular Disease

Heart disease and stroke are two of the leading causes of death in the United States. But following the *Physical Activity Guidelines for Americans* and getting at least 150 minutes a week (2 hours and 30 minutes) of moderate-intensity aerobic activity can put you at a lower risk for these diseases. You can reduce your risk even further with more physical activity. Regular physical activity can also lower your blood pressure and improve your cholesterol levels.

Reduce Your Risk of Type 2 Diabetes and Metabolic Syndrome

Regular physical activity can reduce your risk of developing type 2 diabetes and metabolic syndrome. Metabolic syndrome is a condition in which you have some combination of too much fat around the waist, high blood pressure, low HDL cholesterol, high triglycerides, or high blood sugar. Research shows that lower rates of these conditions are seen with 120 to 150 minutes (2 hours to 2 hours and 30 minutes) a week of at least moderate-intensity aerobic activity. And the more physical activity you do, the lower your risk will be.

Already have type 2 diabetes? Regular physical activity can help control your blood glucose levels.

Reduce Your Risk of Some Cancers

Being physically active lowers your risk for two types of cancer: colon and breast. Research shows that:

- Physically active people have a lower risk of colon cancer than do people who are not active.
- Physically active women have a lower risk of breast cancer than do people who are not active.

Reduce your risk of endometrial and lung cancer. Although the research is not yet final, some findings suggest that your risk of endometrial cancer and lung cancer may be lower if you get regular physical activity compared to people who are not active.

Improve your quality of life. If you are a cancer survivor, research shows that getting regular physical activity not only helps give you a better quality of life, but also improves your physical fitness.

Strengthen Your Bones and Muscles

As you age, it's important to protect your bones, joints and muscles. Not only do they support your body and help you move, but keeping bones, joints and muscles healthy can help ensure that you're able to do your daily activities and be physically active. Research shows that doing **aerobic, muscle-strengthening and bone-strengthening physical activity** of at least a moderately-intense level **can slow the loss of bone density** that comes with age.

Hip fracture is a serious health condition that can have life-changing negative effects, especially if you're an older adult. But research shows that people who do 120 to 300 minutes of at least moderate-intensity aerobic activity each week have a lower risk of hip fracture.

Regular physical activity helps with arthritis and other conditions affecting the joints. If you have arthritis, research shows that doing 130 to 150 (2 hours and 10 minutes to 2 hours and 30 minutes) a week of moderate-intensity, low-impact aerobic activity can not only improve your ability to manage pain and do everyday tasks, but it can also make your quality of life better.

Build strong, healthy muscles. Muscle-strengthening activities can help you increase or maintain your muscle mass and strength. Slowly increasing the amount of weight and number of repetitions you do will give you even more benefits, no matter your age.

Improve Your Mental Health and Mood

Regular physical activity can help keep your thinking, learning, and judgment skills sharp as you age. It can also reduce your risk of depression and may help you sleep better. Research has shown that doing aerobic or a mix of aerobic and muscle-strengthening activities 3 to 5 times a week for 30 to 60 minutes can give you these mental health benefits. Some scientific evidence has also shown that even lower levels of physical activity can be beneficial.

Improve Your Ability to Do Daily Activities and Prevent Falls

A functional limitation is a loss of the ability to do everyday activities such as climbing stairs, grocery shopping, or playing with your grandchildren.

How does this relate to physical activity? If you're a physically active middle-aged or older adult, you have a lower risk of functional limitations than people who are inactive

Already have trouble doing some of your everyday activities? Aerobic and muscle-strengthening activities can help improve your ability to do these types of tasks.

Are you an older adult who is at risk for falls? Research shows that doing **balance** and **muscle-strengthening activities** each week along with **moderate-intensity aerobic activity**, like brisk walking, can help reduce your risk of falling.

Increase Your Chances of Living Longer

Science shows that physical activity can reduce your risk of dying early from the leading causes of death, like heart disease and some cancers. This is remarkable in two ways:

- Only a few lifestyle choices have as large an impact on your health as physical activity. People who are physically active for about 7 hours a week have a 40 percent lower risk of dying early than those who are active for less than 30 minutes a week.

- You don't have to do high amounts of activity or vigorous-intensity activity to reduce your risk of premature death. You can put yourself at lower risk of dying early by doing at least 150 minutes a week of moderate-intensity aerobic activity.

Everyone can gain the health benefits of physical activity—age, ethnicity, shape or size do not matter.

Section 1.3

Facts about Physical Activity

This section contains text excerpted from the following sources:
Text in this section begins with excerpts from "Physical Activity
Guidelines for Americans Midcourse Report," U.S. Department of
Health and Human Services (HHS), December 12, 2012. Reviewed
September 2016; text beginning with the heading "Some Americans
Are Getting Enough, but Too Many Are Not" is excerpted from
"Facts about Physical Activity," Centers for Disease Control
and Prevention (CDC), May 20, 2014.

Regular physical activity in children and adolescents promotes
health and fitness. Compared to those who are inactive, physically
active youth have higher levels of cardiorespiratory fitness and stronger muscles. They also typically have lower body fatness. Their bones
are stronger and they may have reduced symptoms of anxiety and
depression.

Youth who are regularly active also have a better chance of a
healthy adulthood. In the past, chronic diseases, such as heart disease, hypertension, or type 2 diabetes were rare in youth. However,
a growing literature is showing that the incidence of these chronic
diseases and their risk factors are now increasing among children and
adolescents. Regular physical activity makes it less likely that these
risk factors and resulting chronic diseases will develop and more likely
that youth will remain healthy as adults.

Current Levels of Physical Activity among Youth

Despite the importance of regular physical activity in promoting
lifelong health and well-being, current evidence shows that levels of
physical activity among youth remain low, and that levels of physical
activity decline dramatically during adolescence. Opportunities for
regular physical activity are limited in many schools; daily physical
education (PE) is provided in only 4 percent of elementary schools, 8
percent of middle schools, and 2 percent of high schools.

The National Youth Risk Behavior Survey (YRBS), which collects
self-reported physical activity data from high school students across the

United States, found that many youth are not meeting the Guidelines recommendation of 60 minutes of physical activity each day:

- 29 percent of high school students participated in at least 60 minutes per day of physical activity on each of the 7 days before the survey. Boys were more than twice as likely as girls to meet the Guidelines (38% vs. 19%).

- 14 percent of high school students did not participate in 60 or more minutes of any kind of physical activity on any day during the 7 days before the survey.

A separate study of U.S. youth used accelerometers to objectively measure physical activity. This study found that 42 percent of children and only 8 percent of adolescents engaged in moderate- to vigorous-intensity activity on 5 of the past 7 days for at least 60 minutes each day.

The Benefits of Physical Activity for Youth

- Improves cardiorespiratory fitness.
- Strengthens muscles and bones.
- Helps attain/maintain healthy weight.
- Reduces likelihood of developing risk factors for later diseases, such as high blood cholesterol, high blood pressure, and type 2 diabetes, thus increasing the chances that youth will remain healthy as adults.
- May reduce symptoms of anxiety and depression.

Some Americans Are Getting Enough, but Too Many Are Not

- About 1 in 5 (21%) adults meet the 2008 Physical Activity Guidelines.
- Less than 3 in 10 high school students get at least 60 minutes of physical activity every day.
- Physical activity can improve health. People who are physically active tend to live longer and have lower risk for heart disease, stroke, type 2 diabetes, depression, and some cancers. Physical activity can also help with weight control, and may improve academic achievement in students.

- Inactive adults have a higher risk for early death, heart disease, stroke, type 2 diabetes, depression, and some cancers..

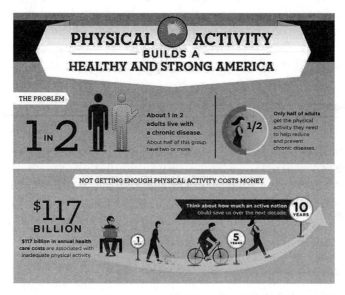

Figure 1.1. *Physical Activity Builds A Healthy and Strong America*

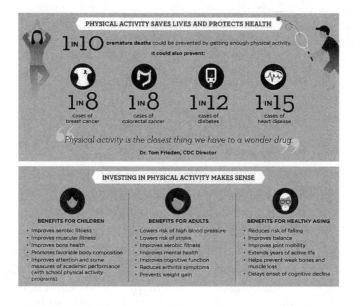

Figure 1.2. *Physical Activity Saves Lives and Protects Health*

Rates of Activity and Inactivity Vary across States and Regions

- Americans living in the South are less likely to be physically active than Americans living in the West, Northeast and Midwest regions of the country.

Some Groups Are More Physically Active than Others

- More non-Hispanic white adults (23%) meet the 2008 Physical Activity Guidelines for aerobic and muscle-strengthening activity than non-Hispanic black adults (18%) and Hispanic adults (16%).

- Men (54%) are more likely than women (46%) to meet the 2008 Physical Activity Guideline for aerobic activity.

- Younger adults are more likely to meet the 2008 Physical Activity Guideline for aerobic activity than older adults.

Physical Activity and Socioeconomic Status

- Adults with more education are more likely to meet the 2008 Physical Activity Guideline for aerobic activity than adults with less education.

- Adults whose family income is above the poverty level are more likely to meet the 2008 Physical Activity Guideline for aerobic activity than adults whose family income is at or near the poverty level.

Chapter 2

Health Burden of Physical Inactivity

Physical activity provides long-term health benefits for everyone! By being active, you will burn calories that you store from eating throughout the day and—it can be as easy as walking the dog or as rigorous as running a marathon. Providing opportunities for children to be active early on puts them on a path to better physical and mental health. It's never too late to jumpstart a healthy lifestyle.

Physical Activity and Obesity

Physical activity, along with proper nutrition, is beneficial to people of all ages, backgrounds, and abilities. And it is important that everyone gets active: over the last 20 years, there's been a significant increase in obesity in the United States. About one-third of U.S. adults (33.8%) are obese and approximately 17% (or 12.5 million) of children and adolescents (aged 2-19 years) are obese.

The health implications of obesity in America are startling:

- If things remain as they are today, one-third of all children born in the year 2000 or later may suffer from diabetes at some point in their lives, while many others are likely to face chronic health problems such as heart disease, high blood pressure, cancer, diabetes, and asthma.

This chapter includes text excerpted from "Why Is It Important?" President's Council on Fitness, Sports & Nutrition, U.S. Department of Health and Human Services (HHS), Aug 31, 2012. Reviewed September 2016.

- Studies indicate that overweight youth may never achieve a healthy weight, and up to 70% of obese teens may become obese adults.

- Even more worrisome, the cumulative effect could be that children born in the year 2000 or later may not outlive their parents.

The impact of obesity doesn't end there. Obesity has personal financial and national economic implications as well. Those who are obese have medical costs that are $1,429 more than those of normal weight on average (roughly 42% higher). And annual direct costs of childhood obesity are $14.3 billion.

By incorporating physical activity into your daily life—30 minutes for adults and 60 minutes for children—as well as healthy eating, you will experience positive health benefits and be on the path for a better future.

The Impact of Physical Activity on Your Health

Regular physical activity can produce long-term health benefits. It can help:

- Prevent chronic diseases such as heart disease, cancer, and stroke (the three leading health-related causes of death)

- Control weight

- Make your muscles stronger

- Reduce fat

- Promote strong bone, muscle, and joint development

- Condition heart and lungs

- Build overall strength and endurance

- Improve sleep

- Decrease potential of becoming depressed

- Increase your energy and self-esteem

- Relieve stress

- Increase your chances of living longer

When you are not physically active, you are more at risk for:

- High blood pressure
- High blood cholesterol
- Stroke
- Type 2 diabetes
- Heart disease
- Cancer

Chapter 3

Physical Activity and Disease Prevention

Chapter Contents

Section 3.1

Physical Fitness and a Healthy Immune System

Exercise has been proven to improve both physical and mental well-being. It keeps a check on obesity, diabetes, high blood pressure, stroke, and stress, among other unhealthy and possibly fatal conditions. A number of studies on colds now also show that regular, moderate exercise can boost an individual's immunity and protect against certain illnesses.

Recent research demonstrates that physical activity triggers physiological changes in the immune system. For example, exercise can increase the production of macrophages, a type of white blood cell that targets and attacks bacteria and other foreign particles in the body, thus reducing the chance of contracting certain illnesses, particularly upper respiratory-tract infections. Exercise also accelerates the circulation of these fighter cells throughout the system, resulting in significantly improved immunity. When a person exercises, the body temperature rises for a short while, and it is believed that this may also prevent bacterial development.

Too much exercise, however, can actually do more harm than good. Though stress-hormones are released more slowly when the body is physically active, thus reducing the probability of falling ill, high-intensity activity over an extended period of time could elevate stress and cause an increase in the number of white blood cells. Conventional cardio routines can cause inflammation, thickening of arteries and heart muscle, arrhythmias, and in some rare cases, stroke and sudden cardiac arrest. This is occasionally seen in athletes participating in marathons and triathlons, in which the extreme activity can make them more prone to infections. It therefore becomes important to keep in mind how much and what type of exercise is ideal for any given individual, as well as the appropriate conditions under which to engage in physical activity. Essentially, giving the body enough time to rest and repair after a challenging fitness routine increases the benefits gained from exercise.

Exercise—A Preventive Medication

Years of research has demonstrated that physical exercise provides numerous preventative health benefits, one of the most important being its effect on insulin and leptin receptor sensitivity by regulating the levels of glucose, insulin, and leptin in the body. This prevents chronic infections and improves overall health. Being physically active can also help reduce the risk of stroke. And sitting too much has been shown to be a risk factor for chronic diseases. Studies demonstrate that people who sit for extended periods of time double their risk for diabetes and heart disease compared to those who sit for shorter durations. Frequent movements, some as simple as standing up and stretching in place every 15 minutes, can help neutralize the negative effects of prolonged inactivity. Ideally, this should be combined with effective aerobic, core, and muscle-strengthening activities two to three times per week.

Exercise for Fighting Cold and Flu

Exercise improves the circulation of certain disease-fighting agents of the immune system throughout the body, which subsequently aids in identifying and countering an illness before it begins to spread. Colds and influenza, among other illness, can be prevented by keeping the body physically engaged. Studies report that moderate-intensity activities, such as a walk for 20 to 30 minutes each day, or biking or going to the gym a few times per week, effectively reduce the chance of getting a cold by boosting the number of white blood cells that fight infections. It is also highly recommended that a person spends two and half hours on vigorous exercise each week to avoid catching the flu.

However, it is best to avoid exercising when one has a cold, particularly when taking medication, such as decongestants, as this may overstress the heart by forcing it to beat too fast. Exercise could also place undue stress on the body if one has a fever with a cold, and it could possibly slow down recovery, as well.

Checking with a Doctor

A doctor should be consulted if a person with a cold exercises and experiences chest congestion and/or coughing and wheezing.

Emergency medical attention is required if the person's breathing becomes labored, or if he or she feels faint or dizzy, has trouble balancing, and feels pressure or tightness in chest. If an asthmatic person has a cold, a doctor's advice should be sought before engaging in strenuous physical activity.

References

1.   Brown, Jim. "How Exercise Affects Immunity," EXOS Knowledge, March 11, 2013.

2.   Mercola, Joseph, D.O. "Do You Exercise Enough to Protect Your Health?" Mercola Peak Fitness, March 28, 2014.

3.   Mercola, Joseph, D.O. "Doctors Prescribe Exercise as 'Best Preventive Drug,'" Mercola Peak Fitness, January 10, 2014.

4.   Robinson, Jennifer. "Exercise and the Common Cold," WebMD, January 20, 2015.

Section 3.2

Peak Longevity Benefit with an Hour of Daily Exercise

This section includes text excerpted from "Study Reports Peak Longevity Benefit with an Hour of Daily Exercise," National Cancer Institute (NCI), April 6, 2015.

A study has found that people who engage in three to five times the recommended minimum level of leisure-time physical activity derive the greatest benefit in terms of mortality reduction when compared with people who do not engage in leisure-time physical activity. *The 2008 Physical Activity Guidelines for Americans*, developed by the U.S. Department of Health and Human Services' (HHS) Physical Activity Guidelines Advisory Committee, recommend a minimum of 2.5 hours of moderate-intensity exercise per week or 1.25 hours of vigorous aerobic activity, but more activity is encouraged for additional health benefits.

Before this study, experts did not know how much additional health benefit might accrue for those doing more exercise. This study confirms that much of the mortality benefit is realized by meeting the minimum recommended levels of physical activity and describes the increased mortality benefit associated with higher levels of physical activity. The study appeared online April 6, 2015, in *JAMA Internal Medicine*.

1. Engaging in one to two times the recommended minimum level of leisure-time physical activity (i.e., 2.5 to 5 hours of moderate-intensity activity, such as walking, or 1.25 to 2.5 hours of vigorous-intensity activity, such as running) provided much of the observed longevity benefits: a 31 percent lower risk of death compared with people who did no leisure-time physical activity.

2. At three to five times the recommended minimum level of leisure-time physical activity the benefit appeared to level off at a 39 percent lower risk of death, compared with those who did no leisure-time physical activity. This level of exercise could be achieved by:

   • walking 7 hours per week

   • biking leisurely 5 hours per week

   • running at a 10 minute/mile pace for 2.25 hours per week

3. At 10 or more times the recommended minimum level of leisure-time physical activity there was no additional mortality benefit, but there was also no increased risk of death.

Section 3.3

Physical Activity Promotes Bone Health

This section includes text excerpted from "Exercise for Your Bone Health," National Institute of Arthritis and Musculoskeletal and Skin Diseases (NIAMS), May 2015.

Why Exercise?

Like muscle, bone is living tissue that responds to exercise by becoming stronger. Young women and men who exercise regularly generally achieve greater peak bone mass (maximum bone density and strength) than those who do not. For most people, bone mass peaks during the third decade of life. After that time, we can begin to lose bone. Women and men older than age 20 can help prevent bone loss with regular exercise. Exercising allows us to maintain muscle strength, coordination, and balance, which in turn helps to prevent falls and related fractures. This is especially important for older adults and people who have been diagnosed with osteoporosis.

The Best Bone Building Exercise

The best exercise for your bones is the weight-bearing kind, which forces you to work against gravity. Some examples of weight-bearing exercises include weight training, walking, hiking, jogging, climbing stairs, tennis, and dancing. Examples of exercises that are not weight-bearing include swimming and bicycling. Although these activities help build and maintain strong muscles and have excellent cardiovascular benefits, they are not the best way to exercise your bones.

Exercise Tips

If you have health problems—such as heart trouble, high blood pressure, diabetes, or obesity—or if you are age 40 or older, check with your doctor before you begin a regular exercise program.

According to the Surgeon General, the optimal goal is at least 30 minutes of physical activity on most days, preferably daily.

Listen to your body. When starting an exercise routine, you may have some muscle soreness and discomfort at the beginning, but this should not be painful or last more than 48 hours. If it does, you may be working too hard and need to ease up. *Stop exercising if you have any chest pain or discomfort,* and see your doctor before your next exercise session.

If you have osteoporosis, ask your doctor which activities are safe for you. If you have low bone mass, experts recommend that you protect your spine by avoiding exercises or activities that flex, bend, or twist it. Furthermore, you should avoid high-impact exercise to lower the risk of breaking a bone. You also might want to consult with an exercise specialist to learn the proper progression of activity, how to stretch and strengthen muscles safely, and how to correct poor posture habits. An exercise specialist should have a degree in exercise physiology, physical education, physical therapy, or a similar specialty. Be sure to ask if he or she is familiar with the special needs of people with osteoporosis.

A Complete Osteoporosis Program

Remember, exercise is only one part of an osteoporosis prevention or treatment program. Like a diet rich in calcium and vitamin D, exercise helps strengthen bones at any age. But proper exercise and diet may not be enough to stop bone loss caused by medical conditions, menopause, or lifestyle choices such as tobacco use and excessive alcohol consumption. It is important to speak with your doctor about your bone health. Discuss whether you might be a candidate for a bone mineral density test. If you are diagnosed with low bone mass, ask what medications might help keep your bones strong.

Section 3.4

The Effect of Physical Activity on the Risk for Coronary Heart Disease

This section includes text excerpted from "What Is Coronary Heart Disease?" National Heart, Lung, and Blood Institute (NHLBI), June 22, 2016.

What Is Coronary Heart Disease?

Coronary heart disease (CHD) is a disease in which a waxy substance called plaque builds up inside the coronary arteries. These arteries supply oxygen-rich blood to your heart muscle.

When plaque builds up in the arteries, the condition is called atherosclerosis. The buildup of plaque occurs over many years.

Over time, plaque can harden or rupture (break open). Hardened plaque narrows the coronary arteries and reduces the flow of oxygen-rich blood to the heart.

If the plaque ruptures, a blood clot can form on its surface. A large blood clot can mostly or completely block blood flow through a coronary artery. Over time, ruptured plaque also hardens and narrows the coronary arteries.

Overview

If the flow of oxygen-rich blood to your heart muscle is reduced or blocked, angina or a heart attack can occur.

Angina is chest pain or discomfort. It may feel like pressure or squeezing in your chest. The pain also can occur in your shoulders, arms, neck, jaw, or back. Angina pain may even feel like indigestion.

A heart attack occurs if the flow of oxygen-rich blood to a section of heart muscle is cut off. If blood flow isn't restored quickly, the section of heart muscle begins to die. Without quick treatment, a heart attack can lead to serious health problems or death.

Over time, CHD can weaken the heart muscle and lead to heart failure and arrhythmias. Heart failure is a condition in which your heart can't pump enough blood to meet your body's needs. Arrhythmias are problems with the rate or rhythm of the heartbeat.

Outlook

Lifestyle changes, medicines, and medical procedures can help prevent or treat coronary heart disease. These treatments may reduce the risk of related health problems.

How Can Coronary Heart Disease Be Prevented or Delayed?

You can prevent and control coronary heart disease (CHD) by taking action to control your risk factors with heart-healthy lifestyle changes and medicines. Examples of risk factors you can control include high blood cholesterol, high blood pressure, and overweight and obesity. Only a few risk factors—such as age, gender, and family history—can't be controlled.

Your risk for CHD increases with the number of risk factors you have. To reduce your risk of CHD and heart attack, try to control each risk factor you have by adopting the following heart-healthy lifestyles:

- Heart-healthy eating
- Maintaining a healthy weight
- Managing stress
- Physical activity
- Quitting smoking

Know your family history of health problems related to CHD. If you or someone in your family has CHD, be sure to tell your doctor. If lifestyle changes aren't enough, you also may need medicines to control your CHD risk factors.

Physical Activity

Routine physical activity and reduction in sedentary lifestyle can improve physical fitness, lower many heart disease risk factors such as bad LDL cholesterol levels and increasing good HDL cholesterol levels in the blood, controlling high blood pressure, and helping you lose excess weight. Physical activity also can lower your risk for type 2 diabetes.

Everyone should try to participate in moderate-intensity aerobic exercise at least 2 hours and 30 minutes per week, or vigorous aerobic exercise for 1 hour and 15 minutes per week. Aerobic exercise, such as brisk walking, is any exercise in which your heart beats faster and you use more oxygen than usual. The more active you are, the more you will benefit. Participate in aerobic exercise for at least 10 minutes at a time spread throughout the week.

Talk with your doctor before you start a new exercise plan. Ask your doctor how much and what kinds of physical activity are safe for you.

Another way you can begin to increase your activity level is by reducing how long you sit at a given time. People who sit for long periods of time have been found to have higher rates of heart disease, diabetes, and death. Reducing sedentary behavior by breaking up how long you sit will benefit your overall health.

Chapter 4

Physical Activity and Mental Health

Chapter Contents

Section 4.1

Physical Activity Can Help the Brain

This section contains text excerpted from the following sources: Text in this section begins with excerpts from "Do Exercise and Physical Activity Protect the Brain?" Go4Life, National Institute on Aging (NIA), August 16, 2013; Text beginning with the heading "Exercise Can Help Treat and Prevent Many Common Health Problems" is excerpted from "Walking to Wellness," U.S. Department of Veterans Affairs (VA), December 7, 2015.

Exercise and physical activity have many benefits. Studies show they are good for our hearts, waistlines, and ability to carry out everyday activities, but what about brain health?

Some studies suggest that exercise also may play a role in reducing risk for Alzheimer disease and age-related cognitive decline, and research in this area is continuing.

Animal studies found that exercise increases both the number of small blood vessels that supply blood to the brain and the number of connections between nerve cells. In addition, exercise raises the level of a protein in an area of the brain important to memory and learning.

Research in humans shows that exercise can stimulate the brain's ability to maintain old network connections and make new ones vital to healthy cognition. For example, in a year-long study, older people exercised daily, walking for 40 minutes or doing stretching and toning exercises. At the end of the study, the walking group showed improved connectivity in the part of the brain engaged in daydreaming, envisioning the future, and recalling the past, as well as improved ability to plan and organize tasks such as cooking a meal.

We don't know yet what prevents Alzheimer disease or age-related cognitive decline, but we do know that a healthy lifestyle that includes a healthy diet, physical activity, appropriate weight, and not smoking can maintain and improve overall health and well-being. Making healthy choices can lower the risk of certain chronic diseases, like heart disease and diabetes. Scientists are very interested in the possibility that a healthy lifestyle also might have a beneficial effect on Alzheimer disease. In the meantime, people of all ages can benefit from taking positive steps to get and stay healthy.

Exercise Can Help Treat and Prevent Many Common Health Problems

Most adults in the United States today do not spend enough time exercising to get optimal benefits. People with anxiety and depression symptoms tend to be even less active than people who do not experience these emotional symptoms. Although there is substantial scientific evidence showing that exercise can help manage anxiety and depression, there are few intervention materials that are especially designed to help people use exercise for emotional health. The benefits of exercise on physical health, including decreased risk of cardiovascular disease, stroke, type 2 diabetes, breast and colon cancer, and osteoporosis are now widely recognized. Additional benefits for older adults include reduced risk of falls and protecting physical and cognitive function. Many scientific reviews support the value of exercise as part of recovery plans for mental illness, treatment for depression, and improved quality of life in varied patient populations.

A Cochrane Database review of 39 controlled clinical trials, a meta-analysis of studies that only included patients with clinically significant depression, and a meta-analysis of 90 articles on depressive symptoms in patients with chronic illness all concluded that aerobic exercise reduces depression symptoms. One study found that exercise could be as effective as adding a second anti-depressant medication and another found less relapse in patients with depression who exercised. Although the smaller number of trials of exercise for anxiety outcomes requires more cautious conclusions, controlled studies have shown that exercise reduces anxiety sensitivity and anxiety symptoms. Exercise also reduces reactivity to stressful stimuli. Positive effects of exercise on sleep in middle aged and older adults with insomnia were recently confirmed in a meta-analysis. A carefully controlled trial found clear dose-response relationships between exercise and improvements in self-reported mental and physical quality of life (QoL) in sedentary women. Reviews have also shown mental health (MH) benefits for cancer survivors and for osteoarthritis pain. Almost everyone could potentially receive multiple benefits from regular exercise.

Exercise Benefits Occur across a Wide Dose Range Achievable by Almost All Adults

Although the public health exercise recommendations for moderate intensity aerobic exercise for at least 10 minutes at a time, accumulating to at least 30 minutes total on at least 5 days each week also seem optimal for MH, exercise of lower intensity and duration also has meaningful physical and mental health benefits. "Incidental" short bursts of moderate intensity activity of less than 10 minutes are positively associated with cardiorespiratory fitness. Exercising for just 10 minutes improves vigor, fatigue, and overall mood. Easy-paced regular walking protects cognition in aging women. Exercise at only 50% of public health recommended levels produces significant improvement in QoL; and even low levels of activity that do not meet recommended guidelines can prevent future depression.

Biological and Psychosocial Mechanisms for Exercise Effects on Mental Health

Potential physiologic mechanisms that are especially relevant to MH include favorable effects of exercise on inflammation, serotonin metabolism, the hypothalamic-pituitary-adrenal axis, autonomic nervous system, endogenous endorphins, and neurotropic factors that could augment learning and extinction processes in cognitive-behavioral therapy. Another theoretical mechanism for exercise in MH is behavioral activation, increasing opportunities for positive interactions with the environment, and positive reinforcement. Some of these effects take weeks or months, but most people want to feel better quickly.

Studies examining the determinants of the increase in positive affect that can last several hours after exercising have identified that self-regulated pace and intensity (rather than prescribed) seem best; pleasant environments and cognitive processes during the experience also may be important. Psychosocial mechanisms that can operate within a single exercise bout, as well as across time, include building self-efficacy and a sense of mastery from meeting a desired goal and persisting in spite of discomfort, inconvenience, and other challenges.

Section 4.2

Physical Activity and Depression

This section includes text excerpted from "Physical Activity Guidelines Advisory Committee Report," Office of Disease Prevention and Health Promotion (ODPHP), U.S. Department of Health and Human Services (HHS), September 15, 2003. Reviewed September 2016.

The American Psychiatric Association (APA) recognizes four types of mood disorders:
1. depression
2. bipolar or manic-depressive disorder
3. mood disorders due to a medical condition
4. substance-induced mood disorders

Depression has an annual prevalence of about 8 percent among women and 4 percent among men worldwide and in the United States. The annual cost of depression in the United States is estimated at $83 billion per year. This condition includes a mild chronic form, *dysthymia*, and a more severe form, *major depressive disorder*. The rate of major depression has increased steadily during the past 50 years, with a lifetime prevalence of about 16%; the rate is higher among Hispanics than whites, and lowest, though still substantial, among African Americans. The lifetime rate of depression among adults aged 30 to 60 years is about twice the rate among people older than age 60 years.

People have a major depressive episode when they have depressed mood or lose interest or pleasure in normal activities most of the time for at least 2 weeks. Other symptoms include abnormalities in appetite, libido, sleep, energy levels, concentration and, often, suicidal thoughts. In some cases, anxiety and motor agitation can be more prominent symptoms than depressed mood. Also, mood disturbance can be less apparent than other features such as irritability, abuse of alcohol, and worsening of comorbid phobias, obsessions, or preoccupation with physical symptoms. Depression is not considered a major depressive episode if it is caused by grief (less than 2 months), drug abuse or medication, or a medical condition such as hyperthyroidism, heart disease, diabetes, multiple sclerosis, hepatitis, or rheumatoid arthritis. Many older patients with symptoms of depression do not meet the full criteria for major depressive disorder. If they have similar, but fewer, symptoms they may have *minor depression*, a sub-syndromal form of depression.

Does Physical Activity Protect Against the Onset of Depression Disorders or Depression Symptoms?

The scientific evidence from prospective cohort studies and randomized controlled trials (RCTs) supports the overall conclusion that regular participation in moderate-to-vigorous physical activity is associated with improved aspects of mental well-being and reduced symptoms of several mental health disorders. Population-based, prospective cohort studies provide substantial evidence that regular physical activity protects against the onset of depression symptoms and major depressive disorder. Evidence is insufficient to draw conclusions about bipolar disorder and other mood disorders. An association between physical activity and reduced symptoms of depression among adults has been generally supported in more than 100 population-based observational studies published since 1995, including nationally representative samples of nearly 190,000 Americans. Most of the studies looked at cross-sectional associations, which indicated that active people on average had nearly 45 percent lower odds of depression symptoms than did inactive people. In the national samples of Americans, active people had approximately 30 percent lower odds of depression.

Does Physical Activity Reduce Symptoms of Depression?

The results of RCTs indicate that participation in physical activity programs reduces depression symptoms in people diagnosed as depressed, healthy adults, and medical patients without psychiatric disorders. A meta-analysis of 14 RCTs of chronic exercise among people diagnosed with depression reported a cumulative, mean reduction in depression symptoms. However, the studies had scientific weaknesses that made it hard to conclude that the reduced depression symptoms were the independent result of exercise, and only 2 of the studies had been published after 1995. Since that review, at least 11 RCTs have used exercise training to reduce depression symptoms in about 500 depressed patients. In 3 studies, depression was identified using cut-point scores on symptom questionnaires that have good predictive validity as screening tests to detect depression.

Section 4.3

Physical Activity and Exercise for Alzheimer Disease

This section contains text excerpted from "Alzheimer's Caregiving Tips," National Institutes of Health (NIH), July 2012. Reviewed September 2016.

Being active and getting exercise helps people with Alzheimer disease (AD) feel better. Exercise helps keep their muscles, joints, and heart in good shape. It also helps people stay at a healthy weight and have regular toilet and sleep habits. You can exercise together to make it more fun.

You want someone with AD to do as much as possible for himself or herself. At the same time, you need to make sure that the person is safe when active.

Getting Started

Here are some tips for helping the person with Alzheimer disease (AD) stay active:

- Be realistic about how much activity can be done at one time. Several 10-minute "mini-workouts" may be best.

- Take a walk together each day. Exercise is good for caregivers, too!

- Make sure the person with Alzheimer disease has an ID bracelet with your phone number if he or she walks alone.

- Check your local TV guide to see if there is a program to help older adults exercise, or watch exercise videos/DVDs made for older people.

- Add music to the exercises if it helps the person with Alzheimer disease. Dance to the music if possible.

- Break exercises into simple, easy-to-follow steps.

- Make sure the person wears comfortable clothes and shoes that fit well and are made for exercise.

- Make sure he or she drinks water or juice after exercise.

Gentle Exercise

Some people with AD may not be able to get around well. This is another problem that becomes more challenging to deal with as the disease gets worse. Some possible reasons for this include:

- Trouble with endurance

- Poor coordination

- Sore feet or muscles

- Illness

- Depression or general lack of interest

Even if people have trouble walking, they may be able to:

- Do simple tasks around the home, such as sweeping and dusting.

- Use a stationary bike.

- Use soft rubber exercise balls or balloons for stretching or throwing back and forth.

- Use stretching bands, which you can buy in sporting goods stores. Be sure to follow the instructions.

- Lift weights or household items such as soup cans.

Chapter 5

Physical Activity and a Healthy Weight

Regular physical activity is important for good health, and it's especially important if you're trying to lose weight or to maintain a healthy weight.

- When losing weight, more physical activity increases the number of calories your body uses for energy or "burns off." The burning of calories through physical activity, combined with reducing the number of calories you eat, creates a "calorie deficit" that results in weight loss.

- Most weight loss occurs because of decreased caloric intake. However, evidence shows the only way to maintain weight loss is to be engaged in regular physical activity.

- Most importantly, physical activity reduces risks of cardiovascular disease and diabetes beyond that produced by weight reduction alone.

Physical activity also helps to:

- Maintain weight.

This chapter contains text excerpted from the following sources: Text in this chapter begins with excerpts from "Physical Activity for a Healthy Weight," Centers for Disease Control and Prevention (CDC), May 15, 2015; Text beginning with the heading "Should I Take Any Precautions before Becoming More Active?" is excerpted from "Getting Started with Physical Activity for a Healthy Weight," Centers for Disease Control and Prevention (CDC), May 15, 2015.

- Reduce high blood pressure.

- Reduce risk for type 2 diabetes, heart attack, stroke, and several forms of cancer.

- Reduce arthritis pain and associated disability.

- Reduce risk for osteoporosis and falls.

- Reduce symptoms of depression and anxiety.

How Much Physical Activity Do I Need?

When it comes to weight management, people vary greatly in how much physical activity they need. Here are some guidelines to follow:

- **To maintain your weight**: Work your way up to 150 minutes of moderate-intensity aerobic activity, 75 minutes of vigorous-intensity aerobic activity, or an equivalent mix of the two each week. Strong scientific evidence shows that physical activity can help you maintain your weight over time. However, the exact amount of physical activity needed to do this is not clear since it varies greatly from person to person. It's possible that you may need to do more than the equivalent of 150 minutes of moderate-intensity activity a week to maintain your weight.

- **To lose weight and keep it off**: You will need a high amount of physical activity unless you also adjust your diet and reduce the amount of calories you're eating and drinking. Getting to and staying at a healthy weight requires both regular physical activity and a healthy eating plan.

What Do Moderate- and Vigorous-Intensity Mean?

Moderate: While performing the physical activity, if your breathing and heart rate is noticeably faster but you can still carry on a conversation—it's probably moderately intense. Examples include:

- Walking briskly (a 15-minute mile).

- Light yard work (raking/bagging leaves or using a lawn mower).

- Light snow shoveling.

- Actively playing with children.

- Biking at a casual pace.

Vigorous: Your heart rate is increased substantially and you are breathing too hard and fast to have a conversation, it's probably vigorously intense. Examples include"

- Jogging/running.

- Swimming laps.

- Rollerblading/inline skating at a brisk pace.

- Cross-country skiing.

- Most competitive sports (football, basketball, or soccer).

- Jumping rope.

How Many Calories Are Used in Typical Activities?

The following table shows calories used in common physical activities at both moderate and vigorous levels.

Table 5.1. Calories Used per Hour in Common Physical Activities

Moderate Physical Activity	Approximate Calories/30 Minutes for a 154 lb Person	Approximate Calories/Hr for a 154 lb Person
Hiking	185	370
Light gardening/yard work	165	330
Dancing	165	330
Golf (walking and carrying clubs)	165	330
Bicycling (<10 mph)	145	290
Walking (3.5 mph)	140	280
Weight lifting (general light workout)	110	220
Stretching	90	180
Vigorous Physical Activity	**Approximate Calories/30 Minutes for a 154 lb Person**	**Approximate Calories/Hr for a 154 lb Person**
Running/jogging (5 mph)	295	590
Bicycling (>10 mph)	295	590
Swimming (slow freestyle laps)	255	510

Table 5.1. Continued

Moderate Physical Activity	Approximate Calories/30 Minutes for a 154 lb Person	Approximate Calories/Hr for a 154 lb Person
Aerobics	240	480
Walking (4.5 mph)	230	460
Heavy yard work (chopping wood)	220	440
Weight lifting (vigorous effort)	220	440
Basketball (vigorous)	220	440

Should I Take Any Precautions before Becoming More Active?

People with chronic diseases, such as a heart condition, arthritis, diabetes, or high blood pressure, should talk to their doctor about what types and amounts of physical activity are appropriate.

Get Motivated!

If you've not been physically active in a while, you may be wondering how to get started again. Lace up those sneakers and find some motivating ideas here.

Here are some tips to help get you started:

- Look for opportunities to reduce sedentary time and to increase active time. For example, instead of watching TV, try taking a walk after dinner.

- Set aside specific times for physical activity in your schedule to make it part of your daily or weekly routine.

- Start with activities, locations, and times you enjoy. For example, some people might like walking in their neighborhood in the mornings; others might prefer an exercise class at a health club after work.

- Try activities with friends or family members to help with motivation and mutual encouragement.

- Start slowly and work your way up to more physically challenging activities. For many people, walking is a particularly good place to begin.

- When necessary, break up your daily activity goal into smaller amounts of time. For example, you could break the 30-minute a day recommendation into three 10-minute sessions or two 15-minute sessions. Just make sure the shorter sessions are at least 10 minutes long.

Strategies for Overcoming Obstacles to Physical Activity

If you're just getting started, you might face certain obstacles that seem difficult to overcome. A few examples of common obstacles and strategies for overcoming them are shown in the following table.

Table 5.2. Strategies for Overcoming Obstacles to Physical Activity

Obstacle	Try This
I just don't have time to be physically active.	Identify available time slots. Monitor your daily activities for one week. Identify at least three 30-minute time slots you could use for physical activity.
I don't have anyone to go with me.	Develop new friendships with physically active people. Join a group, such as the YMCA or a hiking club.
I'm so tired when I get home from work.	Schedule physical activity for times in the day or week when you feel energetic.
I have so much on my "to do" list already, how can I do physical activity too?	Plan ahead. Make physical activity a regular part of your daily or weekly schedule by writing it on your calendar. Keep the appointment with yourself.
I'll probably hurt myself if I try to be more physically active.	Consult with a health professional or educational material to learn how to exercise appropriately considering your age, fitness level, skill level, and health status.
I'm not coordinated enough to be physically active. I can't learn something new at my age!	Select activities requiring no new skills, such as walking, climbing stairs, or jogging.
My job requires me to be on the road, it's impossible for me to exercise.	Stay in places with swimming pools or exercise facilities. Or find a DVD exercise tape that you enjoy and request a DVD player with your room.
I have small children and it's impossible to have time to myself for exercise.	Trade babysitting time with a friend, neighbor, or family member who also has small children. As children get older, family bike rides or walks might be another option.

Chapter 6

Is Physical Inactivity Genetic?

Level of Physical Activity

To understand whether genes can influence physical activity, let's begin by making a distinction between *physical inactivity* and *level of physical activity*. Physical inactivity is a construct of great importance for a proper understanding of the relationships between behavior and risks for a number of diseases and even premature death. Indeed, a sedentary lifestyle, which is dominated by physical inactivity, has been recognized as a major risk factor for hypertension, coronary heart disease, stroke, type 2 diabetes, obesity, and other conditions. The other important concept, level of physical activity, reflects the variation in activity from a small amount of light exercise performed occasionally to a large amount executed every day. Research has clearly shown that an active lifestyle, with even a moderate amount of physical activity almost every day, is quite beneficial in terms of prevention of cardiovascular events, type 2 diabetes, and premature death.

Human variation in degree of physical inactivity or amount of physical activity in a typical day is quite large. For instance, physical inactivity is the way of life in quadriplegic individuals, is almost complete

This chapter includes text excerpted from "Are People Physically Inactive Because of Their Genes?" President's Council on Fitness, Sports, and Nutrition (www.fitness.gov), U.S. Department of Health and Human Services (HHS), June 2006. Reviewed September 2016.

in people who are bedridden for some reasons or who have lost some of their mobility because of disease or senescence, and is pervasive in people who have a sedentary occupation. For instance, the amount of energy expended at rest in the reclining or sitting position is about 1,500 kcal per day in a 165-pound young adult male, but energy expenditure for physical activity of any kind may range from as low as about 100 kcal (for a bedridden patient) to almost 300 kcal or so for a couch potato, a very sedentary individual. In contrast, the range of energy expenditure associated with physical activity is much larger for people who engage in voluntary regular exercise. Thus, a young male may typically expend a total of 400 to 500 kcal when he exercises for about 30 minutes at moderate intensity, while a professional cyclist with the same body mass competing in very demanding races (such as the Tour de France) may expend as many as 6,000 kcal per day.

Even though this enormous range of physical activity level (and related energy expenditure) is best represented by a more or less normal distribution, it is useful for a number of purposes to categorize people in two activity phenotype groups: the physically inactive (or sedentary) group and the physically active group. It is also relevant for research and perhaps clinical purposes to use a third category, based on the distinction between those who are physically active and those who are engaging in very demanding exercise programs. However, for the purpose of this review and considering the dearth of data on the topic in general, only the former is focussed: the physical inactivity and moderate level of physical activity phenotypes (as measured behavioral traits). The fundamental question that is addressed is whether human genetic variation contributes to the observation that there are individuals who are reliably physically inactive and others who readily adopt and maintain a physically active lifestyle.

Challenging the Common Dogma

Research on the determinants of a sedentary lifestyle or level of physical activity is typically rooted in paradigms that incorporate social factors, economic circumstances, time constraint, equipment and facilities, education level, etc. Despite the fact that it is never stated as such, the behaviorists engaged in this field of research assume by and large that biology has little to do with human variation in physical activity level or the adoption of a physically inactive lifestyle. To oversimplify, the underlying assumption is that individuals are born with a blank slate, with an almost infinite ability to learn and adopt desirable behavior. For quite some time, it was expressed that the view that these research paradigms needed to be broadened and enriched to include biological determinants, including genetic factors and epigenetic events as well. Unfortunately, the interest in the biological basis of physical activity does not have a long history.

Several lines of evidence can be invoked to support the hypothesis that biology plays a role among the determinants of physical inactivity and physical activity levels.

- First, current models that do not incorporate biological influences account for only a moderate fraction of the variance in physical activity levels and do not discriminate fully between sedentary and physically active people.

- Second, most people who begin to exercise with the goal of becoming more physically active revert to a sedentary lifestyle. Low adherence rates diminish the public health value of regular physical activity and the preventive and therapeutic potential of regular exercise.

- Third, there are family lines with high rates of sedentary behavior as opposed to others in which all members are quite active as shown by a whole series of twin and family studies.

- Fourth, the heritability coefficients (quantitative indicators of the contribution of genetic inheritance to human variation in a trait) for physical activity level and sedentarism are statistically significant and meaningful from a behavioral perspective.

- Fifth, the genome-wide screening studies in animal models and in one human study have identified several regions on chromosomes that appear to harbor genes and DNA sequence variants that contribute to variation in activity levels among individuals.

- Sixth, a few genes exhibiting DNA sequence differences among people have already been associated with human variation in activity level or physical inactivity.

- Seventh, there is highly suggestive evidence from animal studies that maternal nutritional status and other in utero or perinatal factors cause alterations (epigenetic events) in the levels of gene expression without altering DNA sequence, thus setting the stage for stable changes in physiology.

Evidence from Twin Studies

Much can be learned from observations made in pairs of identical (monozygotic) and fraternal (dizygotic) twins. Quite informative are the studies in which such observations were made on twin brothers or sisters who were separated for a variety of reasons early in life and who have lived apart ever since. Unfortunately no such studies have been reported for physical inactivity or level of physical activity. On the other hand, more than a dozen studies have been conducted with pairs of twin raised together and the findings from these studies have been reviewed elsewhere. To illustrate the major findings from these twin observational studies, the one performed with the largest sample size is relied.

In a large cohort of monozygotic and dizygotic male twin pairs over 18 years of age from the Finnish Twin Registry, information on intensity and duration of activity, years of participation in a given activity, and physical activity on the job was obtained from a questionnaire. A physical activity score was generated from these variables, which was then used to compute correlations within pairs of brothers of each twin type. The correlation for the physical activity score reached 0.57 in 1,537 pairs of monozygotic twins and 0.26 in 3,507 pairs of dizygotic twins. The results indicated that heritability accounted for 62 percent of the physical activity score. Other twin studies have generated higher heritability estimates for indicators of physical activity levels but many more have yielded heritability values in the 40 percent to 50 percent range.

Evidence from Family Studies

Physical activity levels and patterns in children and their parents tend to be similar. A good number of studies have been reported on the relationships between the level of physical activity and a few on the level of sedentarism in parents and their offspring. Only a few examples will be mentioned here.

Detailed analyses of the questionnaire on physical activity habits available on 18,073 individuals living in households from the 1981 Canada Fitness Survey and from a three-day diary obtained in 1,610 subjects from 375 families in Phase 1 of the Québec Family Study generated familial correlations that ranged from 0.2 to 0.3 for various indicators of physical activity. More recently, it was reported that maximal heritabilities reached 25% for an indicator of physical inactivity and 19% for a total physical activity score.

In an interesting study, 100 children, aged four to seven years, and 99 mothers and 92 fathers from the Framingham Children's Study were monitored with an accelerometer for about 10 hours per day for more than one week in children and parents over the course of one year. Active fathers were 3.5 times more likely to have active offspring and active mothers were 2.0 times more likely to have active offspring than inactive fathers or mothers, respectively. When both parents were active, the children were 5.8 times more likely to be active as children of two inactive parents. These results are thus compatible with the notion that genetic or other factors transmitted across generations predispose a child to be active or inactive.

Evidence from Animal Models

Experimental studies in informative animal models provide several examples of how naturally occurring DNA mutations and laboratory-induced changes in key genes may affect physical activity levels and patterns. For example, mice lacking the dopamine transporter gene exhibit marked hyperactivity, whereas dopamine receptor D2-deficient mice are characterized by reduced physical activity levels. Likewise, disruption of genes within the melanin-concentrating hormone pathway leads to hyperactivity.

An intriguing example of the strong effect of a mutation in a single gene on physical activity regulation comes from the fruit fly. In two populations of flies, each exhibiting a distinct activity pattern in terms of food-search behavior, those defined as rovers move about twice the distance while feeding compared to those qualified as sitters. This activity pattern is genetically determined and is regulated by a single gene, dg2, which encodes a cGMP-dependent protein kinase. The activity of this gene product is significantly higher in wild-type rovers than in wild-type and mutant sitters, and activation of this gene reverts foraging behavior from the sitter to rover phenotype. Furthermore, overexpression of the gene in sitters changed their behavior and made them behave more like rovers.

Evidence from Genome-Wide Explorations

The only genome-wide linkage scan for physical activity traits available to date was carried out in the Québec Family Study cohort. The scan was based on 432 DNA markers across the human genome (except the sex chromosomes) that were genotyped in 767 subjects from 207 families. Physical activity measures were derived from a threeday activity diary that yielded three traits of interest—total daily activity, inactivity, and moderate to strenuous activity—and from a questionnaire used to assess weekly physical activity during the past year. The strongest evidence for the presence of a gene influencing physical inactivity scores was detected on chromosome 2. Suggestive linkages with physical inactivity were also reported with markers on chromosomes 7 and 20. Several regions of the genome were linked with indicators of physical activity, including regions on chromosomes 4, 9, 11, 13, and 15.

Are There Epigenetic Effects?

In recent years, a growing body of evidence has emphasized that DNA sequence variation is extremely important in accounting for individual differences in behavior, physiology, and response to drugs or lifestyle interventions. More recently, another and very significant line of evidence indicates that chemical modification of DNA and histone proteins could translate in nongenetic phenotypic differences that often remarkably mimic those associated with DNA sequence variants. These DNA and nucleoprotein alterations have been collectively referred to as "epigenetic events." They begin to occur early after fertilization, are thought to take place in utero and even throughout the lifespan, are typically stable, and influence gene expression. Is there any evidence for a contribution of epigenetics to human variation in physical activity levels or physical inactivity?

No direct evidence exists for a contribution of any epigenetic alterations to physical activity level for the simple reason that the issue has not been considered yet. However, there are experimental data that are highly compatible with the hypothesis that epigenetics can influence the spontaneous level of physical activity. For instance, in one such experiment, performed in a leading New Zealand laboratory, maternal undernutrition throughout pregnancy resulted in differences in postnatal locomotor behavior. Female Wistar rats received only 30% of the ad libitum intake of the control females during pregnancy. The offspring of restricted mothers were significantly smaller at birth. At ages 35 days, 145 days, and 420 days, the voluntary locomotor activity of the offspring of the two groups were assessed. At all ages, the offspring of the undernourished mothers were significantly less active. These results suggested that the effects of undernutrition during pregnancy persisted during postnatal life. This effect persisted even when offspring were overnourished during postnatal life. One possible mechanism for such an effect of maternal undernutrition is via alterations in either the level of production or the sensitivity to endogenous hormones or other secreted factors during pregnancy. It is not unreasonable to hypothesize that chemical modifications superimposed on the DNA, without altering its sequence, could have played a role in the lower spontaneous physical activity level and its persistence throughout the life of the animal exposed to severe undernutrition during fetal life.

Other lines of research suggest that high-fat diets, protein restriction, and other maternal dietary manipulations before and during pregnancy also have considerable consequences on the physiology and behavior of the offspring. The implications of fetal life exposures and epigenetic events on the propensity to be sedentary or physically active remain to be understood.

Summary

Research indicates that the inclination to be physically active or sedentary has a biological foundation. Twin and family studies confirm that physical activity–related traits are characterized by familial aggregation and influenced by genetic factors. Results from animal model studies indicate that single genes can markedly influence physical activity-related behavior. The first molecular genetic studies on physical activity traits in humans have been published during the last few years. They support the notion that it is possible to detect relatively small, yet biologically important genetic effects impacting the tendency to be sedentary or physically active at the molecular level. It is appreciated that the in utero environment and epigenetic events may play a role in postnatal physiology and behavior, but their impact on physical inactivity or physical activity level remains to be determined.

Part Two

Guidelines for Lifelong Physical Fitness

Chapter 7

Understanding the Physical Activity Guidelines for Americans

Physical Activity in Children and Adolescents

Regular physical activity in children and adolescents promotes health and fitness. Compared to those who are inactive, physically active youth have higher levels of cardiorespiratory fitness and stronger muscles. They also typically have lower body fatness. Their bones are stronger and they may have reduced symptoms of anxiety and depression.

Youth who are regularly active also have a better chance of a healthy adulthood. In the past, chronic diseases, such as heart disease, hypertension, or type 2 diabetes were rare in youth. However, a growing literature is showing that the incidence of these chronic diseases and their risk factors are now increasing among children and adolescents. Regular physical activity makes it less likely that these risk factors and resulting chronic diseases will develop and more likely that youth will remain healthy as adults.

This chapter includes text excerpted from "Physical Activity Guidelines for Americans Midcourse Report," Office of Disease Prevention and Health Promotion (ODPHP), U.S. Department of Health and Human Services (HHS), 2012. Reviewed September 2016.

Current Levels of Physical Activity among Youth

Despite the importance of regular physical activity in promoting lifelong health and well-being, current evidence shows that levels of physical activity among youth remain low, and that levels of physical activity decline dramatically during adolescence. Opportunities for regular physical activity are limited in many schools; daily physical education (PE) is provided in only 4 percent of elementary schools, 8 percent of middle schools, and 2 percent of high schools. The National Youth Risk Behavior Survey (YRBS), which collects self-reported physical activity data from high school students across the United States, found that many youth are not meeting the Guidelines recommendation of 60 minutes of physical activity each day:

- 29 percent of high school students participated in at least 60 minutes per day of physical activity on each of the 7 days before the survey. Boys were more than twice as likely as girls to meet the Guidelines (38% vs. 19%).

- 14 percent of high school students did not participate in 60 or more minutes of any kind of physical activity on any day during the 7 days before the survey.

A separate study of U.S. youth used accelerometers to objectively measure physical activity. This study found that 42 percent of children and only 8 percent of adolescents engaged in moderate- to vigorous-intensity activity on 5 of the past 7 days for at least 60 minutes each day.

The Benefits of Physical Activity for Youth

- Improves cardiorespiratory fitness.
- Strengthens muscles and bones.
- Helps attain/maintain healthy weight.
- Reduces likelihood of developing risk factors for later diseases, such as high blood cholesterol, high blood pressure, and type 2 diabetes, thus increasing the chances that youth will remain healthy as adults.
- May reduce symptoms of anxiety and depression.

Physical Activity Guidelines for Americans

In 2008, the U.S. Department of Health and Human Services (HHS) issued the first comprehensive guidelines on physical activity for individuals ages 6 and older. The *2008 Physical Activity Guidelines for Americans* provide information on the amount, types, and intensity of physical activity needed to achieve health benefits across the lifespan

The *Guidelines* provide physical activity guidance for youth ages 6 to 17 and focus on physical activity beyond the light-intensity activities of daily life, such as walking slowly or lifting light objects. As described in the Guidelines, youth can achieve substantial health benefits by doing moderate- and vigorous-intensity physical activity for periods of time that adds up to 60 minutes or more each day. This activity should include aerobic activity as well as age-appropriate muscle- and bone-strengthening activities.

Current science suggests that as with adults, the total amount of physical activity is more important in helping youth achieve health benefits than is any one component (frequency, intensity, or duration) or specific mix of activities (aerobic [e.g., tag, bike riding], muscle-strengthening [e.g., push-ups, climbing trees], or bone strengthening [e.g., hopscotch, tennis]).

Parents and other adults who work with or care for youth should be familiar with the Guidelines, as adults play an important role in providing age-appropriate opportunities for physical activity. They need to foster active play in children and encourage sustained and structured activity in adolescents. In doing so, adults help lay an important foundation for lifelong health, for youth who grow up being physically active are more likely to be active adults.

Key Guidelines for Children and Adolescents

- Children and adolescents should do 60 minute s (1 hour) or more of physical activity daily.

- Aerobic: Most of the 60 or more minute s a day should be either moderate- or vigorous- intensity aerobic physical activity, and should include vigorous-intensity physical activity at least 3 days a week.

- Muscle-strengthening: As part of their 60 or more minutes of daily physical activity, children and adolescents should include muscle-strengthening physical activity on at least 3 days of the week.

- Bone-strengthening: As p art of their 60 or more minutes of daily physical activity, children and adolescents should include bone-strengthening physical activity on at least 3 days of the week.

- It is important to encourage young people to participate in physical activities that are appropriate for their age, that are enjoyable, and that offer variety.

Chapter 8

Prevalence of Self-Reported Physically Active Adults

One in Five Adults Meet Overall Physical Activity Guidelines

About 20 percent of U.S. adults are meeting both the aerobic and muscle strengthening components of the federal government's physical activity recommendations, according to a report published in Morbidity and Mortality Weekly Report, a journal of the Centers for Disease Control and Prevention (CDC).

The data are based on self-reported information from the Behavioral Risk Factor Surveillance System; an annual phone survey of adults aged 18 and over conducted by state health departments.

The *Physical Activity Guidelines for Americans* recommend that adults get at least 2½ hours a week of moderate-intensity aerobic activity such as walking, or one hour and 15 minutes a week of vigorous-intensity aerobic activity, such as jogging, or a combination of both. The guidelines also recommend that adults do muscle-strengthening activities, such as push-ups, sit-ups, or activities using resistance bands or weights. These activities should involve all major muscle groups and be done on two or more days per week.

This chapter includes text excerpted from "One in Five Adults Meet Overall Physical Activity Guidelines," Center for Disease Control and Prevention (CDC), May 2, 2013.

The report finds that nationwide nearly 50 percent of adults are getting the recommended amounts of aerobic activity and about 30 percent are engaging in the recommended muscle-strengthening activity.

"Although only 20 percent of adults are meeting the overall physical activity recommendations, it is encouraging that half the adults in the United States are meeting the aerobic guidelines and a third are meeting the muscle-strengthening recommendations," said Carmen D. Harris, M.P.H, epidemiologist in CDC's physical activity and health branch. "This is a great foundation to build upon, but there is still much work to do. Improving access to safe and convenient places where people can be physically active can help make the active choice the easy choice."

The report also found differences among states and the District of Columbia. The rates of adults meeting the overall guidelines ranged from 27 percent in Colorado to 13 percent in Tennessee and West Virginia. The West (24 percent) and the Northeast (21 percent) had the highest proportion of adults who met the guidelines. Women, Hispanics, older adults and obese adults were all less likely to meet the guidelines.

CDC funds 25 states to address nutrition, physical activity, obesity and other chronic diseases. CDC works with these states to design and improve communities so people can more easily fit physical activity into their lives. Additionally, CDC's Community Transformation Grants program is working to create places that provide safe, accessible ways to be physically active.

Chapter 9

Physical Fitness and Children

Chapter Contents

Section 9.1

How Much Physical Activity Do Children Need?

This section includes text excerpted from "How Much Physical Activity Do Children Need?" Centers for Disease Control and Prevention (CDC), June 4, 2015.

Encourage Your Child to Participate in Activities

This may sound like a lot, but don't worry! Your child may already be meeting the *Physical Activity Guidelines for Americans*. And, you'll soon discover all the easy and enjoyable ways to help your child meet the recommendations. Encourage your child to participate in activities that are age-appropriate, enjoyable and offer variety! Just make sure your child or adolescent is doing three types of physical activity:

- Aerobic Activity

  Aerobic activity should make up most of your child's 60 or more minutes of physical activity each day. This can include either moderate-intensity aerobic activity, such as brisk walking, or vigorous-intensity activity, such as running. Be sure to include vigorous-intensity aerobic activity on at least 3 days per week.

- Muscle Strengthening

  Include muscle strengthening activities, such as gymnastics or push-ups, at least 3 days per week as part of your child's 60 or more minutes.

- Bone Strengthening

  Include bone strengthening activities, such as jumping rope or running, at least 3 days per week as part of your child's 60 or more minutes.

1. On a scale of 0 to 10, where sitting is a 0 and the highest level of activity is a 10, moderate-intensity activity is a 5 or 6. When your son does moderate-intensity activity, his heart

will beat faster than normal and he will breathe harder than normal. Vigorous-intensity activity is a level 7 or 8. When your son does vigorous-intensity activity, his heart will beat much faster than normal and he will breathe much harder than normal.

2. Another way to judge intensity is to think about the activity your child is doing and compare it to the average child. What amount of intensity would the average child use? For example, when your daughter walks to school with friends each morning, she's probably doing moderate-intensity aerobic activity. But while she is at school, when she runs, or chases others by playing tag during recess, she's probably doing vigorous-intensity activity.

What Do You Mean By "Age-Appropriate" Activities?

Some physical activity is better-suited for children than adolescents. For example, children do not usually need formal muscle-strengthening programs, such as lifting weights. Younger children usually strengthen their muscles when they do gymnastics, play on a jungle gym or climb trees. As children grow older and become adolescents, they may start structured weight programs. For example, they may do these types of programs along with their football or basketball team practice.

How Is It Possible for My Child to Meet the Guidelines?

Many physical activities fall under more than one type of activity. This makes it possible for your child to do two or even three types of physical activity in one day! For example, if your daughter is on a basketball team and practices with her teammates everyday, she is not only doing vigorous-intensity aerobic activity but also bone-strengthening. Or, if your daughter takes gymnastics lessons, she is not only doing vigorous-intensity aerobic activity but also muscle- and bone-strengthening! It's easy to fit each type of activity into your child's schedule—all it takes is being familiar with the *Guidelines* and finding activities that your child enjoys.

What Can I Do to Get—and Keep—My Child Active?

As a parent, you can help shape your child's attitudes and behaviors toward physical activity, and knowing these guidelines is a great place to start. Throughout their lives, encourage young people to be physically active for one hour or more each day, with activities ranging from informal, active play to organized sports. Here are some ways you can do this:

- Set a positive example by leading an active lifestyle yourself.

- Make physical activity part of your family's daily routine by taking family walks or playing active games together.

- Give your children equipment that encourages physical activity.

- Take young people to places where they can be active, such as public parks, community baseball fields or basketball courts.

- Be positive about the physical activities in which your child participates and encourage them to be interested in new activities.

- Make physical activity fun. Fun activities can be anything your child enjoys, either structured or non-structured. Activities can range from team sports or individual sports to recreational activities such as walking, running, skating, bicycling, swimming, playground activities or free-time play.

- Instead of watching television after dinner, encourage your child to find fun activities to do on their own or with friends and family, such as walking, playing chase or riding bikes.

- Be safe! Always provide protective equipment such as helmets, wrist pads or knee pads and ensure that activity is age-appropriate.

What If My Child Has a Disability?

Physical activity is important for all children. It's best to talk with a healthcare provider before your child begins a physical activity routine. Try to get advice from a professional with experience in physical activity and disability. They can tell you more about the amounts and types of physical activity that are appropriate for your child's abilities.

Section 9.2

Physical Activity for Preschoolers

Text in this section is excerpted from "Fitness and Your 4- to
5-Year-Old," © 1995–2016. The Nemours Foundation/KidsHealth®.
Reprinted with permission.

By the time kids are 4 to 5 years old, their physical skills like
running, jumping, kicking, and throwing, have come a long way. Now
they'll continue to refine these skills and build on them to learn more
complex ones.

Take advantage of your child's natural tendency to be active. Feeling confident about his or her abilities builds self-esteem, and staying
fit decreases the risk of serious illnesses later in life.

Fitness for Preschoolers

Physical activity guidelines for preschoolers recommend that each
day:

- they get at least 60 minutes of structured (adult-led) physical
  activity

- they get at least 60 minutes of unstructured (free play) physical
  activity

- they not be inactive for more than 1 hour at a time unless
  sleeping

It's important to understand what preschoolers can handle. They
should participate in fun and challenging activities that help build
skills and coordination but aren't beyond their abilities.

Kids this age are learning to hop, skip, and jump forward, and
are eager to show off how they can balance on one foot (for 5 seconds
or longer), catch a ball, or do a somersault. Preschoolers also might
enjoy swimming, hiking, dancing, and riding a tricycle or bicycle with
training wheels.

Many parents look to organized sports to get preschoolers active.
But the average 4- or 5-year-old has not mastered even the basics,

such as throwing, catching, and taking turns. Even simple rules may be hard for them to understand, as any parent who has watched their child run the wrong way during a game knows.

And starting too young can be frustrating for kids and may discourage future participation in sports. So if you decide to sign your preschooler up for soccer or another team sport, be sure to choose a peewee league that focuses on the fundamentals.

No matter what the sport or activity, remember that fitness should be fun. If your child isn't having fun, ask why and try to address the issue or find another activity.

Family Fitness Tips

Walking, playing, running in the backyard, or using playground equipment at a local park can be fun for the entire family.

Other activities to try together, or for a group of preschoolers to enjoy, include:

- playing games such as "Duck, Duck, Goose" or "Follow the Leader," then mixing it up with jumping, hopping, and walking backward

- kicking a ball back and forth

- hitting a ball off a T-ball stand

- playing freeze dance or freeze tag

- pretending to be statues to practice balancing

Kids can be active even when they're stuck indoors. Designate a safe play area and try some active inside games:

- Treasure hunt: Hide "treasures" throughout the house and provide clues to their locations.

- Obstacle course: Set up an obstacle course with chairs, boxes, and toys for the kids to go over, under, through, and around.

- Soft-ball games: Use soft foam balls to play indoor basketball, bowling, soccer, or catch. You can even use balloons to play volleyball or catch.

When to Call the Doctor

If your child refuses to play or join other kids in sports or complains of pain after being active, talk with your doctor.

Kids who enjoy sports and exercise tend to stay active throughout their lives. And staying fit can improve self-esteem, prevent obesity, and decrease the risk of serious illnesses such as high blood pressure, diabetes, and heart disease later in life.

Helping Kids Learn New Skills

Preschoolers develop important motor skills as they grow. New skills your preschooler might show off include hopping, jumping forward, catching a ball, doing a somersault, skipping, and balancing on one foot. Help your child practice these skills by playing and exercising together.

When you go for a walk, your preschooler may complain about being tired but most likely is just bored. A brisk walk can be dull for young kids, so try these tips to liven up your family stroll:

- Make your walk a scavenger hunt by giving your child something to find, like a red door, a cat, a flag, and something square.

- Sing songs or recite nursery rhymes while you walk.

- Mix walking with jumping, racing, hopping, and walking backward.

- Make your walk together a mathematical experience as you emphasize numbers and counting: How many windows are on the garage door? What numbers are on the houses?

These kinds of activities are fun *and* also help to prepare kids for school.

How Much Activity Is Enough?

Physical activity guidelines for preschoolers recommend that each day:

- they get at least 60 minutes of structured (adult-led) physical activity

- they get at least 60 minutes of unstructured (free play) physical activity

- they not be inactive for more than 1 hour at a time unless sleeping
Limit screen—time spent watching TV (including videos and DVDs), on the computer, and playing video games—to no more than 1–2 hours per day.

Structured Play

Preschoolers are likely to get structured play at childcare or in preschool programs through games like "Duck, Duck, Goose" and "London Bridge." Consider enrolling your child in a preschool tumbling or dance class.

Your preschooler can get structured outdoor play at home, too. Play together in the backyard or practice motor skills, such as throwing and catching a ball. Preschoolers also love trips to the playground.

Though many kids love being outdoors, lots of fun things can be organized indoors: a child-friendly obstacle course, a treasure hunt, or forts made out sheets and boxes or chairs. Designate a play area and clear the space of any breakables.

Here are some more ideas for structured play:

- play bounce catch

- use paper airplanes to practice throwing

- balance a beanbag on your heads while walking—make this more challenging by setting up a simple slalom course

- play freeze dance

- play wheelbarrow by holding your child's legs while he or she walks forward on hands

Many parents are eager to enroll their preschool child in organized sports. Although some leagues may be open to kids as young as 4 years old, organized and team sports are not recommended until kids are a little older. Preschoolers can't understand complex rules and often lack the attention span, skills, and coordination needed to play sports.

If you decide to enroll your preschooler in an organized team sport, such as T-ball or soccer, make sure the focus is on helping kids gain basic physical skills, like running, and fundamental social skills, like following rules and taking turns.

If your preschooler is not ready for the team or not interested in sports, consider helping him or her continue to work on fundamental skills—hopping on one foot, catching a ball, doing a somersault, and maybe riding a bicycle or tricycle.

To teach preschoolers to play baseball, start by teaching them basic skills, such as throwing, catching, and hitting off a T-ball stand. Then, if you play a game of wiffle ball, don't worry if your child doesn't tag first base—it's enough to get kids running in the right direction.

Unstructured Play

Unstructured or free play is when kids are left more to their own devices—within a safe environment. During these times, they should be able to choose from a variety of physical activities, such as exploring, playing outside, or dancing around the kitchen.

During pretend play, preschoolers often like to take on a gender-specific role because they are beginning to identify with members of the same gender. A girl might pretend to be her mother by "working" in the garden, while a boy might mimic his dad by pretending to cut the lawn.

It's clear your preschooler is keeping an eye on how you spend your time, so set a good example by exercising regularly. Kids who pick up on this as something parents do will naturally want to do it, too.

Safety Concerns

No matter what type of physical activity your child gets, it's important to keep safety concerns in mind. Remember that preschoolers are still developing coordination, balance, and judgment.

So as preschoolers play, a parent's challenge is to find a balance between letting them try new things and keeping them safe and preventing injuries.

- A child on a tricycle or bike should always wear a helmet.

- If you haven't done so already, it's time to talk about street safety because even the most cautious preschooler may dart into the street after a ball.

- A preschooler in a swimming pool needs constant adult supervision, even if he or she has learned to swim.

It's a tricky age because kids want more independence, and should have some, but cannot be left unsupervised. Preschoolers still need their parents to set limits.

Giving kids safe opportunities to play in both organized and unstructured ways builds a foundation for a fit lifestyle that can carry them through life.

Section 9.3

Fitness Guidelines for School-Aged Youth

This section contains text excerpted from the following sources: Text
under the heading "Active Children and Adolescent" is excerpted
from "Chapter 3: Active Children and Adolescents," Office of Disease
Prevention and Health Promotion (ODPHP), U.S. Department of
Health and Human Services (HHS), October 7, 2008. Reviewed
September 2016; Text under the heading "Youth Physical Activity
Guidelines" is excerpted from "Youth Physical Activity Guidelines
Toolkit," Centers for Disease Control and Prevention (CDC), August
27, 2015; Text under the heading "Explaining the Guidelines" is
excerpted from "Physical Activity Guidelines for Americans: Youth
Physical Activity Recommendations," U.S. Department of Health and
Human Services (HHS), March 10, 2013.

Active Children and Adolescents

Regular physical activity in children and adolescents promotes
health and fitness. Compared to those who are inactive, physically
active youth have higher levels of cardiorespiratory fitness and stronger muscles. They also typically have lower body fatness. Their bones
are stronger, and they may have reduced symptoms of anxiety and
depression.

Youth who are regularly active also have a better chance of a
healthy adulthood. Children and adolescents don't usually develop
chronic diseases, such as heart disease, hypertension, type 2 diabetes,
or osteoporosis. However, risk factors for these diseases can begin to
develop early in life. Regular physical activity makes it less likely
that these risk factors will develop and more likely that children will
remain healthy as adults.

Youth can achieve substantial health benefits by doing moderate-
and vigorous-intensity physical activity for periods of time that add up
to 60 minutes (1 hour) or more each day. This activity should include
aerobic activity as well as age-appropriate muscle- and bone–strengthening activities. Although current science is not complete, it appears
that, as with adults, the total amount of physical activity is more
important for achieving health benefits than is any one component

(frequency, intensity, or duration) or specific mix of activities (aerobic, muscle-strengthening, bone strengthening). Even so, bone-strengthening activities remain especially important for children and young adolescents because the greatest gains in bone mass occur during the years just before and during puberty. In addition, the majority of peak bone mass is obtained by the end of adolescence.

This section provides physical activity guidance for children and adolescents aged 6 to 17, and focuses on physical activity beyond baseline activity.

Parents and other adults who work with or care for youth should be familiar with the *Guidelines* in this section. These adults should be aware that, as children become adolescents, they typically reduce their physical activity. Adults play an important role in providing age-appropriate opportunities for physical activity. In doing so, they help lay an important foundation for lifelong, health-promoting physical activity. Adults need to encourage active play in children and encourage sustained and structured activity as children grow older.

Youth Physical Activity Guidelines

The *Physical Activity Guidelines for Americans*, issued by the U.S. Department of Health and Human Services HHS, recommend that children and adolescents aged 6-17 years should have 60 minutes (1 hour) or more of physical activity each day.

- Children and adolescents should have 60 minutes (1 hour) or more of physical activity daily.

- Aerobic: Most of the 60 or more minutes a day should be either moderate- or vigorous-intensity aerobic physical activity and should include vigorous-intensity physical activity at least 3 days a week.

- Muscle-strengthening: As part of their 60 or more minutes of daily physical activity, children and adolescents should include muscle-strengthening physical activity on at least 3 days of the week.

- Bone-strengthening: As part of their 60 or more minutes of daily physical activity, children and adolescents should include bone-strengthening physical activity on at least 3 days of the week.

- It is important to encourage young people to participate in physical activities that are appropriate for their age, that are enjoyable, and that offer variety.

71

Explaining the Guidelines

Type of Physical

Activity Examples of Activities for Youth

- Moderate–intensity aerobic
  - Active recreation, such as hiking, skateboarding, and rollerblading
  - Bicycle riding
  - Brisk walking
  - Dancing
- Vigorous–intensity aerobic
  - Active games involving running and chasing, such as tag
  - Martial arts
  - Running
  - Sports such as soccer, swimming, and tennis
- Muscle-strengthening
  - Games such as tug-of-war
  - Push-ups or modified push-ups (with knees on floor)
  - Resistance exercises using body weight or resistance bands
  - Sit-ups (curl-ups or crunches)
  - Swinging on playground equipment/bars
- Bone-strengthening
  - Games such as hopscotch
  - Skipping
  - Jumping rope

Chapter 10

Physical Fitness and Teenagers

Chapter Contents

Section 10.1

Statistics on Physical Activity in Teenagers

This section includes text excerpted from "Physical Activity Facts," Centers for Disease Control and Prevention (CDC), June 17, 2015.

Physical Activity Facts

- Regular physical activity in childhood and adolescence improves strength and endurance, helps build healthy bones and muscles, helps control weight, reduces anxiety and stress, increases self-esteem, and may improve blood pressure and cholesterol levels.

- The U.S. Department of Health and Human Services (HHS) recommends that young people aged 6–17 years participate in at least 60 minutes of physical activity daily.

- In 2013, 27.1 percent of high school students surveyed had participated in at least 60 minutes per day of physical activity on all 7 days before the survey, and only 29 percent attended physical education class daily.

- Schools can promote physical activity through comprehensive school physical activity programs, including recess, classroom-based physical activity, intramural physical activity clubs, interscholastic sports, and physical education.

- Schools should ensure that physical education is provided to all students in all grades and is taught by qualified teachers.

- Schools can also work with community organizations to provide out-of-school-time physical activity programs and share physical activity facilities.

Physical Activity and the Health of Young People

Benefits of Regular Physical Activity

Regular physical activity:

- Helps build and maintain healthy bones and muscles.

- Helps reduce the risk of developing obesity and chronic diseases, such as diabetes, cardiovascular disease, and colon cancer.

- Reduces feelings of depression and anxiety and promotes psychological well-being.

- May help improve students' academic performance, including:

    - Academic achievement and grades.

    - Academic behavior, such as time on task.

    - Factors that influence academic achievement, such as concentration and attentiveness in the classroom.

Long-Term Consequences of Physical Inactivity

- Overweight and obesity, which are influenced by physical inactivity and poor diet, can increase one's risk for diabetes, high blood pressure, high cholesterol, asthma, arthritis, and poor health status.

- Physical inactivity increases one's risk for dying prematurely, dying of heart disease, and developing diabetes, colon cancer, and high blood pressure.

Participation in Physical Activity by Young People

- In a nationally representative survey, 77 percent of children aged 9–13 years reported participating in free-time physical activity during the previous 7 days.

- In 2013, only 29 percent percent of high school students had participated in at least 60 minutes per day of physical activity on each of the 7 days before the survey.

- 15.2 percent percent of high school students had not participated in 60 or more minutes of any kind of physical activity on any day during the 7 days before the survey.

- Participation in physical activity declines as young people age.

Table 10.1. Percentage of High School Students Participating in Physical Activity and Physical Education, by Sex, 2013

Type of Activity	Females	Males
Physically active at least 60 minutes/day[a]	17.7%	36.6%
Attended physical education classes daily[b]	24.0%	34.9%

[a]*Any kind of physical activity that increased heart rate and made them breathe hard some of the time for at least 60 minutes per day on each of the 7 days before the survey.*

[b]*Attended physical education classes 5 days in an average week when they were in school.*

Participation in Physical Education Classes

- In 2013, less than half (48 percent) of high school students (64 percent of 9th-grade students but only 35 percent of 12th-grade students) attended physical education classes in an average week.

- The percentage of high school students who attended physical education classes daily decreased from 42 percent in 1991 to 25 percent in 1995 and remained stable at that level until 2013 (29 percent).

- In 2013, 42 percent of 9th-grade students but only 20 percent of 12th-grade students attended physical education class daily.

Section 10.2

Teenagers and Physical Fitness

Text in this section is excerpted from "Fitness and Your 13- to 18-Year-Old," © 1995–2016. The Nemours Foundation/ KidsHealth®. Reprinted with permission.

In the teen years, kids who used to be bundles of nonstop energy might lose interest in physical activity. Between school, studying, friends, and even part-time jobs, they're juggling a lot of interests and responsibilities.

But kids who started out enjoying sports and exercise tend to stay active throughout their lives. So they might just need a little encouragement to keep it going during the teen years.

Immediate benefits include maintaining a healthy weight, feeling more energetic, and promoting a better outlook. Participating in team and individual sports can boost self-confidence, provide chances for social interaction, and offer a chance to have fun. And regular physical activity can help prevent heart disease, diabetes, and other medical problems later in life.

Fitness in the Teen Years

It's recommended that teens get at least 1 hour of physical activity on most, preferably all, days of the week. Yet physical activity tends to lag during the teen years. Many teens drop out of organized sports, and participation in daily physical education classes is a thing of the past.

But given the opportunity and interest, teens can get health benefits from almost any activity they enjoy skateboarding, in-line skating, yoga, swimming, dancing, or kicking a footbag in the driveway. Weight training, under supervision of a qualified adult, can improve strength and help prevent sports injuries.

Teens can work physical activity into everyday routines, such as walking to school, doing chores, or finding an active part-time job. They can be camp counselors, babysitters, or assistant coaches for young sports teams, jobs that come with a chance to be active.

Motivating Teens to Be Active

Teens face many new social and academic pressures in addition to dealing with emotional and physical changes. Studies show that teens on average spend more than 7½ hours a day on various media, including watching TV, listening to music, surfing online, and playing video games. So it's no surprise that they can't seem to find the time to exercise or that parents can't motivate them to be active.

Parents should try to give teens control over how they decide to be physically active. Teens are defining themselves as individuals and want the power to make their own decisions, so they're reluctant to do yet another thing they're told to do. Emphasize that it's not what they do; they just need to be physically active regularly.

Once they get started, many teens enjoy the feelings of well-being, reduced stress, and increased strength and energy they get from exercise. As a result, some begin to exercise regularly without nudging from a parent.

For teens to stay motivated, the activities have to be fun. Support your teen's choices by providing equipment, transportation, and companionship. Peers can play an influential role in teens' lives, so create opportunities for them to be active with their friends.

Help your teen stay active by finding an exercise regimen that fits with his or her schedule. Your teen may not have time to play a team sport at school or in a local league, but many gyms offer teen memberships, and kids might be able to squeeze in a visit before or after school.

Some teens might feel more comfortable doing home exercise videos, which are fine. But while exercise video games (like tennis or bowling) are a good alternative to sedentary activities, they shouldn't replace active play and participation in sports.

And all teens should limit the time spent in sedentary activities, including watching TV, playing video games, and using computers, smartphones, or tablets.

When to Speak with Your Doctor

If you're concerned about your teen's fitness, speak with your doctor. Teens who are overweight or very sedentary might need to start slowly and the doctor can recommend programs or help you devise a fitness plan.

A teen with a chronic health condition or disability should not be excluded from fitness activities. Some activities may need to be changed or adapted, and some may be too risky depending on the condition. Talk to your doctor about which activities are safe for your child.

And some teens may overdo it when it comes to fitness. Young athletes, particularly those involved in gymnastics, wrestling, or dance, may face pressures to lose weight. If your teen refuses to eat certain food groups (such as fats), becomes overly concerned with body image, appears to be exercising compulsively, or has a sudden change in weight, talk with your doctor.

Another dangerous issue is the use of steroids, particularly in sports where size and strength are valued. Talk with your doctor if you suspect your teen is using steroids or other performance-enhancing substances.

Finally, speak with your doctor if your teen complains of pain during sports and exercise.

Fitness for Everyone

Everyone can benefit from being physically fit. Staying fit can help improve self-esteem and decrease the risk of serious illnesses (such as heart disease and stroke) later in life. And regular physical activity can help teens learn to meet the physical and emotional challenges they face every day.

Help your teen commit to fitness by being a positive role model and exercising regularly, too. For fitness activities you can enjoy together, try bike rides, hitting a tennis ball around, going to a local swimming pool, or even playing games like capture the flag and touch football. Not only are you working together to reach your fitness goals, it's a great opportunity to stay connected with your teen.

Chapter 11

Promoting Physical Activity in Children and Teenagers

Chapter Contents

Section 11.1

Motivating Children and Teenagers to Be Active

This section contains text excerpted from the following sources:
Text under the heading "Being Active Every Day" is excerpted
from "Motivating School-Age Kids to Be Active," © 1995–2016. The
Nemours Foundation/KidsHealth®. Reprinted with permission; Text
under the heading "Take Charge of Your Health: A Guide for Teens"
is excerpted from "Take Charge of Your Health: A Guide for Teens,"
National Institute of Diabetes and Digestive and Kidney Diseases
(NIDDK), May 2012. Reviewed September 2016.

Being Active Every Day

Most of us know that kids are supposed to get at least 60 minutes of physical activity a day. And 1 hour spent being active sounds like a pretty easy goal, doesn't it?

But as kids get older, increasing demands on their time can make getting that hour of exercise a challenge. Also, some kids get caught up in sedentary pursuits like watching TV, playing video games, and surfing the Internet. Even doing a lot of studying and reading, while important, can add to a lack of physical activity.

On top of that, during these years kids often come to a fork in the road with sports. Those who are athletic might end up increasing their time and commitment to sports, which is great for their physical fitness. But more casual athletes may lose interest and decide to quit teams and leagues. Unless they find replacement activities, their physical activity levels tend to go way down.

But being active is a key part of good health for all school-age kids. Exercise strengthens their muscles and bones and ensures that their bodies are capable of doing normal kid stuff, like lifting a backpack or running a race. It also helps control their weight and decreases their risk of chronic illnesses, such as high blood pressure and type 2 diabetes.

Keeping Kids Motivated

So how do you get kids motivated to be active, especially those who aren't natural athletes?

Kids can be fit even if they're not winning sports trophies. The key is finding activities they enjoy. The options are many—from inline skating and bike riding to tennis and swimming.

When kids find an activity that's fun, they'll do it a lot, get better at it, feel accomplished, and want to do it even more. Likewise, if they're pushed into activities they don't like, they're unlikely to want to participate and will end up frustrated and will feel like exercising is a chore.

Stick to Basics for 6- to 8-Year-Olds

Expose younger kids to a variety of activities, games, and sports. Keep the focus on fun. A mix of activities at home and at school is often ideal. And be sure to include some free time for kids to make their own decisions about what to do.

At this age, kids are still mastering basic physical skills, such as jumping, throwing, kicking, and catching. It will take a few more years before most can combine these skills the way many 11-year-olds can (for instance, being able to scoop up a baseball, run toward the base, and throw the ball—all in one fluid motion). So if your child is on a sports team, make sure you and the coaches are setting realistic expectations.

Such expectations are also important when it comes to how much kids can handle mentally. Younger kids often are not ready for the pressure of competition, nor can they grasp complex strategy. Look for teams, leagues, and classes that stress the basics and provide encouragement and praise for kids as they improve their skills.

Done correctly, team sports and other group activities can teach kids a lot about teamwork and good sportsmanship.

9- to 12-Year-Olds Are More Coordinated

Older school-age kids usually have mastered basic skills and can start enjoying the benefits of being more coordinated. That means a kid who likes basketball isn't wildly throwing the ball at the basket anymore, but is perfecting the free throw.

They're also better able to understand the rules. Parents of kids involved in team sports might want to talk about handling setbacks and losses, and remind kids that sports should still be fun even as competition heats up.

Whether it's soccer or ballet, if your child doesn't enjoy an activity or feels frustrated by failure, it may be time to switch to something else. That doesn't mean the time spent on those activities was wasted. Instead, ask which ones your child would like to try next. Achieving this transition smoothly, without making a child feel like a failure, can prevent negative feelings about sports and physical activity in general.

Help Kids Find Their Niche

When choosing activities, consider a child's interests, abilities, and body type. A bigger child might be suited for football because size is an advantage. A smaller child might succeed at baseball or might consider a non-team sport.

Also, consider temperament. A mild-mannered boy who might not be comfortable playing football may like the challenge of karate. Likewise, an active girl might not have the patience and control required for ballet, but is well-suited to a fast-paced activity, like soccer.

Personality traits and athletic ability combine to influence a child's attitude toward participation in sports and other physical activities. Which of these three types best describes your child?

Nonathletes: These kids may lack athletic ability, dislike physical activity, or both. By this age, kids are aware of these differences and some may have even been teased about them. The danger for them is not leaving one activity that didn't work out; it's abandoning all physical activity altogether.

Casual athletes: These kids are interested in being active but aren't star players, so are at risk of getting discouraged in a competitive athletic environment. Most kids fall into this category, but in a culture that is obsessed with winning, it's easy to overlook them as athletes. Encourage them to remain active even though they aren't top performers.

Athletes: These kids have athletic ability, are committed to a sport or activity, and are likely to ramp up practice time and intensity of competition. Some are happily settled in a sport or activity by the older school-age years. In this case, a parent can continue to support the child's efforts while still watching for any changes. It's important to ensure that athletes manage schoolwork, get enough rest, and still enjoy the sport. Continue to let your child try out new things and enjoy a variety of physical activities.

Take Charge of Your Health: A Guide for Teens

Get Moving

Being physically active may help you control your weight, increase flexibility and balance, and improve your mood. You don't have to do boring exercise routines. You can be active through daily activities, like taking the stairs instead of the elevator or escalator.

- Be active every day.

- Get outside.

- Have fun with your friends.

- Stay active indoors, too.

Be Active Every Day

Physical activity should be part of your daily life, whether you play sports, take P.E. or other exercise classes, or even get from place to place by walking or bicycling. You should be physically active for 60 minutes a day, but you don't have to do it all at once!

Have Fun with Your Friends

Being active can be more fun with friends or family members. You may also find that you make friends when you join active clubs or community activities. Teach each other new games or activities, and keep things interesting by choosing a different activity each day:

- sports

- active games

- other actions that get you moving, like walking around the mall

Support your friends and challenge them to be healthy with you. You could even take the President's Challenge. Or sign up with your friends for fun, lively events, like charity walks, fun runs, or scavenger hunts.

Get Outside Many teens spend a lot of time indoors on "screen time": watching TV, surfing the web, or playing video games. Too much screen time can lead you to have excess body fat or a higher weight. Instead, be active outdoors to burn calories and get extra vitamin D on a sunny day.

How to Cut Back Your Screen Time

- Tape your favorite shows and watch them later to keep from zoning out and flipping through channels.

- Replace after-school TV and video-game time with physical activities in your home, school, or community.

- Gradually reduce the time you spend using your phone, computer, or TV. Challenge your friends or family members to join you, and see who can spend the least amount of time in front of a screen each week.

- Set up a text-free time with your friends—a length of time when you can be physically active together and agree not to send or respond to text messages.

- Turn off your cell phone before you go to bed.

Stay Active Indoors, Too

- On cold or wet days, screen time is not the only option. Find ways to be active inside:

- Play indoor sports or active games in your building or home, at a local recreation center, or in your school gym.

- Dance to your favorite music by yourself or with friends.

- If you have a gaming system, choose active dance and sports games that track your movement.

Section 11.2

Fitness for Kids Who Don't Like Sports

Text in this section is excerpted from "Fitness for Kids Who Don't Like Sports," © 1995–2016. The Nemours Foundation/ KidsHealth®. Reprinted with permission.

Team sports can boost kids' self-esteem, coordination, and general fitness, and help them learn how to work with other kids and adults.

But some kids aren't natural athletes, and they may tell parents—directly or indirectly—that they just don't like sports. What then?

Why Some Kids Don't Like Teams

Not every child has to join a team, and with enough other activities, kids can be fit without them. But try to find out why your child isn't interested. You might be able to help address deeper concerns or steer your child toward something else.

Tell your child that you'd like to work on a solution together. This might mean making changes and sticking with the team sport or finding a new activity to try.

Here are some reasons why sports might be a turnoff for kids:

Still Developing Basic Skills

Though many sports programs are available for preschoolers, it's not until about age 6 or 7 that most kids have the physical skills, the attention span, and the ability to grasp the rules needed to play organized sports.

Kids who haven't had much practice in a specific sport might need time to reliably perform necessary skills such as kicking a soccer ball on the run or hitting a baseball thrown from the pitcher's mound. Trying and failing, especially in a game situation, might frustrate them or make them nervous.

What you can do: Practice with your child at home. Whether it's shooting baskets, playing catch, or going for a jog together, you'll give your child an opportunity to

build skills and fitness in a safe environment. Your child can try— and, possibly, fail—new things without the self-consciousness of being around peers. And you're also getting a good dose of quality together time.

Coach or League Is Too Competitive

A kid who's already a reluctant athlete might feel extra-nervous when the coach barks out orders or the league focuses heavily on winning.

What you can do: Investigate sports programs before signing your child up for one. Talk with coaches and other parents about the philosophy. Some athletic associations, like the Young Mens Christian Association (YMCA), have non competitive leagues. In some programs, they don't even keep score.

As kids get older, they can handle more competitive aspects such as keeping score and keeping track of wins and losses for the season. Some kids may be motivated by competitive play, but most aren't ready for the increased pressure until they're 11 or 12 years old. Remember that even in more competitive leagues, the atmosphere should remain positive and supportive for all the participants.

Stage Fright

Kids who aren't natural athletes or are a little shy might be uncomfortable with the pressure of being on a team. More self-conscious kids also might worry about letting their parents, coaches, or teammates down. This is especially true if a child is still working on basic skills and if the league is very competitive.

What you can do: Keep your expectations realistic—most kids don't become Olympic medalists or get sports scholarships. Let your child know the goal is to be fit and have fun. If the coach or league doesn't agree, it's probably time to look for something new.

Still Shopping for a Sport

Some kids haven't found the right sport. Maybe a child who doesn't have the hand-eye coordination for baseball has the drive and the build to be a swimmer, a runner, or a cyclist. The idea of an individual sport also can be more appealing to some kids who like to go it alone.

What you can do: Be open to your child's interests in other sports or activities. That can be tough if, for instance, you just loved basketball and wanted to continue the legacy. But by exploring other options, you give your child a chance to get invested in something he or she truly enjoys.

Other Barriers

Different kids mature at different rates, so expect a wide range of heights, weights, and athletic abilities among kids of the same age group. A child who's much bigger or smaller than other kids of the same age—or less coordinated or not as strong—may feel self-conscious and uncomfortable competing with them.

Kids also might be afraid of getting injured or worried that they can't keep up. Kids who are overweight might be reluctant to participate in a sport, for example, while a child with asthma might feel more comfortable with sports that require short outputs of energy, like baseball, football, gymnastics, golf, and shorter track and field events.

What you can do: Give some honest thought to your child's strengths, abilities, and temperament, and find an activity that might be a good match. Some kids are afraid of the ball, so they don't like softball or volleyball but may enjoy an activity like running. If your child is overweight, he or she might lack the endurance to run, but might enjoy a sport like swimming. A child who's too small for the basketball team may enjoy gymnastics or wrestling.

Remember that some kids will prefer sports that focus on individual performance rather than teamwork. The goal is to prevent your child from feeling frustrated, wanting to quit, and being turned off from sports and physical activity altogether.

Try to address your child's concerns. By being understanding and providing a supportive environment, you'll help foster success in whatever activity your child chooses.

Fitness outside of Team Sports

Even kids who once said they hated sports might learn to like team sports as their skills improve or they find the right sport or a league. But even if team sports never thrill your child, there's plenty a kid can do to get the recommended 60 minutes or more of physical activity each day.

Free play can be very important for kids who don't play a team sport. What's free play? It's the activity kids get when they're left to their own devices, like shooting hoops, riding bikes, playing whiffleball, playing tag, jumping rope, or dancing.

Kids might also enjoy individual sports or other organized activities that can boost fitness, such as:

- Swimming
- Horseback riding
- Dance classes
- Inline skating
- Cycling
- Cheerleading
- Skateboarding
- Hiking

- Golf
- Tennis
- Fencing
- Gymnastics
- Martial arts
- Yoga and other fitness classes
- Ultimate Frisbee
- Running

Supporting Your Kid's Choices

Even if the going's tough, work with your child to find something active that he or she likes. Try to remain open-minded. Maybe your child is interested in an activity that is not offered at school. If your daughter wants to try flag football or ice hockey, for example, help her find a local league or talk to school officials about starting up a new team.

You'll need to be patient if your child has difficulty choosing and sticking to an activity. It often takes several tries before kids find one that feels like the right fit. But when something clicks, you'll be glad you invested the time and effort. For your child, it's one big step toward developing active habits that can last a lifetime.

Section 11.3

Tips on Promoting Physical Fitness for Girls

This section includes text excerpted from "Why Physical Activity Is Important," Office on Women's Health (OWH), U.S. Department of Health and Human Services (HHS), March 27, 2015.

Why Physical Activity Is Important

You may wonder if being physically active is really worth the time and effort. Well, lots of girls think so! They know being active is a great way to have fun and hang out with friends. And fitness can do some pretty amazing things for your mind and body. Check out:

What Being Active Does for Your Mental Health

Did you know being physically active can affect how good you feel? It also can affect how well you do your tasks, and even how pleasant you are to be around. That's partly because physical activity gets your brain to make "feel-good" chemicals called endorphins . Regular physical activity may help you by:

- Reducing stress
- Improving sleep
- Boosting your energy
- Reducing symptoms of anxiety and depression
- Increasing your self-esteem
- Making you feel proud for taking good care of yourself
- Improving how well you do at school

What Being Active Does for Your Body

Being physically active is great for your muscles, heart, and lungs. It may even help with nasty PMS symptoms! Some other possible benefits of activity include:

- **Building strong bones.** Your body creates the most bone when you are a kid and a teen. You can learn more about how to build great bones.

- **Promoting a healthy weight.** Obesity is a serious problem among kids in the United States. It can lead to problems with your sleep, knees, heart, emotions, and more, but exercise can help.

- **Helping avoid diabetes.** A lot more young people are getting diabetes than ever before. Regular physical activity can help prevent one type of diabetes.

- **Building healthy habits.** If you get used to being active now, you will more likely keep it up when you're older. You'll thank yourself later!

- **Fighting cancer.** Research shows that exercise may help protect against certain kinds of cancer, including breast cancer.

- **Helping prevent high blood pressure.** The number of kids with high blood pressure is growing. High blood pressure makes your heart and arteries work extra hard to pump blood. It also puts you at risk for things like kidney and eye disease.

Are you worried that exercise will bulk you up? Exercising won't give you big, bulging muscles. It takes a very intense weightlifting program to get a body-builder look. And exercise and other forms of physical activity can help if you need to lose weight or want to stay a healthy weight.

Fitness Basics

Being active may not be as hard as you think. You definitely don't need a gym membership or fancy equipment. Here are some key points to help you build a strong, healthy body:

- **You should aim for at least 60 minutes of activity every day.** You can be active for an hour all at once. Or, you can do a few shorter activities, such as walking to school and playing ball later. (And at least 60 minutes is the right amount from the time you're 6 years old until you turn 18.)

- **You need a mix of different kinds of activities.** Learn about the main types of activity, how they help, and great ways to do them.

- **Most of your 60 minutes should be spent on aerobic activity.** Aerobic activity is anything that gets your heart pumping, such as dancing, running, or swimming laps.

- **How hard you exercise matters, too.** You can learn how to measure your workout to see if it is light, medium, or intense.

- **Focus on fun.** Pick activities you enjoy so you'll be more likely to keep doing them. Also, avoid boredom through variety. We've got ideas for ways to shake up your routine.

- **Start slowly if you haven't been active in a while.** Start with what you can do. Over time, add more days to your activity routine or more time each day. You'll get there!

- **If you have a disability, you should still aim for 60 minutes of activity each day.** Talk with your doctor about what exercises are right for you.

Making Physical Activity Fun

Here are some ways to beat boredom:

- **Join a team.** Playing a sport can be a great way to make friends.

- **Walk or ride a bike to school.** It's good for you and for the environment.

- **Be active while doing something you like.** Maybe march in place while you watch TV or listen to some energizing music.

- **Join a cause.** A walk-a-thon or other fundraiser is a great way to get fit and do something good.

- **Take a class or join a group.** Your local community center may have classes or exercise groups. Check out Girls on the Run External link, which works to boost girls' health and self-respect.

- **Try something new.** Try a DVD or take a class to learn some moves. How about yoga, Pilates, or martial arts?

Got games? Exercise video games (like you play on Xbox or Wii) that get you moving can add to your fitness routine. But for a good workout, make sure to pick options that use your whole body, such as boxing, dancing, or tennis. Also, try not to let this be your only exercise. (And don't forget to get some fresh air!)

Some people love to be active outside. Some people like walking in the calm of nature, or shooting hoops in the playground, for example. If you are one of those people, see our tool below for ways to work out outdoors!

Some people want to stay inside. Maybe your neighborhood isn't safe, or you hate the cold (or heat). If that's you, here are some options:

• Walk up and down stairs

• March in place

• Jump rope

• Tune in to TV or online exercise programs

• Borrow an exercise DVD from your library

• Clean the house with some extra energy

• Pump up some music and dance

Chapter 12

School's Role in Promoting Health and Fitness

Healthy Students Are Better Learners

Health-related factors such as hunger, physical and emotional abuse, and chronic illness can lead to poor school performance. Health-risk behaviors such as early sexual initiation, violence, and physical inactivity are consistently linked to poor grades and test scores and lower educational attainment.

In turn, academic success is an excellent indicator for the overall well-being of youth and a primary predictor and determinant of adult health outcomes. Leading national education organizations recognize the close relationship between health and education, as well as the need to foster health and well-being within the educational environment for all students.

This chapter contains text excerpted from the following sources: Text beginning with the heading "Healthy Students Are Better Learners" is excerpted from "Health and Academics," Centers for Disease Control and Prevention (CDC), February 16, 2016; Text beginning with the heading "Nine Guidelines for Schools" is excerpted from "School Health Guidelines," Centers for Disease Control and Prevention (CDC), August 19, 2015.

Schools Are the Right Place for a Healthy Start

Scientific reviews have documented that school health programs can have positive effects on educational outcomes, as well as health-risk behaviors and health outcomes. Similarly, programs that are primarily designed to improve academic performance are increasingly recognized as important public health interventions.

Schools play a critical role in promoting the health and safety of young people and helping them establish lifelong healthy behaviors. Research also has shown that school health programs can reduce the prevalence of health risk behaviors among young people and have a positive effect on academic performance. Centers for Disease Control and Prevention (CDC) analyzes research findings to develop guidelines and strategies for schools to address health risk behaviors among students and creates tools to help schools implement these guidelines.

Nine Guidelines for Schools

Schools play a critical role in improving the dietary and physical activity behaviors of children and adolescents. Schools can create environments supportive of students' efforts to eat healthy and be active by implementing policies and practices that support healthy eating and regular physical activity and by providing opportunities for students to learn about and practice these behaviors.

The health of students is linked to their academic success. Both physical activity and healthy eating may help improve academic achievement.

Healthy eating and regular physical activity play a powerful role in preventing obesity and chronic diseases, including heart disease, cancer, and stroke—the three leading causes of death among adults aged 18 years or older.

CDC synthesized research and best practices related to promoting healthy eating and physical activity in schools, culminating in nine guidelines. These guidelines were informed by the *Dietary Guidelines for Americans*, the *Physical Activity Guidelines for Americans*, and the *Healthy People 2020* objectives related to healthy eating and physical activity among children, adolescents, and schools. The guidelines serve as the foundation for developing, implementing, and evaluating school-based healthy eating and physical activity policies and practices for students.

Each of the nine guidelines is accompanied by a set of implementation strategies developed to help schools work towards achieving each guideline. Although the ultimate goal is to implement all nine guidelines included in this section, not every strategy will be appropriate for every school, and some schools, due to resource limitations, might need to implement the guidelines incrementally.

1. Use a Coordinated Approach to Develop, Implement, and Evaluate Healthy Eating and Physical Activity Policies and Practices.

Representatives from different segments of the school and community, including parents and students, should work together to maximize healthy eating and physical activity opportunities for students.

Strategies

- Coordinate healthy eating and physical activity policies and practices through a school health council and school health coordinator

- Assess healthy eating and physical activity policies and practices

- Use a systematic approach to develop, implement, and monitor healthy eating and physical activity policies

- Evaluate healthy eating and physical activity policies and practices

2. Establish School Environments That Support Healthy Eating and Physical Activity.

The school environment should encourage all students to make healthy eating choices and be physically active throughout the school day.

Strategies

- Provide access to healthy foods and physical activity opportunities and to safe spaces, facilities, and equipment for healthy eating and physical activity.

- Establish a climate that encourages and does not stigmatize healthy eating and physical activity.

- Create a school environment that encourages a healthy body image, shape, and size among all students and staff members, is accepting of diverse abilities, and does not tolerate weight-based teasing.

The prevalence of obesity among children and adolescents more than tripled from 1980 to 2008. In 2008, more than one third of U.S. children and adolescents aged 6–19 were overweight or obese.

3. Provide a Quality School Meal Program and Ensure That Students Have Only Appealing, Healthy Food and Beverage Choices Offered outside of the School Meal Program.

Schools should model and reinforce healthy dietary behaviors by ensuring that only nutritious and appealing foods and beverages are provided in all food venues in schools, including school meal programs; à la carte service in the cafeteria; vending machines; school stores and snack bars/concessions stands; fundraisers on school grounds; classroom-based activities; staff and parent meetings; and after-school programs.

Strategies

- Promote access to and participation in school meals.

- Provide nutritious and appealing school meals that comply with the *Dietary Guidelines for Americans*.

- Ensure that all foods and beverages sold or served outside of school meal programs are nutritious and appealing.

The *Dietary Guidelines for Americans* (DGA) recommend a diet rich in fruits and vegetables, whole grains, and fat-free and low-fat dairy products for persons aged 2 years or older. The DGA also recommend that children, adolescents, and adults limit their intake of solid fats (major sources of saturated and trans fatty acids), cholesterol, sodium, added sugars, and refined grains.

4. Implement a Comprehensive Physical Activity Program with Quality Physical Education as the Cornerstone.

Children and adolescents should participate in 60 minutes of physical activity every day. A substantial percentage of students' physical activity can be provided through a comprehensive, school-based physical activity program that includes these components: physical education, recess, classroom-based physical activity, walk and bicycle to school, and out-of-school time activities.

The U.S. Department of Health and Human Services (HHS) recommends that children and adolescents engage in 60 minutes or more of physical activity every day.

Strategies

- Require students in grades K–12 to participate in daily physical education that uses a planned and sequential curriculum and instructional practices that are consistent with national or state standards for physical education.

- Provide a substantial percentage of each student's recommended daily amount of physical activity in physical education class.

- Use instructional strategies in physical education that enhance students' behavioral skills, confidence in their abilities, and desire to adopt and maintain a physically active lifestyle.

- Provide ample opportunities for all students to engage in physical activity outside of physical education class.

- Ensure that physical education and other physical activity programs meet the needs and interests of all students.

5. Implement Health Education That Provides Students with the Knowledge, Attitudes, Skills, and Experiences Needed for Lifelong Healthy Eating and Physical Activity.

Health education is integral to the mission of schools, providing students with the knowledge and skills they need to become successful learners and healthy adults.

Strategies

- Require health education from pre-kindergarten through grade 12.

- Implement a planned and sequential health education curriculum that is culturally and developmentally appropriate, addresses a clear set of behavioral outcomes that promote healthy eating and physical activity, and is based on national standards.

- Use curricula that are consistent with scientific evidence of effectiveness in helping students improve healthy eating and physical activity behaviors.

- Use classroom instructional methods and strategies that are interactive, engage all students, and are relevant to their daily lives and experiences.

6. Provide Students with Health, Mental Health, and Social Services to Address Healthy Eating, Physical Activity, and Related Chronic Disease Prevention.

Schools are responsible for students' physical health, mental health, and safety during the school day. Schools should ensure resources are available for identification, follow-up, and treatment of health and mental health conditions related to diet, physical activity, and weight status.

Strategies

- Assess student needs related to physical activity, nutrition, and obesity, and provide counseling and other services to meet those needs.

- Ensure students have access to needed health, mental health, and social services.

- Provide leadership in advocacy and coordination of effective school physical activity and nutrition policies and practices.

Obese children and adolescents are more likely than normal weight children and adolescents to have at least one risk factor for cardiovascular disease, such as high cholesterol, triglycerides, blood pressure, or insulin.

7. Partner with Families and Community Members in the Development and Implementation of Healthy Eating and Physical Activity Policies, Practices, and Programs.

Partnerships among schools, families, and community members can enhance student learning, promote consistent messaging about health behaviors, increase resources, and engage, guide, and motivate students to eat healthily and be active.

Strategies

- Encourage communication among schools, families, and community members to promote adoption of healthy eating and physical activity behaviors among students.

- Involve families and community members on the school health council.

- Develop and implement strategies for motivating families to participate in school-based programs and activities that promote healthy eating and physical activity.

- Access community resources to help provide healthy eating and physical activity opportunities for students.

- Demonstrate cultural awareness in healthy eating and physical activity practices throughout the school.

8. Provide a School Employee Wellness Program That Includes Healthy Eating and Physical Activity Services for All School Staff Members.

School employee wellness programs can improve staff productivity, decrease employee absenteeism, and decrease employee healthcare costs.

Strategies

- Gather data and information to determine the nutrition and physical activity needs of school staff members and assess the availability of existing school employee wellness activities and resources.

- Encourage administrative support for and staff involvement in school employee wellness.

- Develop, implement, and evaluate healthy eating and physical activity programs for all school employees.

9. Employ Qualified Persons, and Provide Professional Development Opportunities for Physical Education, Health Education, Nutrition Services, and Health, Mental Health, and Social Services Staff Members, as Well as Staff Members Who Supervise Recess, Cafeteria Time, and Out-Of-School-Time Programs.

Providing certified and qualified staff with regular professional development opportunities enables them to improve current skills and acquire new ones

Strategies

- Require the hiring of physical education teachers, health education teachers, and nutrition services staff members who are certified and appropriately prepared to deliver quality instruction, programs, and practices.

- Provide school staff with annual professional development opportunities to deliver quality physical education, health education, and nutrition services.

101

- Provide annual professional development opportunities for school health, mental health, and social services staff members, and staff members who lead or supervise out-of-school time programs, recess, and cafeteria time.

Implementing and sustaining school-based healthy eating and physical activity policies and programs will make a powerful contribution toward a healthy future for students in the United States. By adopting these nine guidelines, schools can help ensure that all students have the opportunity to attain their maximum educational potential and pursue a lifetime of good health.

Conclusion

Implementing and sustaining school-based healthy eating and physical activity policies and programs will make a powerful contribution toward a healthy future for students in the United States. By adopting these nine guidelines, schools can help ensure that all students have the opportunity to attain their maximum educational potential and pursue a lifetime of good health.

Chapter 13

Physical Fitness and Adults

Chapter Contents

Section 13.1

Fitness Guidelines for Adults

This section includes text excerpted from "Chapter 4: Active Adults,"
Office of Disease Prevention and Health Promotion (ODPHP),
U.S. Department of Health and Human Services (HHS),
October 7, 2008. Reviewed September 2016.

Active Adults

Adults who are physically active are healthier and less likely to develop many chronic diseases than adults who are inactive. They also have better fitness, including a healthier body size and composition. These benefits are gained by men and women and people of all races and ethnicities who have been studied.

Adults gain most of these health benefits when they do the equivalent of at least 150 minutes of moderate intensity aerobic physical activity (2 hours and 30 minutes) each week. Adults gain additional and more extensive health and fitness benefits with even more physical activity. Muscle-strengthening activities also provide health benefits and are an important part of an adult's overall physical activity plan.

Explaining the Guidelines

The *Physical Activity Guidelines* for adults focus on two types of activity: aerobic and muscle-strengthening.

Aerobic Activity

Aerobic activities, also called endurance activities, are physical activities in which people move their large muscles in a rhythmic manner for a sustained period. Running, brisk walking, bicycling, playing basketball, dancing, and swimming are all examples of aerobic activities. Aerobic activity makes a person's heart beat more rapidly to meet the demands of the body's movement. Over time, regular aerobic activity makes the heart and cardiovascular system stronger and fitter.

The purpose of the aerobic activity does not affect whether it counts toward meeting the Guidelines. For example, physically active occupations can count toward meeting the Guidelines, as can active transportation choices (walking or bicycling). All types of aerobic activities can count as long as they are of sufficient intensity and duration. Time spent in muscle strengthening activities does not count toward the aerobic activity guidelines.

When putting the Guidelines into action, it's important to consider the total amount of activity, as well as how often to be active, for how long, and at what intensity.

Key Guidelines for Adults

- All adults should avoid inactivity. Some physical activity is better than none, and adults who participate in any amount of physical activity gain some health benefits.

- For substantial health benefits, adults should do at least 150 minutes (2 hours and 30 minutes) a week of moderate-intensity, or 75 minutes (1 hour and 15 minutes) a week of vigorous-intensity aerobic physical activity, or an equivalent combination of moderate- and vigorous-intensity aerobic activity. Aerobic activity should be performed in episodes of at least 10 minutes, and preferably, it should be spread throughout the week.

- For additional and more extensive health benefits, adults should increase their aerobic physical activity to 300 minutes (5 hours) a week of moderate-intensity, or 150 minutes a week of vigorous-intensity aerobic physical activity, or an equivalent combination of moderate- and vigorous-intensity activity. Additional health benefits are gained by engaging in physical activity beyond this amount.

- Adults should also do muscle-strengthening activities that are moderate or high intensity and involve all major muscle groups on 2 or more days a week, as these activities provide additional health benefits.

How Much Total Activity a Week?

When adults do the equivalent of 150 minutes of moderate-intensity aerobic activity each week, the benefits are *substantial*. These benefits include lower risk of premature death, coronary heart disease, stroke, hypertension, type 2 diabetes, and depression.

Not all health benefits of physical activity occur at 150 minutes a week. As a person moves from 150 minutes a week toward 300 minutes (5 hours) a week, he or she gains *additional* health benefits. Additional benefits include lower risk of colon and breast cancer and prevention of unhealthy weight gain.

Also, as a person moves from 150 minutes a week toward 300 minutes a week, the benefits that occur at 150 minutes a week become *more extensive*. For example, a person who does 300 minutes a week has an even lower risk of heart disease or diabetes than a person who does 150 minutes a week.

The benefits continue to increase when a person does more than the equivalent of 300 minutes a week of moderate-intensity aerobic activity. For example, a person who does 420 minutes (7 hours) a week has an even lower risk of premature death than a person who does 150 to 300 minutes a week. Current science does not allow identifying an upper limit of total activity above which there are no additional health benefits.

How Many Days a Week and for How Long?

Aerobic physical activity should preferably be spread throughout the week. Research studies consistently show that activity performed on at least 3 days a week produces health benefits. Spreading physical activity across at least 3 days a week may help to reduce the risk of injury and avoid excessive fatigue.

Both moderate- and vigorous-intensity aerobic activity should be performed in episodes of at least 10 minutes. Episodes of this duration are known to improve cardiovascular fitness and some risk factors for heart disease and type 2 diabetes.

How Intense?

The Guidelines for adults focus on two levels of intensity: moderate-intensity activity and vigorous–intensity activity. To meet the Guidelines, adults can do either moderate-intensity or vigorous-intensity aerobic activities, or a combination of both. It takes less time to get the same benefit from vigorous-intensity activities as from moderate-intensity activities. A general rule of thumb is that 2 minutes of moderate-intensity activity counts the same as 1 minute of vigorous-intensity activity. For example, 30 minutes of moderate-intensity activity a week is roughly the same as 15 minutes of vigorous-intensity activity.

There are two ways to track the intensity of aerobic activity: absolute intensity and relative intensity.

- **Absolute intensity** is the amount of energy expended per minute of activity. The energy expenditure of light-intensity activity, for example, is 1.1 to 2.9 times the amount of energy expended when a person is at rest. Moderate-intensity activities expend 3.0 to 5.9 times the amount of energy expended at rest. The energy expenditure of vigorous-intensity activities is 6.0 or more times the energy expended at rest.

- **Relative intensity** is the level of effort required to do an activity. Less fit people generally require a higher level of effort than fitter people to do the same activity. Relative intensity can be estimated using a scale of 0 to 10, where sitting is 0 and the highest level of effort possible is 10. Moderate intensity activity is a 5 or 6. Vigorous-intensity activity is a 7 or 8.

Examples of Different Aerobic Physical Activities and Intensities

Moderate Intensity

- Walking briskly (3 miles per hour or faster, but not race-walking)
- Water aerobics
- Bicycling slower than 10 miles per hour
- Tennis (doubles)
- Ballroom dancing
- General gardening

Vigorous Intensity

- Racewalking, jogging, or running
- Swimming laps
- Tennis (singles)
- Aerobic dancing
- Bicycling 10 miles per hour or faster
- Jumping rope
- Heavy gardening (continuous digging or hoeing, with heart rate increases)
- Hiking uphill or with a heavy backpack

Muscle-Strengthening Activity

Muscle-strengthening activities provide additional benefits not found with aerobic activity. The benefits of muscle-strengthening activity include increased bone strength and muscular fitness. Muscle-strengthening activities can also help maintain muscle mass during a program of weight loss.

Muscle-strengthening activities make muscles do more work than they are accustomed to doing. That is, they overload the muscles. Resistance training, including weight training, is a familiar example of muscle-strengthening activity. Other examples include working with resistance bands, doing calisthenics that use body weight for resistance (such as push-ups, pull-ups, and sit-ups), carrying heavy loads, and heavy gardening (such as digging or hoeing).

Muscle-strengthening activities count if they involve a moderate to high level of intensity or effort and work the major muscle groups of the body: the legs, hips, back, chest, abdomen, shoulders, and arms. muscle strengthening activities for all the major muscle groups should be done at least 2 days a week.

No specific amount of time is recommended for muscle strengthening, but muscle-strengthening exercises should be performed to the point at which it would be difficult to do another repetition without help. When resistance training is used to enhance muscle strength, one set of 8 to 12 repetitions of each exercise is effective, although two or three sets may be more effective. Development of muscle strength and endurance is progressive over time. Increases in the amount of weight or the days a week of exercising will result in stronger muscles.

Meeting the Guidelines

Adults have many options for becoming physically active, increasing their physical activity, and staying active throughout their lives. In deciding how to meet the Guidelines, adults should think about how much physical activity they're already doing and how physically fit they are. Personal health and fitness goals are also important to consider. Examples provided later in the section illustrate how to include these goals in decisions to be active.

In general, healthy men and women who plan prudent increases in their weekly amounts of physical activity do not need to consult a healthcare provider before becoming active.

Inactive Adults

Inactive adults or those who don't yet do 150 minutes of physical activity a week should work gradually toward this goal. The initial amount of activity should be at a light or moderate intensity, for short periods of time, with the sessions spread throughout the week. The good news is that "some is better than none."

People gain some health benefits even when they do as little as 60 minutes a week of moderate-intensity aerobic physical activity.

To reduce risk of injury, it is important to increase the amount of physical activity gradually over a period of weeks to months. For example, an inactive person could start with a walking program consisting of 5 minutes of slow walking several times each day, 5 to 6 days a week. The length of time could then gradually be increased to 10 minutes per session, 3 times a day, and the walking speed could be increased slowly.

Muscle-strengthening activities should also be gradually increased over time. Initially, these activities can be done just 1 day a week starting at a light or moderate level of effort. Over time, the number of days a week can be increased to 2, and then possibly to more than 2. Each week, the level of effort (intensity) can be increased slightly until it becomes moderate to high.

Active Adults

Adults who are already active and meet the minimum Guidelines (the equivalent of 150 minutes of moderate-intensity aerobic activity every week) can gain additional and more extensive health and fitness benefits by increasing physical activity above this amount. Most American adults should increase their aerobic activity to exceed the minimum level and move toward 300 minutes a week. Adults should also do muscle-strengthening activities on at least 2 days each week.

One time-efficient way to achieve greater fitness and health goals is to substitute vigorous-intensity aerobic activity for some moderate-intensity activity. Using the 2-to-1 rule of thumb, doing 150 minutes of vigorous-intensity aerobic activity a week provides about the same benefits as 300 minutes of moderate intensity activity.

Adults are encouraged to do a variety of activities, as variety probably reduces risk of injury caused by doing too much of one kind of activity (this is called an overuse injury).

Highly Active Adults

Adults who are highly active should maintain their activity level. These adults are also encouraged to do a variety of activities.

Special Considerations

Flexibility Activities

Flexibility is an important part of physical fitness. Some types of physical activity, such as dancing, require more flexibility than others. Stretching exercises are effective in increasing flexibility, and thereby can allow people to more easily do activities that require greater flexibility. For this reason, flexibility activities are an appropriate part of a physical activity program, even though they have no known health benefits and it is unclear whether they reduce risk of injury. Time spent doing flexibility activities by themselves does not count toward meeting the aerobic or muscle-strengthening Guidelines.

Warm-Up and Cool-Down

Warm-up and cool-down activities are an acceptable part of a person's physical activity plan. Commonly, the warm-up and cool-down involve doing an activity at a slower speed or lower intensity. A warm-up before moderate- or vigorous-intensity aerobic activity allows a gradual increase in heart rate and breathing at the start of the episode of activity. A cool-down after activity allows a gradual decrease at the end of the episode. Time spent doing warm-up and cool-down may count toward meeting the aerobic activity Guidelines if the activity is at least moderate intensity (for example, walking briskly as a warm-up before jogging). A warm-up for muscle-strengthening activity commonly involves doing exercises with lighter weight.

Physical Activity in a Weight-Control Plan

Along with appropriate dietary intake, physical activity is an important part of maintaining healthy weight, losing weight, and keeping extra weight off once it has been lost. Physical activity also helps reduce abdominal fat and preserve muscle during weight loss. Adults should aim for a healthy, stable body weight. The amount of physical activity necessary to achieve this weight varies greatly from person to person.

The first step in achieving or maintaining a healthy weight is to meet the minimum level of physical activity in the Guidelines. For some people this will result in a stable and healthy body weight, but for many it may not.

The health benefits of physical activity are generally independent of body weight. The good news for people needing to lose weight is that regular physical activity provides major health benefits, no matter how their weight changes over time.

Adults should strongly consider walking as one good way to get aerobic physical activity. Many studies show that walking has health benefits and a low risk of injury. It can be done year-round and in many settings.

People who are at a healthy body weight but slowly gaining weight can either gradually increase the level of physical activity (toward the equivalent of 300 minutes a week of moderate-intensity aerobic activity), or reduce caloric intake, or both, until their weight is stable. By regularly checking body weight, people can find the amount of physical activity that works for them.

Many adults will need to do more than the 150 minutes a week of moderate-intensity aerobic physical activity as part of a program to lose weight or keep it off. These adults should do more physical activity and/or further reduce their caloric intake. Some people will need to do the equivalent of 300 or more minutes of moderate-intensity physical activity a week to meet their weight-control goals. Combined with restricting caloric intake, these adults should gradually increase minutes or the intensity of aerobic physical activity per week, to the point at which the physical activity is effective in achieving a healthy weight.

It is important to remember that all activities—both baseline and physical activity—"count" for energy balance. Active choices, such as taking the stairs rather than the elevator or adding short episodes of walking to the day, are examples of activities that can be helpful in weight control.

For weight control, vigorous-intensity activity is far more time-efficient than moderate-intensity activity. For example, an adult who weighs 165 pounds (75 kg) will burn 560 calories from 150 minutes of brisk walking at 4 miles an hour (these calories are in addition to the calories normally burned by a body at rest). That person can burn the same number of additional calories in 50 minutes by running 5 miles at a 10 minutes-per-mile pace.

Achieving Target Levels of Physical Activity: The Possibilities Are Endless

Ways to get the equivalent of 150 minutes (2 hours and 30 minutes) of moderate-intensity aerobic physical activity a week plus muscle-strengthening activities:

- Thirty minutes of brisk walking (moderate intensity) on 5 days, exercising with resistance bands (muscle strengthening) on 2 days;

- Twenty-five minutes of running (vigorous intensity) on 3 days, lifting weights on 2 days (muscle strengthening);

- Thirty minutes of brisk walking on 2 days, 60 minutes (1 hour) of social dancing (moderate intensity) on 1 evening, 30 minutes of mowing the lawn (moderate intensity) on 1 afternoon, heavy gardening (muscle strengthening) on 2 days;

- Thirty minutes of an aerobic dance class on 1 morning (vigorous intensity), 30 minutes of running on 1 day (vigorous intensity), 30 minutes of brisk walking on 1 day (moderate intensity), calisthenics (such as sit-ups, push-ups) on 3 days (muscle strengthening);

- Thirty minutes of biking to and from work on 3 days (moderate intensity), playing softball for 60 minutes on 1 day (moderate intensity), using weight machines on 2 days (muscle-strengthening on 2 days); and

- Forty-five minutes of doubles tennis on 2 days (moderate intensity), lifting weights after work on 1 day (muscle strengthening), hiking vigorously for 30 minutes and rock climbing (muscle strengthening) on 1 day.

Ways to Be Even More Active

For adults who are already doing at least 150 minutes of moderate-intensity physical activity, here are a few ways to do even more. Physical activity at this level has even greater health benefits.

- Forty-five minutes of brisk walking every day, exercising with resistance bands on 2 or 3 days;

- Forty-five minutes of running on 3 or 4 days, circuit weight training in a gym on 2 or 3 days;

- Thirty minutes of running on 2 days, 45 minutes of brisk walking on 1 day, 45 minutes of an aerobics and weights class on 1 day, 90 minutes (1 hour and 30 minutes) of social dancing on 1 evening, 30 minutes of mowing the lawn, plus some heavy garden work on 1 day;

- Ninety minutes of playing soccer on 1 day, brisk walking for 15 minutes on 3 days, lifting weights on 2 days; and

- Forty-five minutes of stationary bicycling on 2 days, 60 minutes of basketball on 2 days, calisthenics on 3 days.

Section 13.2

How Much Physical Activity Do Adults Need?

This section includes text excerpted from "How Much Physical Activity Do Adults Need?" Centers for Disease Control and Prevention (CDC), June 4, 2015.

Physical Activity

Physical activity is anything that gets your body moving. According to the *2008 Physical Activity Guidelines for Americans*, you need to do two types of physical activity each week to improve your health—aerobic and muscle-strengthening.

For Important Health Benefits

Adults need at least:

- 2 hours and 30 minutes (150 minutes) of moderate-intensity aerobic activity (i.e., brisk walking) every week and

- muscle-strengthening activities on 2 or more days a week that work all major muscle groups (legs, hips, back, abdomen, chest, shoulders, and arms).

  OR

- 1 hour and 15 minutes (75 minutes) of vigorous-intensity aerobic activity (i.e., jogging or running) every week and

- muscle-strengthening activities on 2 or more days a week that work all major muscle groups (legs, hips, back, abdomen, chest, shoulders, and arms).

OR

- An equivalent mix of moderate- and vigorous-intensity aerobic activity and

- muscle-strengthening activities on 2 or more days a week that work all major muscle groups (legs, hips, back, abdomen, chest, shoulders, and arms).

10 minutes at a time is fine

We know 150 minutes each week sounds like a lot of time, but it's not. That's 2 hours and 30 minutes, about the same amount of time you might spend watching a movie. The good news is that you can spread your activity out during the week, so you don't have to do it all at once. You can even break it up into smaller chunks of time during the day. It's about what works best for you, as long as you're doing physical activity at a moderate or vigorous effort for at least 10 minutes at a time.

For Even Greater Health Benefits

Older adults should increase their activity to:

- 5 hours (300 minutes) each week of moderate-intensity aerobic activity and

- weight training muscle-strengthening activities on 2 or more days a week that work all major muscle groups (legs, hips, back, abdomen, chest, shoulders, and arms).

OR

- 2 hours and 30 minutes (150 minutes) each week of vigrous-intensity aerobic activity and

- weight training muscle-strengthening activities on 2 or more days a week that work all major muscle groups (legs, hips, back, abdomen, chest, shoulders, and arms).

OR

- An equivalent mix of moderate- and vigorous-intensity aerobic activity and

- muscle-strengthening activities on 2 or more days a week that work all major muscle groups (legs, hips, back, abdomen, chest, shoulders, and arms).

Aerobic Activity—What Counts?

Aerobic activity or "cardio" gets you breathing harder and your heart beating faster. From pushing a lawn mower, to taking a dance class, to biking to the store—all types of activities count. As long as you're doing them at a moderate or vigorous intensity for **at least 10 minutes at a time.**

Intensity is how hard your body is working during aerobic activity.

How do you know if you're doing light, moderate, or vigorous intensity aerobic activities?

For most people, light daily activities such as shopping, cooking, or doing the laundry doesn't count toward the guidelines. Why? Your body isn't working hard enough to get your heart rate up.

Moderate-intensity aerobic activity means you're working hard enough to raise your heart rate and break a sweat. One way to tell is that you'll be able to talk, but not sing the words to your favorite song. Here are some examples of activities that require moderate effort:

- Walking fast
- Doing water aerobics
- Riding a bike on level ground or with few hills
- Playing doubles tennis
- Pushing a lawn mower

Vigorous-intensity aerobic activity means you're breathing hard and fast, and your heart rate has gone up quite a bit. If you're working at this level, you won't be able to say more than a few words without pausing for a breath. Here are some examples of activities that require vigorous effort:

- Jogging or running
- Swimming laps
- Riding a bike fast or on hills
- Playing singles tennis
- Playing basketball

You can do moderate- or vigorous-intensity aerobic activity, or a mix of the two each week. A rule of thumb is that **1 minute of vigorous-intensity activity is about the same as 2 minutes of moderate-intensity activity.**

Some people like to do vigorous types of activity because it gives them about the same health benefits in half the time. If you haven't been very active lately, increase your activity level slowly. You need to feel comfortable doing moderate-intensity activities before you move on to more vigorous ones. The guidelines are about doing physical activity that is right for you.

Muscle-Strengthening Activities—What Counts?

Besides aerobic activity, you need to do things to strengthen your muscles at least 2 days a week. These activities should work all the major muscle groups of your body (legs, hips, back, chest, abdomen, shoulders, and arms).

To gain health benefits, muscle-strengthening activities need to be done to the point where it's hard for you to do another repetition without help. A **repetition** is one complete movement of an activity, like lifting a weight or doing a sit-up. Try to do 8–12 repetitions per activity that count as 1 set. Try to do at least **1 set** of muscle-strengthening activities, but to gain even more benefits, do 2 or 3 sets.

You can do activities that strengthen your muscles on the same or different days that you do aerobic activity, whatever works best. Just keep in mind that muscle-strengthening activities don't count toward your aerobic activity total.

There are many ways you can strengthen your muscles, whether it's at home or the gym. You may want to try the following:

- Lifting weights

- Working with resistance bands

- Doing exercises that use your bodyweight for resistance (i.e., push ups, sit ups)

- Heavy gardening (i.e., digging, shoveling)

- Yoga

Section ·13.3

Women, Physical Fitness, and Heart Health

This section contains text excerpted from the following sources: Text
under the heading "Benefits of Physical Activity" is excerpted from
"Benefits of Physical Activity," National Heart, Lung, and Blood
Institute (NHLBI), June 22, 2016; Text under the heading "How
Does Heart Disease Affect Women?" is excerpted from "Heart Disease
in Women," National Heart, Lung, and Blood Institute (NHLBI),
April 21, 2014; Text under the heading "Facts on Women and Heart
Disease" is excerpted from "Women and Heart Disease Fact Sheet,"
Centers for Disease Control and Prevention (CDC), June 16, 2016.

Benefits of Physical Activity

Physical activity has many health benefits. These benefits apply to
people of all ages and races and both sexes.

For example, physical activity helps you maintain a healthy weight
and makes it easier to do daily tasks, such as climbing stairs and
shopping.

Physically active adults are at lower risk for depression and declines
in cognitive function as they get older. (Cognitive function includes
thinking, learning, and judgment skills.) Physically active children
and teens may have fewer symptoms of depression than their peers.

Physical activity also lowers your risk for many diseases, such as
coronary heart disease (CHD), diabetes, and cancer.

Physical Activity Strengthens Your Heart and Improves Lung Function

When done regularly, moderate- and vigorous-intensity physical
activity strengthens your heart muscle. This improves your heart's
ability to pump blood to your lungs and throughout your body. As a
result, more blood flows to your muscles, and oxygen levels in your
blood rise.

Capillaries, your body's tiny blood vessels, also widen. This allows
them to deliver more oxygen to your body and carry away waste
products.

117

Physical Activity Reduces Coronary Heart Disease Risk Factors

When done regularly, moderate- and vigorous-intensity aerobic activity can lower your risk for CHD. CHD is a condition in which a waxy substance called plaque builds up inside your coronary arteries. These arteries supply your heart muscle with oxygen-rich blood.

Plaque narrows the arteries and reduces blood flow to your heart muscle. Eventually, an area of plaque can rupture (break open). This causes a blood clot to form on the surface of the plaque.

If the clot becomes large enough, it can mostly or completely block blood flow through a coronary artery. Blocked blood flow to the heart muscle causes a heart attack.

Certain traits, conditions, or habits may raise your risk for CHD. Physical activity can help control some of these risk factors because it:

- Can lower blood pressure and triglyceride. Triglycerides are a type of fat in the blood.

- Can raise HDL cholesterol levels. HDL sometimes is called "good" cholesterol.

- Helps your body manage blood sugar and insulin levels, which lowers your risk for type 2 diabetes.

- Reduces levels of C-reactive protein (CRP) in your body. This protein is a sign of inflammation. High levels of CRP may suggest an increased risk for CHD.

- Helps reduce overweight and obesity when combined with a reduced-calorie diet. Physical activity also helps you maintain a healthy weight over time once you have lost weight.

- May help you quit smoking. Smoking is a major risk factor for CHD.

Inactive people are more likely to develop CHD than people who are physically active. Studies suggest that inactivity is a major risk factor for CHD, just like high blood pressure, high blood cholesterol, and smoking.

Physical Activity Reduces Heart Attack Risk

For people who have CHD, aerobic activity done regularly helps the heart work better. It also may reduce the risk of a second heart attack in people who already have had heart attacks.

Vigorous aerobic activity may not be safe for people who have CHD. Ask your doctor what types of activity are safe for you.

How Does Heart Disease Affect Women?

In the United States, 1 in 4 women dies from heart disease. In fact, coronary heart disease (CHD)—the most common type of heart disease—is the #1 killer of both men and women in the United States.

Other types of heart disease, such as coronary microvascular disease (MVD) and broken heart syndrome, also pose a risk for women. These disorders, which mainly affect women, are not as well understood as CHD. However, research is ongoing to learn more about coronary MVD and broken heart syndrome.

This section focuses on CHD and its complications. However, it also includes general information about coronary MVD and broken heart syndrome.

Coronary Heart Disease

Coronary heart disease (CHD) is a disease in which plaque builds up on the inner walls of your coronary arteries. These arteries carry oxygen-rich blood to your heart. When plaque builds up in the arteries, the condition is called atherosclerosis.

Plaque is made up of fat, cholesterol, calcium, and other substances found in the blood. Over time, plaque can harden or rupture (break open).

Hardened plaque narrows the coronary arteries and reduces the flow of oxygen-rich blood to the heart. This can cause chest pain or discomfort called angina.

If the plaque ruptures, a blood clot can form on its surface. A large blood clot can mostly or completely block blood flow through a coronary artery. This is the most common cause of a heart attack. Over time, ruptured plaque also hardens and narrows the coronary arteries.

Plaque also can develop within the walls of the coronary arteries. Tests that show the insides of the coronary arteries may look normal in people who have this pattern of plaque. Studies are under way to see whether this type of plaque buildup occurs more often in women than in men and why.

In addition to angina and heart attack, CHD can cause other serious heart problems. The disease may lead to heart failure, irregular heartbeats called arrhythmias, and sudden cardiac arrest (SCA).

119

Coronary Microvascular Disease

Coronary MVD is heart disease that affects the heart's tiny arteries. This disease is also called cardiac syndrome X or nonobstructive CHD. In coronary MVD, the walls of the heart's tiny arteries are damaged or diseased.

Women are more likely than men to have coronary MVD. Many researchers think that a drop in estrogen levels during menopause combined with other heart disease risk factors causes coronary MVD.

Although death rates from heart disease have dropped in the last 30 years, they haven't dropped as much in women as in men. This may be the result of coronary MVD.

Standard tests for CHD are not designed to detect coronary MVD. Thus, test results for women who have coronary MVD may show that they are at low risk for heart disease.

Research is ongoing to learn more about coronary MVD and its causes.

Broken Heart Syndrome

Women are also more likely than men to have a condition called broken heart syndrome. In this recently recognized heart problem, extreme emotional stress can lead to severe (but often short-term) heart muscle failure.

Broken heart syndrome is also called stress-induced cardiomyopathy or takotsubo cardiomyopathy.

Doctors may misdiagnose broken heart syndrome as a heart attack because it has similar symptoms and test results. However, there's no evidence of blocked heart arteries in broken heart syndrome, and most people have a full and quick recovery.

Researchers are just starting to explore what causes this disorder and how to diagnose and treat it. Often, patients who have broken heart syndrome have previously been healthy.

Facts on Women and Heart Disease

- Heart disease is the leading cause of death for women in the United States, killing 289,758 women in 2013—that's about **1 in every 4** female deaths.

- Although heart disease is sometimes thought of as a "man's disease," around the same number of women and men die each year of heart disease in the United States. Despite increases in awareness over the past decade, **only 54** percent of women recognize that heart disease is their **number 1 killer**.

- Heart disease is the **leading cause** of death for African American and white women in the United States. Among Hispanic women, heart disease and cancer cause roughly the same number of deaths each year. For American Indian or Alaska Native and Asian or Pacific Islander women, heart disease is second only to cancer.

- About 5.8 percent of all white women, 7.6 percent of black women, and 5.6 percent of Mexican American women have coronary heart disease.

- Almost **two-thirds** (64 percent) of women who die suddenly of coronary heart disease have **no previous symptoms**. Even if you have no symptoms, you may still be at risk for heart disease.

Symptoms

While some women have no symptoms, others experience angina (dull, heavy to sharp chest pain or discomfort), pain in the neck/jaw/throat or pain in the upper abdomen or back. These may occur during rest, begin during physical activity, or be triggered by mental stress.

Women are more likely to describe chest pain that is sharp, burning and more frequently have pain in the neck, jaw, throat, abdomen or back.

Sometimes heart disease may be silent and not diagnosed until a woman experiences signs or symptoms of a heart attack, heart failure, an arrhythmia, or stroke.

These symptoms may include:

- **Heart Attack:** Chest pain or discomfort, upper back pain, indigestion, heartburn, nausea/vomiting, extreme fatigue, upper body discomfort, and shortness of breath.

- **Arrhythmia:** Fluttering feelings in the chest (palpitations).

- **Heart Failure:** Shortness of breath, fatigue, swelling of the feet/ankles/legs/abdomen.

- **Stroke:** Sudden weakness, paralysis (inability to move) or numbness of the face/arms/legs, especially on one side of the body. Other symptoms may include: confusion, trouble speaking or understanding speech, difficulty seeing in one or both eyes, shortness of breath, dizziness, loss of balance or coordination, loss of consciousness, or sudden and severe headache.

Risk Factors

High blood pressure, high LDL cholesterol, and smoking are key risk factors for heart disease. About half of Americans (49%) have at least one of these three risk factors.

Several other medical conditions and lifestyle choices can also put people at a higher risk for heart disease, including:

- Physical inactivity

- Diabetes

- Overweight and obesity

- Poor diet

- Excessive alcohol use

Section 13.4

Physical Activity for Pregnant and Postpartum Women

This section contains text excerpted from the following sources: Text in this section begins with excerpts from "Chapter 7: Additional Considerations for Some Adults," Office of Disease Prevention and Health Promotion (ODPHP), U.S. Department of Health and Human Services (HHS), October 7, 2008. Reviewed September 2016; Text under the heading "Aren't There Risks Involved with Physical Activity and Pregnancy?" is excerpted from "Healthy Pregnant or Postpartum Women," Center for Disease Control and Prevention (CDC), June 4, 2015.

All Americans should be physically active to improve overall health and fitness and to prevent many adverse health outcomes. However, some people have conditions that raise special issues about recommended types and amounts of physical activity. This section provides guidance on physical activity for healthy women who are pregnant

Physical Activity for Women during Pregnancy and the Postpartum Period

Physical activity during pregnancy benefits a woman's overall health. For example, moderate-intensity physical activity by healthy women during pregnancy maintains or increases cardiorespiratory fitness.

Strong scientific evidence shows that the risks of moderate-intensity activity done by healthy women during pregnancy are very low, and do not increase risk of low birth weight, preterm delivery, or early pregnancy loss. Some evidence suggests that physical activity reduces the risk of pregnancy complications, such as preeclampsia and gestational diabetes, and reduces the length of labor, but this evidence is not conclusive.

During a normal postpartum period, regular physical activity continues to benefit a woman's overall health. Studies show that moderate-intensity physical activity during the period following the birth of a child increases a woman's cardiorespiratory fitness and improves her mood. Such activity does not appear to have adverse effects on breast milk volume, breast milk composition, or infant growth.

Physical activity also helps women achieve and maintain a healthy weight during the postpartum period, and when combined with caloric restriction, helps promote weight loss.

Key Guidelines for Women during Pregnancy and the Postpartum Period

- Healthy women who are not already highly active or doing vigorous-intensity activity should get at least 150 minutes (2 hours and 30 minutes) of moderate-intensity aerobic activity per week during pregnancy and the postpartum period. Preferably, this activity should be spread throughout the week.

- Pregnant women who habitually engage in vigorous-intensity aerobic activity or are highly active can continue physical activity during pregnancy and the postpartum period, provided that they remain healthy and discuss with their healthcare provider how and when activity should be adjusted over time.

Explaining the Guidelines

Women who are pregnant should be under the care of a healthcare provider with whom they can discuss how to adjust amounts of physical activity during pregnancy and the postpartum period. Unless a woman has medical reasons to avoid physical activity during pregnancy, she can begin or continue moderate-intensity aerobic physical activity during her pregnancy and after the baby is born.

When beginning physical activity during pregnancy, women should increase the amount gradually over time. The effects of vigorous-intensity aerobic activity during pregnancy have not been studied carefully, so there is no basis for recommending that women should begin vigorous-intensity activity during pregnancy.

Women who habitually do vigorous-intensity activity or high amounts of activity or strength training should continue to be physically active during pregnancy and after giving birth. They generally do not need to drastically reduce their activity levels, provided that they remain healthy and discuss with their healthcare provider how to adjust activity levels during this time.

During pregnancy, women should avoid doing exercises involving lying on their back after the first trimester of pregnancy. They should also avoid doing activities that increase the risk of falling or abdominal trauma, including contact or collision sports, such as horseback riding, downhill skiing, soccer, and basketball.

Aren't There Risks Involved with Physical Activity and Pregnancy?

According to scientific evidence, the risks of moderate-intensity aerobic activity, such as brisk walking, are very low for healthy pregnant women. Physical activity does not increase your chances of low-birth weight, early delivery, or early pregnancy loss. It's also not likely that the composition or amount of your breast milk or your baby's growth will be affected by physical activity.

Section 13.5

Overweight Adults Can Improve Quality of Life through Exercise

This section includes text excerpted from "Overweight, Obesity, and Weight Loss Fact Sheet," Office on Women's Health (OWH), U.S. Department of Health and Human Services (HHS), July 16, 2012. Reviewed September 2016.

How Do I Know If I'm Overweight or Obese?

Find out your body mass index (BMI). BMI is a measure of body fat based on height and weight. People with a BMI of 25 to 29.9 are considered overweight. People with a BMI of 30 or more are considered obese.

What Causes Someone to Become Overweight or Obese?

You can become overweight or obese when you eat more calories than you use. A calorie is a unit of energy in the food you eat. Your body needs this energy to function and to be active. But if you take in more energy than your body uses, you will gain weight.

Many factors can play a role in becoming overweight or obese. These factors include:

- Behaviors, such as eating too many calories or not getting enough physical activity

- Environment and culture

- Genes

Overweight and obesity problems keep getting worse in the United States. Some cultural reasons for this include:

- Bigger portion sizes

- Little time to exercise or cook healthy meals

- Using cars to get places instead of walking

What Are the Health Effects of Being Overweight or Obese?

Being overweight or obese can increase your risk of:

- Heart disease
- Stroke
- Type 2 diabetes
- High blood pressure

- Breathing problems
- Arthritis
- Gallbladder disease
- Some kinds of cancer

But excess body weight isn't the only health risk. The places where you store your body fat also affect your health. Women with a "pear" shape tend to store fat in their hips and buttocks. Women with an "apple" shape store fat around their waists. If your waist is more than 35 inches, you may have a higher risk of weight-related health problems.

What Is the Best Way for Me to Lose Weight?

The best way to lose weight is to use more calories than you take in. You can do this by following a healthy eating plan and being more active. Before you start a weight-loss program, talk to your doctor.

Safe weight-loss programs that work well:

- Offer low-calorie eating plans with a wide range of healthy foods.

- Encourage you to be more physically active.

- Teach you about healthy eating and physical activity.

- Adapt to your likes and dislikes and cultural background.

- Help you keep weight off after you lose it.

How Can Physical Activity Help?

The *2008 Physical Activity Guidelines for Americans* state that an active lifestyle can lower your risk of early death from a variety of causes. There is strong evidence that regular physical activity can also lower your risk of:

- Heart disease
- Stroke
- High blood pressure

- Unhealthy cholesterol levels
- Type 2 diabetes
- Metabolic syndrome

- Colon cancer
- Breast cancer
- Falls
- Depression

Regular activity can help prevent unhealthy weight gain and also help with weight loss, when combined with lower calorie intake. If you are overweight or obese, losing weight can lower your risk for many diseases. Being overweight or obese increases your risk of heart disease, high blood pressure, stroke, type 2 diabetes, breathing problems, osteoarthritis, gallbladder disease, sleep apnea (breathing problems while sleeping), and some cancers.

Regular physical activity can also improve your cardiorespiratory (heart, lungs, and blood vessels) and muscular fitness. For older adults, activity can improve mental function.

Physical activity may also help:

- Improve functional health for older adults

- Reduce waistline size

- Lower risk of hip fracture

- Lower risk of lung cancer

- Lower risk of endometrial cancer

- Maintain weight after weight loss

- Increase bone density

- Improve sleep quality

Health benefits are gained by doing the following each week:

- 2 hours and 30 minutes of moderate-intensity aerobic physical activity

or

- 1 hour and 15 minutes of vigorous-intensity aerobic physical activity

or

- A combination of moderate and vigorous-intensity aerobic physical activity

and

- Muscle-strengthening activities on 2 or more days

127

This physical activity should be in addition to your routine activities of daily living, such as cleaning or spending a few minutes walking from the parking lot to your office.

If you want to lose a substantial (more than 5 percent of body weight) amount of weight, you need a high amount of physical activity unless you also lower calorie intake. This is also the case if you are trying to keep the weight off. Many people need to do more than 300 minutes of moderate-intensity activity a week to meet weight-control goals.

Moderate activity

During moderate-intensity activities you should notice an increase in your heart rate, but you should still be able to talk comfortably. An example of a moderate-intensity activity is walking on a level surface at a brisk pace (about 3 to 4 miles per hour). Other examples include ballroom dancing, leisurely bicycling, moderate housework, and waiting tables.

Vigorous activity

If your heart rate increases a lot and you are breathing so hard that it is difficult to carry on a conversation, you are probably doing vigorous-intensity activity. Examples of vigorous-intensity activities include jogging, bicycling fast or uphill, singles tennis, and pushing a hand mower.

Chapter 14

Physical Fitness and the Elderly

Chapter Contents

Section 14.1

Fitness for the Elderly: What the Research Says

This section includes text excerpted from "Structured Physical Activity Program Can Help Maintain Mobility in Vulnerable Older People," National Institute on Aging (NIA), May 27, 2014.

A carefully structured, moderate physical activity program can reduce risk of losing the ability to walk without assistance, perhaps the single most important factor in whether vulnerable older people can maintain their independence, a study has found.

Older people who lose their mobility have higher rates of disease, disability, and death. A substantial body of research has shown the benefits of regular physical activity for a variety of populations and health conditions. But none has identified a specific intervention to prevent mobility disability.

In this large clinical study, researchers found that a regular, balanced, and moderate physical activity program followed for an average of 2.6 years reduced the risk of major mobility disability by 18 percent in an elderly, vulnerable population. Participants receiving the intervention were better able to maintain their ability to walk without assistance for 400 meters, or about a quarter of a mile, the primary measure of the study. Results of the large clinical trial, conducted by researchers at the University of Florida, Gainesville and Jacksonville, and colleagues at seven other clinics across the country, were published online on May 27, 2014, in the *Journal of the American Medical Association* (JAMA). The researchers were supported by the National Institute on Aging (NIA) and the National Heart, Lung, and Blood Institute (NHLBI) of the National Institutes of Health (NIH).

"We are gratified by these findings," said Richard J. Hodes, M.D., director of the NIA, which was the primary sponsor of the trial. "They show that participating in a specific, balanced program of aerobic, resistance, and flexibility training activities can have substantial positive benefits for reducing risk of mobility disability. These are actionable results that can be applied today to make a difference for many frail older people and their families."

The Lifestyle Interventions and Independence for Elders (LIFE) trial included 1,635 sedentary men and women aged 70–89 at risk of disability, who were randomly assigned to a program of structured, moderate-intensity physical activity or to a health education program focused on topics related to successful aging. The diverse participants were recruited from urban, suburban, and rural communities.

Led by Marco Pahor, M.D., of the University of Florida, the study was also conducted at field sites at Northwestern University in Chicago; Pennington Biomedical Research Center in Baton Rouge, Louisiana; Stanford University in Palo Alto, California; Tufts University in Boston; the University of Pittsburgh; Wake Forest University in Winston-Salem, North Carolina; and Yale University in New Haven, Connecticut. Data management and analysis were coordinated by Wake Forest University.

Participation in the study averaged 2.6 years. The physical activity group of 818 people gradually worked up to the goal of 150 minutes of weekly activity, including 30 minutes of brisk walking, 10 minutes of lower extremity strength training, 10 minutes of balance training, and large muscle flexibility exercises. Their programs took place at a clinic twice a week and at home three or four times a week. The 817 people in the comparison group participated in weekly health education workshops for the first 26 weeks, followed by monthly sessions thereafter. They also performed five to 10 minutes of upper body stretching and flexibility exercises in each session. Participants in both groups were assessed every six months at clinic visits.

Adherence to the program was measured by attendance at sessions and by questionnaires in which participants recorded the number of hours per week that they were physically active. In addition, participants' activity was recorded for one week during each year of the trial through an accelerometer, a small belt device that measures physical activity.

"At the beginning of this trial, all the participants were at high risk for mobility disability," said Evan Hadley, M.D., director of the NIA Division of Geriatrics and Clinical Gerontology. "At the start, they were able to walk about a quarter of a mile without a cane, walker, or help of another person. But they did have sedentary lifestyles and low scores on some standard physical tests that measure risk for disability. The study shows it is never too late for exercise to have a positive effect for a significant portion of frail older people."

Principal investigator Pahor noted that participants attended more sessions and stayed in the study longer than anticipated. He also noted that people in the intervention group were very enthusiastic about the exercise program. "When we finished the exercise program at our site, the people were so disappointed that the classes were over," he said. "We know that many of them are continuing to exercise and we are so pleased that they have kept up with this."

In 2011, NIA launched Go4Life®, a national exercise and physical activity campaign, based on previously demonstrated benefits of exercise for healthy community-dwelling adults age 50 and older. The LIFE study adds to that evidence with findings that older people vulnerable to disability can also be included among those who could reap rewards from regular physical activity. Go4Life® emphasizes endurance, strength, flexibility, and balance exercises.

Section 14.2

Fitness Guidelines for the Elderly

This section includes text excerpted from "Chapter 5:
Active Older Adults," Office of Disease Prevention and
Health Promotion (ODPHP), U.S. Department of Health
and Human Services (HHS), August 26, 2016.

Active Older Adults

Regular physical activity is essential for healthy aging. Adults aged 65 years and older gain substantial health benefits from regular physical activity, and these benefits continue to occur throughout their lives. Promoting physical activity for older adults is especially important because this population is the least physically active of any age group.

Older adults are a varied group. Most, but not all, have one or more chronic conditions, and these conditions vary in type and severity. All have experienced a loss of physical fitness with age, some more than others. This diversity means that some older adults can run several miles, while others struggle to walk several blocks.

This section provides guidance about physical activity for adults aged 65 years and older. The section focuses on physical activity beyond baseline activity. The Guidelines seek to help older adults select types and amounts of physical activity appropriate for their abilities. The

Guidelines for older adults are also appropriate for adults younger than age 65 who have chronic conditions and those with a low level of fitness.

Explaining the Guidelines

Like the Guidelines for other adults, those for older adults mainly focus on two types of activity: aerobic and muscle-strengthening. In addition, these Guidelines discuss the addition of balance training for older adults at risk of falls.

Aerobic Activity

People doing aerobic activities move large muscles in a rhythmic manner for a sustained period. Brisk walking, jogging, biking, dancing, and swimming are all examples of aerobic activities. This type of activity is also called endurance activity.

Aerobic activity makes a person's heart beat more rapidly to meet the demands of the body's movement.

Over time, regular aerobic activity makes the heart and cardiovascular system stronger and fitter.

When putting the Guidelines into action, it's important to consider the total amount of activity, as well as how often to be active, for how long, and at what intensity.

Key Guidelines for Older Adults

- All older adults should avoid inactivity. Some physical activity is better than none, and older adults who participate in any amount of physical activity gain some health benefits.

- For substantial health benefits, older adults should do at least 150 minutes (2 hours and 30 minutes) a week of moderate-intensity, or 75 minutes (1 hour and 15 minutes) a week of vigorous-intensity aerobic physical activity, or an equivalent combination of moderate- and vigorous-intensity aerobic activity. Aerobic activity should be performed in episodes of at least 10 minutes, and preferably, it should be spread throughout the week.

- For additional and more extensive health benefits, older adults should increase their aerobic physical activity to 300 minutes (5 hours) a week of moderate-intensity, or 150 minutes a week of vigorous-intensity aerobic physical activity, or an equivalent combination of moderate- and vigorous-intensity activity. Additional health benefits are gained by engaging in physical activity beyond this amount.

- Older adults should also do muscle-strengthening activities that are moderate or high intensity and involve all major muscle groups on 2 or more days a week, as these activities provide additional health benefits.

- When older adults cannot do 150 minutes of moderate-intensity aerobic activity a week because of chronic conditions, they should be as physically active as their abilities and conditions allow.

- Older adults should do exercises that maintain or improve balance if they are at risk of falling.

- Older adults should determine their level of effort for physical activity relative to their level of fitness.

- Older adults with chronic conditions should understand whether and how their conditions affect their ability to do regular physical activity safely.

How Much Total Activity a Week?

Older adults should aim to do at least 150 minutes (2 hours and 30 minutes) of moderate-intensity physical activity a week, or an equivalent amount (75 minutes or 1 hour and 15 minutes) of vigorous-intensity activity. Older adults can also do an equivalent amount of activity by combining moderate- and vigorous-intensity activity. As is true for younger people, greater amounts of physical activity provide additional and more extensive health benefits to people aged 65 years and older.

No matter what its purpose—walking the dog, taking a dance or exercise class, or bicycling to the store—aerobic activity of all types counts toward the Guidelines.

How Many Days a Week and for How Long?

Aerobic physical activity should be spread throughout the week. Research studies consistently show that activity performed on at least 3 days a week produces health benefits. Spreading physical activity across at least 3 days a week may help to reduce the risk of injury and avoid excessive fatigue.

Episodes of aerobic activity count toward meeting the Guidelines if they last at least 10 minutes and are performed at moderate or vigorous intensity. These episodes can be divided throughout the day or week. For example, a person who takes a brisk 15-minute walk twice a day on every day of the week would easily meet the minimum Guideline for aerobic activity.

Table 14.1. Examples of Aerobic and Muscle-Strengthening Physical Activities for Older Adults.

Aerobic	Muscle-Strengthening
• Walking • Dancing • Swimming • Water aerobics • Jogging • Aerobic exercise classes • Bicycle riding (stationary or on a path) • Some activities of gardening, such as raking and pushing a lawn mower • Tennis • Golf (without a cart)	• Exercises using exercise bands, weight machines, hand-held weights • Calisthenic exercises (body weight provides resistance to movement) • Digging, lifting, and carrying as part of gardening • Carrying groceries • Some yoga exercises • Some Tai chi exercises

How Intense?

Older adults can meet the Guidelines by doing relatively moderate-intensity activity, relatively vigorous-intensity activity, or a combination of both. Time spent in light activity (such as light housework) and sedentary activities (such as watching TV) do not count.

The relative intensity of aerobic activity is related to a person's level of cardiorespiratory fitness.

- **Moderate-intensity activity** requires a medium level of effort. On a scale of 0 to 10, where sitting is 0 and the greatest effort possible is 10, moderate-intensity activity is a 5 or 6 and produces noticeable increases in breathing rate and heart rate.

- **Vigorous-intensity activity** is a 7 or 8 on this scale and produces large increases in a person's breathing and heart rate.

A general rule of thumb is that 2 minutes of moderate-intensity activity count the same as 1 minute of vigorous-intensity activity. For example, 30 minutes of moderate-intensity activity a week is roughly same as 15 minutes of vigorous-intensity activity.

Muscle-Strengthening Activities

At least 2 days a week, older adults should do muscle-strengthening activities that involve all the major muscle groups. These are the muscles of the legs, hips, chest, back, abdomen, shoulders, and arms.

Muscle-strengthening activities make muscles do more work than they are accustomed to during activities of daily life. Examples of muscle-strengthening activities include lifting weights, working with resistance bands, doing calisthenics using body weight for resistance (such as push-ups, pull-ups, and sit-ups), climbing stairs, carrying heavy loads, and heavy gardening.

Muscle-strengthening activities count if they involve a moderate to high level of intensity, or effort, and work the major muscle groups of the body. Whatever the reason for doing it, any muscle-strengthening activity counts toward meeting the Guidelines. For example, muscle-strengthening activity done as part of a therapy or rehabilitation program can count.

No specific amount of time is recommended for muscle strengthening, but muscle-strengthening exercises should be performed to the point at which it would be difficult to do another repetition without help. When resistance training is used to enhance muscle strength, one set of 8 to 12 repetitions of each exercise is effective, although two or three sets may be more effective. Development of muscle strength and endurance is progressive over time. This means that gradual increases in the amount of weight or the days per week of exercise will result in stronger muscles.

Balance Activities for Older Adults at Risk of Falls

Older adults are at increased risk of falls if they have had falls in the recent past or have trouble walking. In older adults at increased risk of falls, strong evidence shows that regular physical activity is safe and reduces the risk of falls. Reduction in falls is seen for participants in programs that include balance and moderate-intensity muscle-strengthening activities for 90 minutes (1 hour and 30 minutes) a week plus moderate-intensity walking for about 1 hour a week. Preferably, older adults at risk of falls should do balance training 3 or more days a week and do standardized exercises from a program demonstrated to reduce falls. Examples of these exercises include backward walking, sideways walking, heel walking, toe walking, and standing from a sitting position. The exercises can increase in difficulty by progressing from holding onto a stable support (like furniture) while doing the exercises to doing them without support. It's not known whether different combinations of type, amount, or frequency of activity can reduce falls to a greater degree. Tai chi exercises also may help prevent falls.

Meeting the Guidelines

Older adults have many ways to live an active lifestyle that meets the Guidelines. Many factors influence decisions to be active, such as personal goals, current physical activity habits, and health and safety considerations.

Healthy older adults generally do not need to consult a healthcare provider before becoming physically active. However, healthcare providers can help people attain and maintain regular physical activity by providing advice on appropriate types of activities and ways to progress at a safe and steady pace.

Adults with chronic conditions should talk with their healthcare provider to determine whether their conditions limit their ability to do regular physical activity in any way. Such a conversation should also help people learn about appropriate types and amounts of physical activity.

Inactive Older Adults

Older adults should increase their amount of physical activity gradually. It can take months for those with a low level of fitness to gradually meet their activity goals. To reduce injury risk, inactive or insufficiently active adults should avoid vigorous aerobic activity at first. Rather, they should gradually increase the number of days a week and duration of moderate-intensity aerobic activity. Adults with a very low level of fitness can start out with episodes of activity less than 10 minutes and slowly increase the minutes of light-intensity aerobic activity, such as light-intensity walking.

Older adults who are inactive or who don't yet meet the Guidelines should aim for at least 150 minutes a week of relatively moderate-intensity physical activity. Getting at least 30 minutes of relatively moderate-intensity physical activity on 5 or more days each week is a reasonable way to meet these Guidelines. Doing muscle-strengthening activity on 2 or 3 nonconsecutive days each week is also an acceptable and appropriate goal for many older adults.

Active Older Adults

Older adults who are already active and meet the Guidelines can gain additional and more extensive health benefits by moving beyond the 150 minutes a week minimum to 300 or more minutes a week of relatively moderate-intensity aerobic activity. Muscle-strengthening activities should also be done at least 2 days a week.

Older Adults with Chronic Conditions

Older adults who have chronic conditions that prevent them from doing the equivalent of 150 minutes of moderate-intensity aerobic activity a week should set physical activity goals that meet their abilities. They should talk with their healthcare provider about setting physical activity goals. They should avoid an inactive lifestyle. Even 60 minutes (1 hour) a week of moderate-intensity aerobic activity provides some health benefits.

Section 14.3

Benefits of Exercise for the Elderly

This section includes text excerpted from "Exercise: Benefits of Exercise: Health Benefits," NIHSeniorHealth, National Institutes of Health (NIH), January 2015.

One of the Healthiest Things You Can Do

Like most people, you've probably heard that physical activity and exercise are good for you. In fact, being physically active on a regular basis is one of the healthiest things you can do for yourself. Studies have shown that exercise provides many health benefits and that older adults can gain a lot by staying physically active. Even moderate exercise and physical activity can improve the health of people who are frail or who have diseases that accompany aging.

Being physically active can also help you stay strong and fit enough to keep doing the things you like to do as you get older. Making exercise and physical activity a regular part of your life can improve your health and help you maintain your independence as you age.

Be as Active as Possible

Regular physical activity and exercise are important to the physical and mental health of almost everyone, including older adults. Staying physically active and exercising regularly can produce long-term health benefits and even improve health for some older people who already have diseases and disabilities. That's why health experts say that older adults should aim to be as active as possible.

Being Inactive Can Be Risky

Although exercise and physical activity are among the healthiest things you can do for yourself, some older adults are reluctant to exercise. Some are afraid that exercise will be too hard or that physical activity will harm them. Others might think they have to join a gym or have special equipment. Yet, studies show that "taking it easy" is risky. For the most part, when older people lose their ability to do things on their own, it doesn't happen just because they've aged. It's usually because they're not active. Lack of physical activity also can lead to more visits to the doctor, more hospitalizations, and more use of medicines for a variety of illnesses.

Prevent or Delay Disease

Scientists have found that staying physically active and exercising regularly can help prevent or delay many diseases and disabilities. In some cases, exercise is an effective treatment for many chronic conditions. For example, studies show that people with arthritis, heart disease, or diabetes benefit from regular exercise. Exercise also helps people with high blood pressure, balance problems, or difficulty walking.

Manage Stress, Improve Mood

Regular, moderate physical activity can help manage stress and improve your mood. And, being active on a regular basis may help reduce feelings of depression. Studies also suggest that exercise can improve or maintain some aspects of cognitive function, such as your ability to shift quickly between tasks, plan an activity, and ignore irrelevant information.

Section 14.4

Exercises for Elderly

This section contains text excerpted from the following sources: Text
beginning with the heading "Start out Slowly" is excerpted from
"Exercise: How to Get Started: Safety First," NIHSeniorHealth,
National Institutes of Health (NIH), October 2015; Text under the
heading "Endurance Exercises: Endurance Exercises" is excerpted
from "Exercise: Exercises to Try," NIHSeniorHealth, National
Institutes of Health (NIH), January 2015.

Start out Slowly

Most older adults, regardless of age or condition, will do just fine
increasing their physical activity to a moderate level. However, if you
haven't been active for a long time, it's important to start out at a low
level of effort and work your way up slowly.

When to Check with Your Doctor

If you are at high risk for any chronic diseases such as heart disease
or diabetes, or if you smoke or are obese, you should check first with
your doctor before becoming more physically active.

Other reasons to check with your doctor before you exercise include:

- any new, undiagnosed symptom
- chest pain
- irregular, rapid, or fluttery heartbeat
- severe shortness of breath.

Check with your doctor if you have:

- ongoing, significant, and undiagnosed weight loss
- infections, like pneumonia, accompanied by fever which can
  cause rapid heart beat and dehydration
- an acute blood clot

- a hernia that is causing symptoms such as pain and discomfort.
- foot or ankle sores that won't heal
- persistent pain or problems walking after a fall—you might have a fracture and not know it
- eye conditions such as bleeding in the retina or a detached retina. Also consult your doctor after a cataract removal or lens implant, or after laser treatment or other eye surgery.
- a weakening in the wall of the heart's major outgoing blood vessel called an abdominal aortic aneurysm
- a narrowing of one of the heart's valves called critical aortic stenosis
- joint swelling.

If You've Had Hip Replacement

If you have had hip repair or replacement:

- check with your doctor before doing lower-body exercises.
- don't cross your legs.
- don't bend your hips farther than a 90-degree angle.
- avoid locking the joints in your legs into a strained position.

Discuss Your Activity Level

Your activity level is an important topic to discuss with your doctor as part of your ongoing preventive healthcare. Talk about exercise at least once a year if your health is stable, and more often if your health is getting better or worse over time so that you can adjust your exercise program. Your doctor can help you choose activities that are best for you and reduce any risks.

When to Stop Exercising

Stop exercising if you:

- have pain or pressure in your chest, neck, shoulder, or arm
- feel dizzy or sick to your stomach
- break out in a cold sweat

- have muscle cramps

- feel severe pain in joints, feet, ankles, or legs.

Endurance Exercises

To get all of the benefits of physical activity, try all four types of exercise—endurance, strength, balance, and flexibility.

Increasing Your Breathing and Heart Rate

Endurance exercises are activities that increase your breathing and heart rate for an extended period of time. Examples are walking, jogging, swimming, raking, sweeping, dancing, and playing tennis. Endurance exercises will make it easier for you to walk farther, faster, or uphill. They also should make everyday activities such as gardening, shopping, or playing a sport easier.

How Much, How Often?

Refer to your starting goals, and build up your endurance gradually. If you haven't been active for a long time, it's especially important to work your way up over time. It may take a while to go from a long-standing inactive lifestyle to doing some of the activities listed below.

For example, start out with 5 or 10 minutes at a time, and then build up to at least 30 minutes of moderate-intensity endurance activity. Doing less than 10 minutes at a time won't give you the desired heart and lung benefits. Try to build up to at least 150 minutes (2 ½ hours) of moderate endurance activity a week. Being active at least 3 days a week is best.

Going Further

When you're ready to do more, build up the amount of time you spend doing endurance activities first, then build up the difficulty of your activities. For example, gradually increase your time to 30 minutes over several days to weeks (or even months, depending on your condition) by walking longer distances. Then walk more briskly or up steeper hills.

Safety Tips

- Do a little light activity, such as easy walking, before and after your endurance activities to warm up and cool down.

- Drink liquids when doing any activity that makes you sweat.
- Dress appropriately for the heat and cold. Dress in layers if you're outdoors so you can add or remove clothes as needed.
- Wear proper shoes.
- When you're out walking, watch out for low-hanging branches and uneven sidewalks.
- Walk during the day or in well-lit areas at night, and be aware of your surroundings.
- To prevent injuries, use safety equipment such as helmets for biking.
- Endurance activities should not make you breathe so hard that you can't talk and should not cause dizziness, or chest pain or pressure, or a feeling like heartburn.

Indoor Endurance Activities

Don't let bad weather stop you from exercising. Here are some options for exercising indoors.

- going to a gym or fitness center and using the treadmill, elliptical machine, stationary bike, or rowing machine
- swimming laps
- joining a water aerobics class
- dancing
- performing martial arts
- bowling

Outdoor Endurance Activities

Use your exercise program as a chance to get outside and enjoy nature. Here are some ideas for being active outdoors.

- biking, hand-crank bicycling, or tandem biking
- horseback riding
- sailing
- jogging or running
- skating
- snorkeling

Endurance Activities around the House

You don't need to leave your house to be active. Check out these ways to exercise at home.

- gardening
- heavy housework
- sweeping
- raking
- shoveling snow

Walking or Rolling

Walking or wheelchair rolling are simple ways to be active. You can do it alone, with friends, even with your dog! Try one of these types of walking or rolling to get active today.

- Nordic walking
- hiking
- walking the dog
- mall walking
- wheelchair rolling
- race walking

Sports

Sports are a great way to motivate yourself to be active. Competition and teamwork can inspire you to work harder and to keep up your commitment to exercise. Try one of these sports.

- tennis
- golf
- pickleball
- hockey
- seated volleyball
- wheelchair basketball

Section 14.5

Making Exercise a Habit

This section includes text excerpted from "Exercise: How to Stay Active: Make Exercise a Habit," NIHSeniorHealth, National Institutes of Health (NIH), June 2016.

Once you've started exercising, it's important to keep going because physical activity needs to be done on a regular basis to produce maximum benefits.

A Regular Part of Your Day

One of the best ways to stay physically active is to make it a lifelong habit. Set yourself up to succeed right from the start by seeking to make exercise a regular part of your day. When it becomes a normal part of your everyday routine, like brushing your teeth, then you'll be less likely to stop and will find it easier to start up again if you're interrupted for some reason. If you can stick with an exercise routine or physical activity for at least 6 months, it's a good sign that you're on your way to making physical activity a regular habit.

Ways to Make Exercise a Habit

Here are a few ways to help you make exercise a regular part of your daily life.

- Make it a priority.
- Make it easy.
- Make it safe.
- Make it social.
- Make it interesting and fun.
- Make it an active decision.

1. Make It a Priority

Many of us lead busy lives, and it's easy to put physical activity at the bottom of the "to do" list. Remember, though, being active is one of the most important things you can do each day to maintain and improve your health. Make it a point to include physical activities throughout your day. Try being active first thing in the morning before you get busy. Think of your time to exercise as a special appointment, and mark it on your calendar.

2. Make It Easy

If it's difficult, costs too much, or is too inconvenient, you probably won't be active. You are more likely to exercise if it's easy to do. Put your 2-pound weights next to your easy chair so you can do some lifting while you watch TV. Walk up and down the soccer field during your grandchild's game.

Do more of the activities you already like and know how to do. Walk the entire mall or every aisle of the grocery store when you go shopping. When you go out to get the mail, walk around the block. Join a gym or fitness center that's close to home. You can be active all at once, or break it up into smaller amounts throughout the day.

3. Make It Safe

Exercise and moderate physical activity, such as brisk walking, are safe for almost all older adults. Even so, avoiding injury is an important thing to keep in mind, especially if you're just starting a new activity or you haven't been active for a long time. Talk to your doctor if you have an ongoing health condition or certain other health problems or if you haven't seen your doctor for a while. Ask how physical activity can help you, whether you should avoid certain activities, and how to modify exercises to fit your situation.

You may feel some minor discomfort or muscle soreness when you start to exercise. This should go away as you get used to the activities. However, if you feel sick to your stomach or have strong pain, you've done too much. Go easier and then gradually build up.

4. Make It Social

Enlist a friend or family member. Many people agree that having an "exercise buddy" keeps them going. Take a yoga class with a neighbor. If you don't already have an exercise partner, find one by joining a walking club at your local mall or an exercise class at a nearby senior center. Take a walk during lunch with a co-worker.

5. Make It Interesting and Fun

Do things you enjoy and pick up the pace a bit. If you love the outdoors, try biking, fishing, jogging, or hiking. Listen to music or a book on CD while walking, gardening, or raking. Plan a hiking trip at a nearby park.

Most people tend to focus on one activity or type of exercise and think they're doing enough. The goal is to be creative and choose exercises from each of the four categories—endurance, strength, balance, and flexibility. Mixing it up will help you reap the benefits of each type of exercise, as well as reduce boredom and risk of injury.

6. Make Exercise an Active Decision

Seize opportunities. Choose to be active in many places and many ways. Multi-task the active way.

- When you unload the groceries, strengthen your arms by lifting the milk carton or a 1-pound can a few times before you put it away. When you go shopping, build your endurance by parking the car at the far end of the parking lot and walking briskly to the store. Or, get off the bus one or two stops earlier than usual.

- Instead of calling or e-mailing a colleague at work, go in person—and take the stairs.

- Take a few extra trips up and down the steps at home to strengthen your legs and build endurance.

- Try to do some of your errands on foot rather than in the car.

- While you're waiting in line, practice your balancing skills by standing on one foot for a few seconds, then the other. Gradually build up your time. While you're talking on the phone, stand up and do a few leg raises or toe stands to strengthen your legs. Take advantage of small bits of "down time" to do an exercise or two. For example, while you're waiting for the coffee to brew or for your spouse to get ready to go out, do a few wall push-ups or calf stretches

Part Three

Start Moving

Chapter 15

Ways to Add Physical Activity to Your Life

Chapter Contents

Section 15.1

Get Active

This section contains text excerpted from the following sources:
Text in the begining is excerpted from "Get Active," Let's Move!
WhiteHouse.gov, June 5, 2013; Text under the heading "Take Action:
Get Started" is excerpted from "Get Active," U.S. Department of
Health and Human Services (HHS), March 23, 2016.

Physical activity is an essential component of a healthy lifestyle. In combination with healthy eating, it can help prevent a range of chronic diseases, including heart disease, cancer, and stroke, which are the three leading causes of death. Physical activity helps control weight, builds lean muscle, reduces fat, promotes strong bone, muscle and joint development, and decreases the risk of obesity. Children need 60 minutes of play with moderate to vigorous activity every day to grow up to a healthy weight.

If this sounds like a lot, consider that eight to 18 year old adolescents spend an average of 7.5 hours a day using entertainment media including TV, computers, video games, cell phones and movies in a typical day, and only one-third of high school students get the recommmended levels of physical activity. To increase physical activity, today's children need safe routes to walk and bike ride to school, parks, playgrounds and community centers where they can play after school, and activities like sports, dance or fitness programs that are exciting and challenging enough to keep them engaged.

Let's Move! aims to increase opportunities for kids to be physically active, both in and out of school and to create new opportunities for families to move together.

- **Active Families**: Engage in physical activity each day: a total of 60 minutes for children, 30 minutes for adults.

- **Active Schools:** A variety of opportunities are available for schools to add more physical activity into the school day, including additional physical education classes, before–and after school programs, recess, and opening school facilities for student and family recreation in the late afternoon and evening.

- **Active Communities:** Mayors and community leaders can promote physical fitness by working to increase safe routes for kids to walk and ride to school; by revitalizing parks, playgrounds, and community centers; and by providing fun and affordable sports and fitness programs.

Let's Move! supports the Presidential Active Lifestyle Award (PALA+) challenge, which helps individuals commit to regular physical activity and healthy eating—and rewards them for it. The challenge is for anyone, from students to seniors, but it's geared toward people who want to set themselves on the road to a healthier life through positive changes to physical activity and eating behaviors.

For kids and teens (that's anyone between 6 and 17 years), your goals are:

- **Physical activity:** You need to be active 60 minutes a day, at least 5 days a week, for 6 out of 8 weeks. As an alternative, you can count your daily activity steps using a pedometer (girls' goal: 11,000; boys' goal: 13,000).

- **Healthy eating:** Each week, you'll also focus on a healthy eating goal. There are eight to choose from, and each week you will add a new goal while continuing with your previous goals. By the end of the six weeks, you'll be giving your body more of the good stuff it needs.

For adults (that's anyone aged 18 and older), your goals are:

- **Physical activity:** You need to be active 30 minutes a day, at least 5 days a week, for 6 out of 8 weeks. As an alternative, you can count your daily activity steps using a pedometer (goal: 8,500).

- **Healthy eating:** Each week, you'll also focus on a healthy eating goal. There are eight to choose from, and each week you will add a new goal while continuing with your previous goals. By the end of the six weeks, you'll be giving your body more of the good stuff it needs.

Take Action: Get Started

I'm just getting started.

Start out slowly and add new physical activities little by little. After a few weeks or months, do them longer and more often.

153

Choose activities that you enjoy.

Team up with a friend or join a class. Ask your family and friends to be active with you. Play games like tennis or basketball, or take a class in dance or martial arts.

Everyday activities can add up to an active lifestyle. You can:

- Go for a brisk walk around the neighborhood
- Ride a bicycle to work or just for fun
- Play outdoor games with your children

Have fun with your family.

If you have children, you can be a role model for making healthy choices. Encourage your whole family to get active outside. Go for a hike or organize a family soccer game.

Build Muscles

Try some of these activities a few days a week:

- Crunches (sit-ups)
- Heavy gardening, like digging or shoveling
- Doing push-ups on the floor or against the wall
- Lifting small weights – you can even use bottled water or cans of food as weights

Track Progress

Use a pedometer.

A pedometer clips onto your belt or waistband and counts the number of steps you take. Make it your goal to take at least 10,000 steps a day. Increase the number of steps you take each day until you reach your goal.

A pedometer counts the number of steps you take.

Be realistic.

Remember, it's not all or nothing. Even 10 minutes of activity is better than none! Try walking for 10 minutes a day a few days a week.

Find a time that works for you. See if you can fit in 10 minutes of activity before work or after dinner.

Add More Activity

I'm doing a little, but I'm ready to get more active.

You may already be feeling the benefits of getting active, such as sleeping better or getting toned. Here are 2 ways to add more activity to your life.

- Be active for longer each time. If you are walking 3 days a week for 30 minutes, try walking for an additional 10 minutes or more each day.

- Be active more often. If you are riding your bike to work 2 days a week, try riding your bike to work 4 days a week.

Find time in your schedule.

Look at your schedule for the week. Find a few 30-minute time periods you can use for more physical activity. Put them in your calendar.

Challenge Yourself

I'm already physically active, and I want to keep it up.

If you are already active for 2 hours and 30 minutes each week, you can get even more health benefits by stepping up your routine.

Getting more physical activity can further lower your risk for:

- Heart disease

- Type 2 diabetes

- Breast cancer

- Colorectal cancer

Do more vigorous activities.

In general, 15 minutes of vigorous activity has the same benefits as 30 minutes of moderate activity. Try jogging for 15 minutes instead of walking for 30 minutes.

Mix it up.

Mix vigorous activities with moderate ones. Try joining a fitness group or gym class. Don't forget to do muscle-strengthening activities 2 days a week.

Section 15.2

Exercise Opportunities in Your Daily Life

This section includes text excerpted from "Tips for Increasing Physical Activity," ChooseMyPlate.gov, U.S. Department of Agriculture (USDA), June 10, 2015.

Make Physical Activity a Regular Part of the Day

Choose activities that you enjoy and can do regularly. Fitting activity into a daily routine can be easy—such as taking a brisk 10 minute walk to and from the parking lot, bus stop, or subway station. Or, join an exercise class. Keep it interesting by trying something different on alternate days. Every little bit adds up and doing something is better than doing nothing.

Make sure to do at least 10 minutes of activity at a time, shorter bursts of activity will not have the same health benefits. For example, walking the dog for 10 minutes before and after work or adding a 10 minute walk at lunchtime can add to your weekly goal. Mix it up. Swim, take a yoga class, garden or lift weights. To be ready anytime, keep some comfortable clothes and a pair of walking or running shoes in the car and at the office.

More Ways to Increase Physical Activity

At Home

- Join a walking group in the neighborhood or at the local shopping mall. Recruit a partner for support and encouragement.

- Push the baby in a stroller.

- Get the whole family involved—enjoy an afternoon bike ride with your kids.

- Walk up and down the soccer or softball field sidelines while watching the kids play.

- Walk the dog—don't just watch the dog walk.

- Clean the house or wash the car.
- Walk, skate, or cycle more, and drive less.
- Do stretches, exercises, or pedal a stationary bike while watching television.
- Mow the lawn with a push mower.
- Plant and care for a vegetable or flower garden.
- Play with the kids—tumble in the leaves, build a snowman, splash in a puddle, or dance to favorite music.
- Exercise to a workout video.

At Work

- Get off the bus or subway one stop early and walk or skate the rest of the way.
- Replace a coffee break with a brisk 10-minute walk. Ask a friend to go with you.
- Take part in an exercise program at work or a nearby gym.
- Join the office softball team or walking group.

At Play

- Walk, jog, skate, or cycle.
- Swim or do water aerobics.
- Take a class in martial arts, dance, or yoga.
- Golf (pull cart or carry clubs).
- Canoe, row, or kayak.
- Play racquetball, tennis, or squash.
- Ski cross-country or downhill.
- Play basketball, softball, or soccer.
- Hand cycle or play wheelchair sports.
- Take a nature walk.
- Most important—have fun while being active!

Chapter 16

Make a Fitness Plan and Stick with It

Chapter Contents

Section 16.1

Designing Your Own Fitness Plan

This section includes text excerpted from "Getting Started and Staying Active," Office on Women's Health (OWH), U.S. Department of Health and Human Services (HHS), March 27, 2015.

Getting Started and Staying Active

Are you new to physical activity? Start with small steps, like getting off the bus a couple of blocks early or taking the stairs instead of the elevator.

Do you think, "I don't have time to work out" or "Exercise is too boring!"? You may have lots of reasons not to be active. But there are so many more reasons to get fit!

Here's some info to help you get and stay active:

- Learn how to make a personal fitness plan—and stick to it!

- Get tips for making fitness fun.

- Check out some great ways to beat your obstacles.

How to Make a Fitness Plan

Use the three steps and tips below to make a personal fitness plan that's right for you.

1. Set Goals

- **Be specific.**

  Saying something like "I'll be active three days a week" works better than "I'll exercise more."

- **Be realistic.**

  If you try to increase your activity a lot all at once, you may get overwhelmed.

- **Go slow.**

  Try tackling just one goal at a time instead of several. After sticking with your goal for a couple of weeks, see if you can add another one.

2. Pick Small Steps

- **Break your goal into smaller steps.**

  That way it will feel more doable. If you said "I'll be active three days a week," for example, start by figuring out which days might work.

- **Pick items you enjoy.**

  You are more likely to stick with activities you enjoy. If you decide to walk, for example, ask a friend to join you to make it more fun.

- **Enter a few steps on your calendar.**

  Pick days. That way you won't forget and you'll make sure you have enough time.

3. Monitor Your Progress

- **Check your list.**

  See what you've done in the past week.

- **Did you skip a lot of your fitness time?**

  Don't give up! Creating new habits does not happen fast. This is a chance to see what gets in your way and then find solutions. For example, maybe you need to exercise in the morning instead of at night.

- **Did you succeed a lot of the time?**

  Celebrate! Reward yourself! Tell your friends and family! You might inspire them.

Section 16.2

Goal Setting

This section includes text excerpted from "Physical Activity:
Strength Training for Older Adults," Centers for Disease Control and
Prevention (CDC), December 3, 2008. Reviewed September 2016.

If you want to make positive, lasting change in your life, it helps to
spend some time thinking about motivation. What are your reasons
for wanting to exercise? What are your personal goals? What obstacles
do you anticipate and how might you overcome them? It's also a good
idea to visualize your success and consider how you might celebrate
your achievements.

Visualizing Your Goals

Believing in yourself—believing that you can leap barriers and achieve
your goals—is the ticket to success. One of the most powerful tools for
building self-confidence is visualization. This easy technique involves
imagining the accomplishment of the changes or goals you're working to
achieve. It is a process of "training" purely within the mind. By visualizing in detail your successful execution of each step in a given activity,
you create, modify, or strengthen brain pathways that are important in
coordinating your muscles for the visualized activity. This prepares you to
perform the activity itself. The technique is useful in many areas of life—
from avoiding anxiety during a stressful situation to performing well
during competition. You may find it a powerful tool in physical fitness.

1. Identify the goal you want to visualize—for example, walking
    a golf course.

2. Find a comfortable place to sit and relax.

3. Eliminate all distractions—turn off the phone, television, etc.

4. Close your eyes and focus on feeling relaxed. Free your mind of
    intruding thoughts.

5. Now, imagine yourself on the golf course. Create a picture
    in your mind of the place—the sights, sounds, and smells.

Imagine a perfect day, warm and sunny, with a gentle breeze. Picture yourself with your favorite golfing friends, talking and laughing. Now visualize yourself starting on your way, passing the golf carts, and setting off to walk the whole course.

6. Take a moment to feel the pleasure and excitement of achieving this goal.

7. Then imagine yourself walking from hole to hole, enjoying the sunshine, the views, the fresh air, the good company and excellent play.

8. Finally, visualize yourself finishing the course and feeling great, both physically and emotionally.

Define Your Goals

When taking on any challenge, it's a good idea to define your goals. You should identify what you want to accomplish and how you will carry out your plan. This is important when making positive change and will help you succeed. Before starting your exercise program, set short-term and long-term goals. These goals should be SMART: specific, measurable, attainable, relevant, and time based.

For example, a specific short-term goal may be to start strength training; the long-term goal may be easing the symptoms of arthritis, improving balance, or controlling your weight. This goal is easily measurable: Have you or have you not begun the program? Indeed, this is an attainable goal, as long as your doctor approves, and this goal is certainly relevant to living a long, healthy life. Your goal should be time based: you should buy the equipment you need and set your exercise schedule within the next five days. Start the program within the following two to three days.

The goals and time frame are entirely up to you. You may want to focus your long-term goals on improving a specific health condition, such as reducing pain from arthritis, controlling diabetes, increasing bone density to help combat osteoporosis, or increasing muscle mass to help with balance or weight control. Or your goal may be to bowl or play tennis. Your success depends on setting goals that are truly important to you—and possessing a strong desire to achieve them.

Identifying Your Short-Term Goals

Identify at least two or three of your own short-term goals and write them down. Remember that each goal should be S-M-A-R-T—specific, measurable, attainable, relevant, and time based. Setting these short-term goals will help motivate you to make the program a regular part of your life.

Examples

1. I will talk to my doctor about starting this program.

2. I will buy the equipment I need and get ready to exercise within two weeks.

3. I will look at my calendar and schedule two or three 45-minute blocks of time for exercise each week.

4. I will invite my spouse/friend/family member to join me in these exercises.

Identifying Your Long-Term Goals

Identify at least two or three long-term goals and write them down. Are there activities that you want to do more easily over the long-term? Are there things that you haven't done in some time that you want to try again? Listing these goals will help you stay with the program, see your progress, and enjoy your success. (Don't forget to use the S-M-A-R-T technique.)

Examples

1. I will do each exercise two or three times each week. Within three months, I will do each exercise with five-pound weights.

2. After 12 weeks of the program, I will take the stairs instead of the elevator.

3. I will play golf.

4. I will reduce some of the pain and stiffness from arthritis.

Stay Motivated

Consider these factors that motivate people to begin and stick with their exercise program. Then identify which ones motivate you.

- **Pleasure:** People often really enjoy strength-training exercises; they find them less taxing than aerobic workouts and love the results.

- **Health and fitness benefits:** Strength training increases muscle mass and bone density. It makes you feel strong and energized, alleviates stress and depression, and gives you a better night's sleep. And it can help prevent the onset of certain chronic diseases or ease their symptoms.

- **Improvements in appearance:** Lifting weights firms the body, trims fat, and can boost metabolism by as much as 15 percent which helps with weight control.

- **Social opportunities:** Exercising with friends or family gives you a chance to visit and chat while you work out.

- **Thrills:** People who start strength training later in life often find that they are willing and able to try new, exciting activities, such as parasailing, windsurfing, or kayaking.

Celebrate Your Achievements

Making any major lifestyle change can be trying. A great way to motivate yourself to keep with the program is to properly celebrate your achievements. This may be as important as setting goals and visualizing success. When you accomplish one of your short-term or long-term goals, make sure that you reward yourself well!

1. Buy yourself new workout clothes or shoes.

2. Make plans with good friends to see a movie or go hiking.

3. Go on a weekend getaway.

4. Treat yourself to a new piece of exercise equipment.

5. Plan a dinner at your favorite restaurant.

6. Get tickets to your favorite theater production or athletic event.

7. Pamper yourself with a massage, manicure, or pedicure.

8. Enroll in a class, such as ballroom dancing, yoga, or pottery making.

Chapter 17

Overcoming Barriers to Exercise

You know that physical activity is good for you. So what is stopping you from getting out there and getting at it? Maybe you think that working out is boring, joining a gym is costly, or doing one more thing during your busy day is impossible. Physical activity can be part of your daily life, and his chapter offers ideas to beat your roadblocks to getting active.

Why Should I Be Physically Active?

You may know that regular physical activity can help you control your weight. But do you know why? Physical activity burns calories. When you burn more calories than you eat each day, you will take off pounds. You can also avoid gaining weight by balancing the number of calories you burn with the number of calories you eat. Regular physical activity may also help prevent or delay the onset of chronic diseases like type 2 diabetes, heart disease, high blood pressure, and stroke. If you have one of these health problems, physical activity may improve your condition. Regular physical activity may also increase your energy and boost your mood.

This chapter includes text excerpted from "Tips to Help You Get Active," National Institute of Diabetes and Digestive and Kidney Diseases (NIDDK), January 2009. Reviewed September 2016.

If you are a man and over age 40 or a woman and over age 50, or have a chronic health problem, talk to your healthcare provider before starting a vigorous physical activity program. You do not need to talk to your provider before starting an activity like walking.

What Is Standing in My Way?

Personal Barriers

Barrier: Between work, family, and other demands, I am too busy to exercise.

Solutions: Make physical activity a priority. Carve out some time each week to be active, and put it on your calendar. Try waking up a half hour earlier to walk, scheduling lunchtime workouts, or taking an evening fitness class.

Build physical activity into your routine chores. Rake the yard, wash the car, or do energetic housework. That way you do what you need to do around the house and move around too. Make family time physically active. Plan a weekend hike through a park, a family softball game, or an evening walk around the block.

Barrier: By the end of a long day, I am just too tired to work out.

Solutions: Think about the other health benefits of physical activity. Regular physical activity may help lower cholesterol and blood pressure. It may also lower your odds of having heart disease, type 2 diabetes, or cancer. Research shows that people who are overweight, active, and fit live longer than people who are not overweight but are inactive and unfit. Also, physical activity may lift your mood and increase your energy level.

Do it just for fun. Play a team sport, work in a garden, or learn a new dance. Make getting fit something fun.

Train for a charity event. You can work to help others while you work out.

Barrier: Getting on a treadmill or stationary bike is boring.

Solutions: Meet a friend for workouts. If your buddy is on the next bike or treadmill, your workout will be less boring.

Watch TV or listen to music or an audio book while you walk or pedal indoors. Check out music or audio books from your local library.

Get outside. A change in scenery can relieve your boredom. If you are riding a bike outside, be sure to wear a helmet and learn safe rules of the road.

Barrier: I am afraid I will hurt myself.

Solutions: Start slowly. If you are starting a new physical activity program, go slow at the start. Even if you are doing an activity that you once did well, start up again slowly to lower your risk of injury or burnout.

Choose moderate-intensity physical activities. You are not likely to hurt yourself by walking 30 minutes per day. Doing vigorous physical activities may increase your risk for injury, but moderate-intensity physical activity carries a lower risk.

Take a class. A knowledgeable group fitness instructor should be able to teach you how to move with proper form and lower risk for injury. The instructor can watch your actions during class and let you know if you are doing things right.

Choose water workouts. Whether you swim laps or try water aerobics, working out in the water is easy on your joints and helps reduce sore muscles and injury.

Work with a personal trainer. A certified personal trainer should be able to show you how to warm up, cool down, use fitness equipment like treadmills and dumbbells, and use proper form to help lower your risk for injury. Personal training sessions may be cheap or costly, so find out about fees before making an appointment.

Barrier: I have never been into sports.

Solutions: Find a physical activity that you enjoy. You do not have to be an athlete to benefit from physical activity. Try yoga, hiking, or planting a garden.

Choose an activity that you can stick with, like walking. Just put one foot in front of the other. Use the time you spend walking to relax, talk with a friend or family member, or just enjoy the scenery.

Barrier: I do not want to spend a lot of money to join a gym or buy workout gear.

Solutions: Choose free activities. Take your children to the park to play or take a walk.

Find out if your job offers any discounts on memberships. Some companies get lower membership rates at fitness or community centers.

Other companies will even pay for part of an employee's membership fee. Check out your local recreation or community center. These centers may cost less than other gyms, fitness centers, or health clubs.

Choose physical activities that do not require any special gear. Walking requires only a pair of sturdy shoes. To dance, just turn on some music.

Barrier: I do not have anyone to watch my kids while I work out.

Solutions: Do something physically active with your kids. Kids need physical activity too. No matter what age your kids are, you can find an activity you can do together. Dance to music, take a walk, run around the park, or play basketball or soccer together.

Take turns with another parent to watch the kids. One of you minds the kids while the other one works out.

Hire a babysitter.

Look for a fitness or community center that offers child care. Centers that offer child care are becoming more popular. Cost and quality vary, so get all the information up front.

Barrier: My family and friends are not physically active.

Solutions: Do not let that stop you. Do it for yourself. Enjoy the rewards you get from working out, such as better sleep, a happier mood, more energy, and a stronger body.

Join a class or sports league where people count on you to show up. If your basketball team or dance partner counts on you, you will not want to miss a workout, even if your family and friends are not involved.

Barrier: I would be embarrassed if my neighbors or friends saw me exercising.

Solutions: Ask yourself if it really matters. You are doing something positive for your health and that is something to be proud of. You may even inspire others to get physically active too.

Invite a friend or neighbor to join you. You may feel less self-conscious if you are not alone.

Go to a park, nature trail, or fitness or community center to be physically active.

Place Barriers

Barrier: My neighborhood does not have sidewalks.

Solutions: Find a safe place to walk. Instead of walking in the street, walk in a friend or family member's neighborhood that has sidewalks. Walk during your lunch break at work. Find out if you can walk at a local school track.

Work out in the yard. Do yard work or wash the car. These count as physical activity too.

Barrier: The winter is too cold / summer is too hot to be active outdoors.

Solutions: Walk around the mall. Join a mall-walking group to walk indoors year-round. Join a fitness or community center. Find one that lets you pay only for the months or classes you want, instead of the whole year.

Exercise at home. Work out to fitness videos or DVDs. Check a different one out from the library each week for variety.

Barrier: I do not feel safe exercising by myself.

Solutions: Join or start a walking group. You can enjoy added safety and company as you walk.

Take an exercise class at a nearby fitness or community center.

Work out at home. You don't need a lot of space. Turn on the radio and dance or follow along with a fitness show on TV.

Health Barriers

Barrier: I have a health problem (diabetes, heart disease, asthma, arthritis) that I do not want to make worse.

Solutions: Talk with your healthcare professional. Most health problems are helped by physical activity. Find out what physical activities you can safely do and follow advice about length and intensity of workouts.

Start slowly. Take it easy at first and see how you feel before trying more challenging workouts. Stop if you feel out of breath, dizzy, faint, or nauseated, or if you have pain.

Barrier: I have an injury and do not know what physical activities, if any, I can do.

Solutions: Talk with your healthcare professional. Ask your doctor or physical therapist about what physical activities you can safely perform. Follow advice about length and intensity of workouts.

Start slowly. Take it easy at first and see how you feel before trying more challenging workouts. Stop if you feel pain.

Work with a personal trainer. A knowledgeable personal trainer should be able to help you design a fitness plan around your injury.

What Can I Do to Break through My Roadblocks?

What are the top two or three roadblocks to physical activity that you face? What can you do to break through these barriers? Write down a list of the barriers you face and solutions you can use to overcome them.

You have thought about ways to beat your roadblocks to physical activity. Now, create your roadmap for adding physical activity to your life by following these three steps:

1. **Know your goal.** Set up short-term goals, like walking 10 minutes a day, three days a week. Once you are comfortable, try to do more. Try 15 minutes instead of 10 minutes. Then walk on more days a week while adding more minutes to your walk. You can try different activities too. To add variety, you can do low-impact aerobics or water aerobics for 30 minutes, two days a week. Then walk on a treadmill or outdoors for 30 minutes, one day a week. Then do yoga or lift weights for two days. Track your progress by writing down your goals and what you have done each day, including the type of activity and how long you spent doing it. Seeing your progress in black and white can help keep you motivated.

2. **See your healthcare provider if necessary.** If you are a man and over age 40 or a woman and over age 50, or have a chronic health problem such as heart disease, high blood pressure, diabetes, osteoporosis, or obesity, talk to your healthcare provider before starting a vigorous physical activity program. You do not need to talk to your provider before starting an activity like walking.

3. **Answer questions about how physical activity will fit into your life.** Think about answers to the following four questions. You can write your answers on a sheet of paper. Your answers will be your roadmap to your physical activity program.

   • **What physical activities will you do?** List the activities you would like to do, such as walking, energetic yard work or housework, joining a sports league, exercising with a video, dancing, swimming, bicycling, or taking a class at a fitness or community center. Think about sports or other activities that you enjoyed doing when you were younger. Could you enjoy one of these activities again?

- **When will you be physically active?** List the days and times you could do each activity on your list, such as first thing in the morning, during lunch break from work, after dinner, or on Saturday afternoon. Look at your calendar or planner to find the days and times that work best.

- **Who will remind you to get off the couch?** List the people—your spouse, sibling, parent, or friends—who can support your efforts to become physically active. Give them ideas about how they could be supportive, like offering encouraging words, watching your kids, or working out with you.

- **When will you start your physical activity program?** Set a date when you will start getting active. The date might be the first meeting of an exercise class you have signed up for, or a date you will meet a friend for a walk. Write the date on your calendar. Then stick to it. Before you know it, physical activity will become a regular part of your life.

Chapter 18

Measuring Physical Activity Intensity and Physical Fitness

Chapter Contents

Section 18.1

Measuring Physical Activity Intensity

This section includes text excerpted from "Measuring Physical Activity Intensity," Centers for Disease Control and Prevention (CDC), June 4, 2015.

How Much Physical Activity Do You Need?

Regular physical activity helps improve your overall health and fitness, and reduces your risk for many chronic diseases.

Fitting regular exercise into your daily schedule may seem difficult at first, but the *2008 Physical Activity Guidelines for Americans* are more flexible than ever, giving you the freedom to reach your physical activity goals through different types and amounts of activities each week. It's easier than you think!

Measuring Physical Activity

Here are some ways to understand and measure the intensity of aerobic activity: relative intensity and absolute intensity.

Relative Intensity

The level of effort required by a person to do an activity. When using relative intensity, people pay attention to how physical activity affects their heart rate and breathing.

The **talk test** is a simple way to measure relative intensity. In general, if you're doing moderate-intensity activity you can talk, but not sing, during the activity. If you're doing vigorous-intensity activity, you will not be able to say more than a few words without pausing for a breath.

Absolute Intensity

The amount of energy used by the body per minute of activity. The list below has examples of activities classified as moderate-intensity or vigorous-intensity based upon the amount of energy used by the body while doing the activity.

Moderate Intensity

- Walking briskly (3 miles per hour or faster, but not race-walking)
- Water aerobics
- Bicycling slower than 10 miles per hour
- Tennis (doubles)
- Ballroom dancing
- General gardening

Vigorous Intensity

- Race walking, jogging, or running
- Swimming laps
- Tennis (singles)
- Aerobic dancing
- Bicycling 10 miles per hour or faster
- Jumping rope
- Heavy gardening (continuous digging or hoeing)
- Hiking uphill or with a heavy backpack

Section 18.2

Target Heart Rates

This section contains text excerpted from the following sources: Text beginning with the heading "Target Heart Rate" is excerpted from "Target Heart Rate and Estimated Maximum Heart Rate," Centers for Disease Control and Prevention (CDC), August 10, 2015; Text under the heading "Tracking Your Target Heart Rate" is excerpted from "Your Guide To Physical Activity and Your Heart," National Heart, Lung, and Blood Institute (NHLBI), June 2006. Reviewed September 2016.

Target Heart Rate

One way of monitoring physical activity intensity is to determine whether a person's pulse or heart rate is within the target zone during physical activity.

For moderate-intensity physical activity, a person's target heart rate should be 50 to 70 percent of his or her maximum heart rate. This maximum rate is based on the person's age. An estimate of a person's maximum age-related heart rate can be obtained by subtracting the person's age from 220. For example, for a 50-year-old person, the estimated maximum age-related heart rate would be calculated as 220 - 50 years = 170 beats per minute (bpm). The 50 percent and 70 percent levels would be:

- 50 percent level: 170 x 0.50 = 85 bpm, and

- 70 percent level: 170 x 0.70 = 119 bpm

Thus, moderate-intensity physical activity for a 50-year-old person will require that the heart rate remains between 85 and 119 bpm during physical activity.

For vigorous-intensity physical activity, a person's target heart rate should be 70 to 85 percent of his or her maximum heart rate. To calculate this range, follow the same formula as used above, except change "50 and 70 percent" to "70 and 85 percent." For example, for a 35-year-old person, the estimated maximum age-related heart rate would be calculated as 220 – 35 years = 185 beats per minute (bpm). The 70% and 85% levels would be:

- 70% level: 185 x 0.70 = 130 bpm, and

- 85% level: 185 x 0.85 = 157 bpm

Thus, vigorous-intensity physical activity for a 35-year-old person will require that the heart rate remains between 130 and 157 bpm during physical activity.

Taking Your Heart Rate

Generally, to determine whether you are exercising within the heart rate target zone, you must stop exercising briefly to take your pulse. You can take the pulse at the neck, the wrist, or the chest. Taking the pulse at the wrist is recommended. You can feel the radial pulse on the artery of the wrist in line with the thumb. Place the tips of the index and middle fingers over the artery and press lightly. Do not use the thumb. Take a full 60-second count of the heartbeats, or take for 30 seconds and multiply by 2. Start the count on a beat, which is counted as "zero." If this number falls between 85 and 119 bpm in the case of the 50-year-old person, he or she is active within the target range for moderate-intensity activity.

Tracking Your Target Heart Rate

As you become more physically active, how will you know whether you're improving your heart and lung fitness? The best way is to track your target heart rate during your activity. Your target heart rate is a percentage of your maximum heart rate, which is the fastest your heart can beat, based on your age. Unless you're in excellent physical condition, any physical activity that boosts your heart rate above 75 percent of your maximum rate is likely to be too strenuous. By the same token, any activity that increases your heart rate to less than 50 percent of your maximum rate gives your heart and lungs too little conditioning.

Table 18.1. Target Heart Rate

Finding Your Target Heart Rate Zone		
Age	Target Heart Rate Zone: 50–75%	Maximum Heart Rate: 100%
20	100–150 beats per min.	200 beats per min.
25	98–146 beats per min.	195 beats per min.
30	95–142 beats per min.	190 beats per min.
35	93–138 beats per min.	185 beats per min.

Table 18.1. Continued

Finding Your Target Heart Rate Zone		
Age	Target Heart Rate Zone: 50–75%	Maximum Heart Rate: 100%
40	90-135 beats per min.	180 beats per min.
45	88-131 beats per min.	175 beats per min.
50	85-127 beats per min.	170 beats per min.
55	83-123 beats per min.	165 beats per min.
60	80-120 beats per min.	160 beats per min.
65	78-116 beats per min.	155 beats per min.
70	75-113 beats per min.	150 beats per min.

Section 18.3

Perceived Exertion

This section includes text excerpted from "Perceived
Exertion (Borg Rating of Perceived Exertion Scale)," Centers
for Disease Control and Prevention (CDC), August 11, 2015.

Borg Rating of Perceived Exertion Scale

The Borg Rating of Perceived Exertion (RPE) is a way of measuring
physical activity intensity level. Perceived exertion is how hard you
feel like your body is working. It is based on the physical sensations
a person experiences during physical activity, including increased
heart rate, increased respiration or breathing rate, increased sweating,
and muscle fatigue. Although this is a subjective measure, a person's
exertion rating may provide a fairly good estimate of the actual heart
rate during physical activity*.

* *A high correlation exists between a person's perceived exertion rating times 10
and the actual heart rate during physical activity; so a person's exertion rating may
provide a fairly good estimate of the actual heart rate during activity. For example,
if a person's rating of perceived exertion (RPE) is 12, then 12 x 10 = 120; so the heart
rate should be approximately 120 beats per minute. Note that this calculation is*

only an approximation of heart rate, and the actual heart rate can vary quite a bit depending on age and physical condition. The Borg Rating of Perceived Exertion is also the preferred method to assess intensity among those individuals who take medications that affect heart rate or pulse.

Practitioners generally agree that perceived exertion ratings between 12 to 14 on the Borg Scale suggests that physical activity is being performed at a moderate level of intensity. During activity, use the Borg Scale to assign numbers to how you feel (see instructions below). Self-monitoring how hard your body is working can help you adjust the intensity of the activity by speeding up or slowing down your movements.

Through experience of monitoring how your body feels, it will become easier to know when to adjust your intensity. For example, a walker who wants to engage in moderate-intensity activity would aim for a Borg Scale level of "somewhat hard" (12–14). If he describes his muscle fatigue and breathing as "very light" (9 on the Borg Scale) he would want to increase his intensity. On the other hand, if he felt his exertion was "extremely hard" (19 on the Borg Scale) he would need to slow down his movements to achieve the moderate-intensity range.

Instructions for Borg Rating of Perceived Exertion (RPE) Scale

While doing physical activity, rate your perception of exertion. This feeling should reflect how heavy and strenuous the exercise feels to you, combining all sensations and feelings of physical stress, effort, and fatigue. Do not concern yourself with any one factor such as leg pain or shortness of breath, but try to focus on your total feeling of exertion.

Look at the rating scale below while you are engaging in an activity; it ranges from 6 to 20, where 6 means "no exertion at all" and 20 means "maximal exertion." Choose the number from below that best describes your level of exertion. This will give you a good idea of the intensity level of your activity, and you can use this information to speed up or slow down your movements to reach your desired range.

Try to appraise your feeling of exertion as honestly as possible, without thinking about what the actual physical load is. Your own feeling of effort and exertion is important, not how it compares to other people's. Look at the scales and the expressions and then give a number.

Table 18.2. Level of Exertion

#	Level of Exertion
6	No exertion at all
7	
7.5	Extremely light (7.5)
8	
9	Very light
10	
11	Light
12	
13	Somewhat hard
14	
15	Hard (heavy)
16	
17	Very hard
18	
19	Extremely hard
20	Maximal exertion

9 corresponds to "very light" exercise. For a healthy person, it is like walking slowly at his or her own pace for some minutes

13 on the scale is "somewhat hard" exercise, but it still feels OK to continue.

17 "very hard" is very strenuous. A healthy person can still go on, but he or she really has to push him- or herself. It feels very heavy, and the person is very tired.

19 on the scale is an extremely strenuous exercise level. For most people this is the most strenuous exercise they have ever experienced.

Section 18.4

Burning Calories

This section contains text excerpted from the following sources: Text
beginning with the heading "What Are Calories?" is excerpted from
"A Calorie Is a Calorie, or Is It?" Department of Health and Human
Services (HHS), January 15, 2005. Reviewed September 2016; Text
under the heading "Calories Burned during Physical Activities" is
excerpted from "Calories Burned during Physical Activities," U.S.
Department of Veterans Affairs (VA), March 16, 2014.

What Are Calories?

A calorie is the amount of heat needed to raise the temperature of
a liter of water 1 degree. Sure, it was hard to understand when your
science teacher explained it. Relax. It is just a scientific way to measure energy. That said, what do you need to know about calories? Just
a few things: Think about what you regularly eat, what your calorie
needs are, and how to count calories. It takes approximately 3,500
calories below your calorie needs to lose a pound of body fat. It takes
approximately 3,500 calories above your calorie needs to gain a pound.

At this point, you know how many excess calories it takes to gain a
pound or deficit calories to lose a pound (3,500), and you know about
how many calories you need. You are already on the road to a Healthier
You! The next thing you need to learn is how to count calories so you
can determine how many you eat each day. At first, this may seem
like too much trouble, but once you get familiar with portion size and
the number of calories in your favorite foods, you'll be able to estimate
how many calories you eat each day, easily, without weighing your
food and without taking too much of your valuable time.

How Many Calories Do You Eat Each Day?

Calories count and they come from both food and beverages. When
eating packaged foods (for example, frozen, canned, and some prepared foods from the grocery store), counting your calories is easy, as
it is on the Nutrition Facts label. When eating foods that do not have
a Nutrition Facts label, such as fresh fruits and vegetables, or when

eating at home or in restaurants, determining calories is more difficult. If you can't count calories because there is no Nutrition Facts label, you should pay attention to portion size.

Use the Nutrition Facts label. Most packaged foods have a Nutrition Facts label. You can use this tool to make smart food choices and to find out how many calories and nutrients you are actually eating. To use the label effectively to count calories, you need to check serving size, servings per container, and calories. Look at the serving size and the number of servings per container. How many servings are you consuming? If you are eating 2 servings, you are eating double the calories and the nutrients listed on the Nutrition Facts label.

Portion size is the amount of food eaten at one time. Serving size is the amount stated on the Nutrition Facts label. Sometimes, the portion size and serving size match; sometimes, they don't. For example, if the label says that 1 serving size is 6 cookies and you eat 3, you've eaten ½ of a serving of cookies. More importantly, you have just reduced by half the calories listed on the Nutrition Facts label. Remember that the serving size on the Nutrition Facts label is not a recommended amount to eat; it's a simple and easy way for letting you know the calories and nutrients in a certain amount of a food. If the label helps you be more aware of how much you eat or drink—all the better!

When eating foods without a Nutrition Facts label, pay attention to how your portion size compares to a recommended amount of food from each food group.

Some foods prepared at the grocery store and other foods such as produce items may not have food packaging that provides nutritional information, but this information can sometimes be obtained in the store by request. Many restaurants have nutrition information on the foods they serve available at the restaurant or on their Website. As grocery stores increase the number of prepared products that have nutrition information, it will become easier for you to make lower-calorie choices to help you control your calories every day. Don't be afraid to ask for nutrition information if you don't see it displayed at the grocery store or on the menu when eating out.

The serving size of this food is 1 cup, and there are 2 servings in this container. There are 260 calories per serving of this food. If you eat the entire container of this product, you will eat 2 servings. That means you need to double the calories (260 calories x 2 = 520 calories) to know how many calories you are eating. If you eat 2 servings, you will have eaten over 500 calories!

Now, you've learned how to use food packaging to help you figure out how many calories you are eating. Estimating how many calories you are getting from these foods can be challenging at first. But since one of the best ways to manage your weight is to be aware of foods and beverages high in calories, being able to keep track of where your calories are coming from is an important skill that will help you for the rest of your life.

Calories Burned during Physical Activities

The following table gives the number of calories you burn doing 10 minutes of each physical activity listed. The calories will vary depending on a number of factors including weight, age, and environmental conditions. The figures given are for men ranging in weight from 175–250 lbs. and women ranging from 140–200 lbs. If you weigh more than this, you will burn more calories per minute.

Table 18.3. Calories Burned in 10 Minutes

Light Activity	Male	Female
Ballroom Dancing	35–50	28–40
Cleaning, Sweeping at moderate effort	26–38	21–30
Washing Dishes	29–42	23–30
Tai Chi	35–50	28–40
Moderate Activity		
Bicycling at <10 miles per hour	46–66	37–53
Step Aerobics	64–91	51–73
Cleaning Gutters	58–83	46–66
Mowing the Lawn	64–91	51–73
Raking Leaves	44–63	35–50
Walking at 4 miles per hour	58–83	46–66
Shoveling Snow	61–88	49–70
Bowling	44–63	35–50
Golf, Walking and Pulling Clubs	61–88	49–70
Slow Lap-Swimming	63–90	54–72
Vigorous Activity		
Jogging (9 min/mile)	149–213	119–170

Table 18.3. Continued

Light Activity	Male	Female
Basketball	75–108	60–86
Carrying Groceries Upstairs	87–125	70–100

Section 18.5

Body Mass Index (BMI)

This section includes text excerpted from "About Adult BMI,"
Centers for Disease Control and Prevention (CDC), May 15, 2015.

What Is Body Mass Index (BMI)?

Body mass index (BMI) is a person's weight in kilograms divided by the square of height in meters. BMI does not measure body fat directly, but research has shown that BMI is moderately correlated with more direct measures of body fat obtained from skinfold thickness measurements, bioelectrical impedance, densitometry (underwater weighing), dual energy X-ray absorptiometry (DXA) and other methods.

Furthermore, BMI appears to be as strongly correlated with various metabolic and disease outcome as are these more direct measures of body fatness. In general, BMI is an inexpensive and easy-to-perform method of screening for weight category, for example underweight, normal or healthy weight, overweight, and obesity.

How Is BMI Used?

A high BMI can be an indicator of high body fatness. BMI can be used as a screening tool but is not diagnostic of the body fatness or health of an individual.

To determine if a high BMI is a health risk, a healthcare provider would need to perform further assessments. These assessments might include skinfold thickness measurements, evaluations of diet, physical activity, family history, and other appropriate health screenings.

What Are the BMI Trends for Adults in the United States?

The prevalence of adult BMI greater than or equal to 30 kg/m² (obese status) has greatly increased since the 1970s. Recently, however, this trend has leveled off, except for older women. Obesity has continued to increase in adult women who are age 60 years and older.

Why Is BMI Used to Measure Overweight and Obesity?

BMI can be used for population assessment of overweight and obesity. Because calculation requires only height and weight, it is inexpensive and easy to use for clinicians and for the general public. BMI can be used as a screening tool for body fatness but is not diagnostic.

What Are Some of the Other Ways to Assess Excess Body Fatness besides BMI?

Other methods to measure body fatness include skinfold thickness measurements (with calipers), underwater weighing, bioelectrical impedance, dual-energy X-ray absorptiometry (DXA), and isotope dilution. However, these methods are not always readily available, and they are either expensive or need to be conducted by highly trained personnel. Furthermore, many of these methods can be difficult to standardize across observers or machines, complicating comparisons across studies and time periods.

How Is BMI Calculated?

BMI is calculated the same way for both adults and children. The calculation is based on the following formulas:

Table 18.4. BMI Calculated

Measurement Units	Formula and Calculation
Kilograms and meters (or centimeters)	Formula: weight (kg) / [height (m)]² With the metric system, the formula for BMI is weight in kilograms divided by height in meters squared. Because height is commonly measured in centimeters, divide height in centimeters by 100 to obtain height in meters. Example: Weight = 68 kg, Height = 165 cm (1.65 m) Calculation: $68 \div (1.65)^2 = 24.98$

Table 18.4. Continued

Measurement Units	Formula and Calculation
Pounds and inches	Formula: weight (lb) / [height (in)]^2 x 703 Calculate BMI by dividing weight in pounds (lbs) by height in inches (in) squared and multiplying by a conversion factor of 703. Example: Weight = 150 lbs, Height = 5'5" (65") Calculation: [150 ÷ (65)^2] x 703 = 24.96

How Is BMI Interpreted for Adults?

For adults 20 years old and older, BMI is interpreted using standard weight status categories. These categories are the same for men and women of all body types and ages.

The standard weight status categories associated with BMI ranges for adults are shown in the following table.

Table 18.5. BMI Interpreted

BMI	Weight Status
Below 18.5	Underweight
18.5–24.9	Normal or Healthy Weight
25.0–29.9	Overweight
30.0 and Above	Obese

For example, here are the weight ranges, the corresponding BMI ranges, and the weight status categories for a person who is 5' 9".

Table 18.6. Corresponding BMI Ranges

Height	Weight Range	BMI	Weight Status
5' 9"	124 lbs or less	Below 18.5	Underweight
	125 lbs to 168 lbs	18.5 to 24.9	Normal or Healthy Weight
	169 lbs to 202 lbs	25.0 to 29.9	Overweight
	203 lbs or more	30 or higher	Obese

For children and teens, the interpretation of BMI depends upon age and sex.

Is BMI Interpreted the Same Way for Children and Teens as It Is for Adults?

BMI is interpreted differently for children and teens, even though it is calculated using the same formula as adult BMI. Children and teen's BMI need to be age and sex-specific because the amount of body fat changes with age and the amount of body fat differs between girls and boys. The Centers for Disease Control and Prevention (CDC) BMI-for-age growth charts take into account these differences and visually show BMI as a percentile ranking. These percentiles were determined using representative data of the U.S. population of 2- to 19-year-olds that was collected in various surveys from 1963–65 to 1988–94.

Obesity among 2- to 19-year-olds is defined as a BMI at or above the 95th percentile of children of the same age and sex in this 1963 to 1994 reference population. For example, a 10-year-old boy of average height (56 inches) who weighs 102 pounds would have a BMI of 22.9 kg/m². This would place the boy in the 95th percentile for BMI—meaning that his BMI is greater than that of 95 percent of similarly aged boys in this reference population—and he would be considered to have obesity.

How Good Is BMI as an Indicator of Body Fatness?

The correlation between the BMI and body fatness is fairly strong, but even if 2 people have the same BMI, their level of body fatness may differ.

In general,

- At the same BMI, women tend to have more body fat than men.

- At the same BMI, Blacks have less body fat than do Whites, and Asians have more body fat than do Whites

- At the same BMI, older people, on average, tend to have more body fat than younger adults.

- At the same BMI, athletes have less body fat than do non-athletes.

The accuracy of BMI as an indicator of body fatness also appears to be higher in persons with higher levels of BMI and body fatness. While, a person with a very high BMI (e.g., 35 kg/m²) is very likely to have high body fat, a relatively high BMI can be the results of either high body fat or high lean body mass (muscle and bone). A trained healthcare provider should perform appropriate health assessments in order to evaluate an individual's health status and risks.

If an Athlete or Other Person with a Lot of Muscle Has a BMI over 25, Is That Person Still Considered to Be Overweight?

According to the BMI weight status categories, anyone with a BMI between 25 and 29.9 would be classified as overweight and anyone with a BMI over 30 would be classified as obese.

However, athletes may have a high BMI because of increased muscularity rather than increased body fatness. In general, a person who has a high BMI is likely to have body fatness and would be considered to be overweight or obese, but this may not apply to athletes. A trained healthcare provider should perform appropriate health assessments in order to evaluate an individual's health status and risks.

Chapter 19

Choosing Physical Fitness Partners

Chapter Contents

Section 19.1

Exercising with Your Loved One

This section includes text excerpted from "Help a Loved One Get More Active: Quick Tips," Office of Disease Prevention and Health Promotion (ODPHP), U.S. Department of Health and Human Services (HHS), March 23, 2016.

Lots of people struggle to fit physical activity into their busy lives. If someone you care about is having a hard time getting active, you can help. Here are some tips to get you started.

Suggest Activities You Can Do Together

- Start small. Try taking a walk after dinner twice a week, or do crunches (sit-ups) while you watch TV.

- Mix it up. Learn new stretches and warm-up exercises.

- Join a fitness class. Choose an activity that's new for both of you.

Make It Part of Your Regular Routine

- Meet up at the local gym or recreation center on your way home from work.

- Wake up a bit earlier so you can go for a brisk walk together before breakfast.

- Pick a certain time for physical activity, like right after your favorite TV show.

- Ride your bikes or walk to the store or coffee shop.

Be Understanding

What are your loved one's reasons for not being more active? Maybe he or she feels overwhelmed or embarrassed. Ask what you can do to be supportive.

Recognize Small Efforts

- Be patient. Change takes time.

- Remember, some physical activity is better than none!

- Offer encouragement and praise. ("Great job doing your crunches today!")

- Point out positive choices. ("I'm glad we're walking to the park instead of driving.")

Choose Healthy Gifts

For birthdays or special rewards, choose gifts that encourage your loved one to be more active. Some ideas include:

- New sneakers or workout clothes

- A basketball or balance ball

- Hand weights

- A yoga mat

- A pedometer (a tool that counts the number of steps you take)

- Gift certificate to a gym or exercise class

Section 19.2

Making Exercise Fun for the Whole Family

This section includes text excerpted from "Active Families," WhiteHouse.gov, August 23, 2016.

Active Families

Engaging in physical activity as a family can be a fun way to get everyone moving. Studies show that kids who believe they are competent and have the skills to be physically active are more likely to be active. And those who feel supported by friends and families to become active, or surrounded by others interested in physical activity, are more likely to participate.

Children need 60 minutes of play with moderate to vigorous activity every day, but it doesn't have to occur at once. It all adds up! And remember, sleep is just as important and is an essential part of living an active life. A recent study found that with each extra hour of sleep, the risk of a child being overweight or obese dropped by nine percent.

Here are a few activities and steps that you and your family can consider to get started on a path to a healthier lifestyle:

- Give children toys that encourage physical activity like balls, kites, and jump ropes.

- Encourage children to join a sports team or try a new physical activity.

- Limit TV time and keep the TV out of a child's bedroom.

- Facilitate a safe walk to and from school a few times a week.

- Take the stairs instead of the elevator.

- Walk around the block after a meal.

- Make a new house rule: no sitting still during television commercials.

- Find time to spend together doing a fun activity: family park day, swim day or bike day.

- Issue a family challenge to see who can be the first to achieve a Presidential Active Lifestyle Award by committing to physical activity five days a week, for six weeks. Adults and children can both receive the award!

- Talk to your children's principal or write a letter to your district superintendent to incorporate more physical education in schools.

- Encourage schools to hold recess prior to lunch to increase physical activity before mealtime.

- Volunteer to help with afterschool physical activity programs or sports teams.

- Be sure that children get the sleep they need. Most children under age five need to sleep for 11 hours or more per day, children age five to 10 need 10 hours of sleep or more per day, and children over age 10 need at least nine hours per day.

Find Places to Get Moving Outside

Regular exercise in nature is proven to improve children's physical and mental health. Outdoor activity helps kids maintain a healthy weight, boosts their immunity and bone health, and lowers stress.

Kids need at least 60 minutes of active and vigorous play each day to stay healthy, and one of the easiest and most enjoyable ways to meet this goal is by playing outside.

Have Fun outside and Get Exercise

Getting outside isn't just a great way to get exercise, it's also a lot of fun! Find affordable physical activities that will bring the whole family together and start enjoying the great outdoors.

Let's Explore

Traveling by foot is a fun, easy and affordable way to get moving and get outside. From a walk around the block to a mountain hike there are a lot of new places to explore. Activities like hiking and walking have been shown to improve cardiovascular health and build stronger bones. Stay healthy by making physical activity a part of your family's routine.

Let's Ride

Biking is a fun, family-friendly activity that can help improve endurance and balance. Use your bike as a means of "active transport" to get places faster while also getting healthier. Explore your community by bike with your family and get everyone active.

Let's Swim

When the weather is warm, there is no better way to cool off—or get fit—than by splashing around. Swimming burns more calories per hour than almost any other activity, and has been shown to improve cardiovascular health and lead to greater strength and flexibility. It's also low-impact, making it an ideal activity for people with disabilities or those recovering from an injury.

Let's Play

Getting active outside can help to improve coordination, balance, and agility. Keep kids healthy mentally and physically by making time for play each day.

Chapter 20

Joining a Gym

If you're looking to get in shape, a membership at a gym, fitness center, health spa, or sports club could be a good option. But joining a gym often means signing a contract, and not all contracts are the same. To avoid a problem down the road, find out more about the business and what you're committing to before you sign up. People have told the Federal Trade Commission (FTC) about high-pressure sales tactics, misrepresentations about facilities and services, broken cancellation policies, and lost membership fees when gyms go out of business.

Check out the Facilities

Plan a visit at a time you would normally be using the gym to see how crowded it is, whether the facilities are clean and well-maintained, and whether the equipment is in good shape. Ask about the:

- **Number of members.** Many gyms set no membership limits. It might not be crowded when you visit, but be packed during peak hours or after a membership drive.

- **Hours of operation.** Do they suit your schedule? Some fitness centers restrict men's use to certain days and women's to others. Some may limit lower-cost memberships to certain hours.

This chapter includes text excerpted from "Joining a Gym," Federal Trade Commission (FTC), July 15, 2012. Reviewed September 2016.

- **Instructors and trainers.** Some places hire trainers and instructors who have special qualifications. If you're looking for professionals to help you, ask about their qualifications and how long they've been on the staff.

- **Classes.** Will you need to pay extra for certain activities, or are they included in your membership fees?

Know What You're Agreeing To

Some gyms will ask you to join—and pay—the first time you visit and will offer incentives like special rates to get you to sign on the spot. It's best to wait a few days before deciding. Take the contract home and read it carefully. Before you sign, find out:

Is Everything the Salesperson Promised Written in the Contract?

If a problem comes up after you join, the contract is what counts. If something isn't written in the contract, it's going to be difficult to prove your case.

Is There A "Cooling-Off" or Trial Period?

Some gyms give customers several days to reconsider after they've signed a contract. Others might let you join for a trial period. Even if it costs a little more each month, if you're not enjoying the membership or using it as much as you planned, you will have saved yourself years of payments.

Can You Cancel Your Membership or Get a Refund?

What happens if you need to cancel your membership because of a move or an injury, or if you find you just aren't using it? Will they refund your money? Knowing the gym's cancellation policies is especially important if you choose a long-term membership.

What happens if the gym goes out of business? You can check with your state Attorney General to see what your rights are according to your state's laws.

Is the Price Right?

Break down the cost to weekly and even daily figures to get a better idea of what you will pay to use the facility. Include possible finance charges if you pay by credit. Can you afford it?

If you signed up for a special introductory rate, make sure you know the terms of your contract once the discounted rate ends.

Find out What Other People Think

Search for Reviews Online

Do a search online to see what other people are saying about the location you're interested in. You might search the name of the gym with words like "reviews" or "complaints." Are people having the same kinds of issues with their contracts or the facilities?

Check for Complaints and Find out Your Rights

Contact your state Attorney General or local consumer protection office to find out whether state laws regulate health club memberships, and whether the office has gotten any complaints about the business.

Chapter 21

Personal Trainers and Equipment

Personal Trainers

Personal trainers are individuals who help people achieve their health and fitness goals through various exercise programs. They work with one client at a time, either at a gym or at the client's home, to provide total focused attention. They chart specific workouts and exercise programs, assess fitness levels, discuss health goals, and sometimes provide diet advice to complement the fitness regimen. Personal trainers choose their career out of passion and zeal to help people pursue a healthy lifestyle.

The Role of a Personal Trainer

The primary role of a personal trainer is to help people realize their fitness goals and assist them through the process. Personal trainers have the knowledge and experience, as well as detailed information about their individual clients, to provide maximum health and exercise benefits.

A few of the roles of personal trainers are listed below:

- Personal trainers always screen their client's medical history and fitness level in order to chart safe and effective workout programs.

"Personal Trainers and Equipment," © 2017 Omnigraphics. Reviewed September 2016.

- Trainers help motivate their clients by supporting and understanding them.

- They help keep the individual on track and carefully monitor progress.

- They can offer general advice on diet and nutrition.

- They modify the type and difficulty of exercise in response to the individual's fitness level.

- They plan safe and effective workouts that are also fun and interesting, so that the exercise regimen doesn't become monotonous.

- They keep up-to-date with the current standards and practices of the industry.

Choosing a Personal Trainer

Personal trainers can be found at the gym or online. But the best way to find a trainer is usually by talking to friends, asking at the gym, or consulting others who have had good experiences with a particular trainer.

Before deciding on a personal trainer, certain specifics should be kept in mind to ensure safe and effective results:

Certification

Before choosing a personal trainer, make sure he or she is qualified to manage your fitness routine. Ensure that the trainer is certified by a recognized organization or association. A few reputable associations include:

- Aerobics and Fitness Association of America (AFAA)

- American Council on Exercise (ACE)

- National Academy of Sports Medicine (NASM)

- National Strength and Conditioning Association (NSCA)

Questions

Never hesitate to ask questions of the trainer before deciding on hiring him or her. This will help make sure you are with the right person to help you accomplish your fitness and health goals. The following are a few questions that will help you to identify the right trainer:

- How much will it cost to hire the trainer, including cancellation fees and extra charges, if any?
- Is the trainer certified from a recognized organization?
- How much experience does he or she have?
- Does the trainer carry liability insurance?
- How does the trainer stay current on the latest trends and practices?
- What feedback can the trainer provide from previous clients?
- Can a mutually agreeable schedule be worked out?
- Does the trainer work with a network of health professionals, such as physicians, dietitians, and physiotherapists?

Compatibility

A vital consideration in choosing a personal trainer is the rapport between the individuals. Each client has his or her own method or style of working. Some want rigorous workouts while others may prefer something less strenuous. And some people need positive reinforcement each time they reach even smaller goals. Ensure that your trainer can adapt to your preferences and needs.

Expertise and Competence

When choosing a trainer, you need to have confidence in his or her professional ability. Ask for proof of results and feedback from clients the trainer has worked with, and follow up with those clients to determine whether the trainer is a suitable match for you. Take the time to investigate, and make a decision only when you are satisfied that this particular trainer is right for you.

Benefits of a Personal Trainer

Hiring a personal trainer entails an investment of both money and time, as well as a considerable amount of work on the part of the client. But for many individuals, these benefits can make the investment worthwhile:

Achieving Health Goals

When working with a personal trainer, you may find that your health and fitness goals are easier to achieve. He or she will help you design a realistic exercise plan that suits your body, as well as your schedule and budget.

Focused Attention

Personal training provides focused, specialized attention. Your trainer will concentrate only on you as you work out and will help you get through the most challenging times. The trainer will be well-aware of your physical condition and what works best for you, and the program he or she creates for you will be designed to meet your specific needs.

Motivation

Reaching a specific goal requires considerable motivation, and meeting challenges and overcoming hurdles is an important part of the process. Many people who embark on an exercise regimen on their own find that they become discouraged during the difficult times and lack the will to continue. A personal trainer can help keep you motivated and will guide you through the inevitable ups and downs of the exercise program.

Accountability

Achieving desirable results from an exercise program requires consistency and accountability. A personal trainer not only provides motivation but can also hold you accountable to the program you have planned together. With a trainer, there is a set time for workouts, an established exercise routine, and a set of rules to follow while working out.

Necessary and Relevant Information

Because of their knowledge of the latest fitness practices and techniques, personal trainers are able to provide the latest reliable information to help you achieve the best results. There is a daunting amount of health and fitness information available on the internet and in health magazines, newspapers, and books. A personal trainer will be able to sort through the data and extract the information that will best apply to your fitness program.

Correct Technique and Injury Prevention

Any workout should follow the right techniques to accomplish the desired goals safely. Fitness trainers know how the body works and are able to advise on methods that will deliver the best results while avoiding injury. A personal trainer will help you do the right workouts and do the workouts right.

Equipment for the Personal Gym

There is an overwhelming amount of home gym equipment available in the marketplace, some of it very expensive and each claiming to provide miraculous results. It is important to know what kind of equipment you will need for your training before you make a significant investment. You can seek the help of your trainer in this regard.

Some of the basic equipment that can help build your own personal gym is listed below:

Barbell and Plate Set

A barbell is a long metal rod, intended to be lifted with both hands, to which plates of various weights are secured at each end. This is a necessary piece of equipment that helps in strength training, body building, and muscle toning.

Weight Bench

This is a sturdy, padded bench, often with upright supports to hold the barbell, which helps make the best use of the barbell and plate set. It is considered a must-have for a personal gym and can help build the upper body through exercises like the bench press, done by lying on the bench and lifting the barbell straight up. In addition, some benches include attachments for leg lifts and other lower-body exercises.

Dumbbells

Dumbbells are short versions of the barbell that are meant to be lifted with one hand. Some have fixed weights and some come with interchangeable plates. And since they're relatively small pieces of equipment, they are mobile and can be used easily in a small space.

Racks

Storage racks are designed to keep the gym neat and organized by holding barbells, dumbbells, weight plates, and other equipment. They can be expensive, but many people consider them indispensable for their home gyms.

Treadmill

This is a device with a motorized rolling belt that is used for walking and running while remaining in one place. It's another fairly expensive piece of equipment, but it provides a convenient and efficient cardiovascular workout and helps build strength and endurance. The treadmill can be placed in one corner of a room, and most of them don't take up much space.

Points to Remember

- Personal trainers work with clients in gyms or in their homes to help guide them toward their health and fitness goals.

- Personal trainers should be certified, and clients need to ask pertinent questions before committing to a particular trainer.

- By choosing to work out with a personal trainer, you will remain motivated, accountable, and well-focused, thereby ensuring the best possible results.

- The purchase of expensive gym equipment is not required; even the most basic equipment will help you start the training.

References

1. Cavazos, Miguel. "Duties & Responsibilities of Fitness Personal Trainer" LiveStrong.com, January 5, 2015.

2. "Personal Trainers–How to Choose One," Better Health Channel, February, 2015.

3. "Benefits of Personal Training" UNT Health Science Center, August 11, 2016.

4. Halvorson, Ryan. "30 Essential Pieces of Equipment for the Successful Personal Training Studio," Idea Health and Fitness Association, July 1, 2012.

5. "Scope of Practice: Your Role as a NFPT Certified Personal Trainer," National Federation of Professional Trainers, n.d.

6. Laidler, Scott. "How to Create the Perfect Home Gym," The Telegraph, May 19, 2015.

Chapter 22

Tips for Buying Exercise Equipment

When daily trips to the gym aren't possible or gym memberships seem a little too expensive, home exercise equipment might seem like a good alternative. But before you spring for new equipment, make sure you're not buying the fitness fiction of quick, easy results. When shopping, look for equipment that suits your lifestyle and budget, and shop around to get the best price.

What the Ads Say

Home exercise equipment can be a great way to shape up—but only if you use it regularly. Ads promising quick, easy results are selling a line, not a reality. Here are some claims to watch for:

It's Quick, Easy, and Effortless

Whether they're promoting shoes, clothing, or equipment, some advertisers say their products offer a quick, easy way to shape up and lose weight—without sound science to back it up. There's no such thing

---

This chapter includes text excerpted from "Tips for Buying Exercise Equipment," Federal Trade Commission (FTC), July 15, 2012. Reviewed September 2016.

as a no-work, no-sweat way to a fit, healthy body. To get the benefits of exercise, you have to do the work.

We Promise to Fix Your Problem Areas

Promises that you can effortlessly burn a spare tire or melt fat from your hips and thighs are tempting, but spot reduction—losing weight in a specific place—takes regular exercise that still works the whole body to burn extra calories.

Look at These Before-And-After Photos

They may be "satisfied customers," but their experiences may not reflect the results most users get. And celebrity endorsements? They're no proof the product will work as claimed, either. As for the chiseled models in the ads, is that six-pack the result of the product they're promoting, months in the gym and years of healthy habits, or an altered photo?

What to Do before You Buy Exercise Equipment

You've done your job and looked at any claims with a skeptical, savvy eye. But you're not quite finished. Before you buy any equipment, here are a few tips to make sure your new gear won't wind up collecting dust:

Start Working Out

Don't expect the equipment to change your habits. Are you ready to act on your good intentions? If you're not active already, start now.

Find the Right Equipment

Take a test drive Before you buy, give different equipment a test drive at a local gym, recreation center, retailer, or even a friend's place.

Read reviews. Check out consumer and fitness magazines that rate exercise equipment to get an idea of how a product performs, and whether it's likely to help you achieve your goal, whether it's building strength, increasing flexibility, improving endurance, or enhancing your health. You also can check out user reviews online. Just don't put all your trust in any one review. Try typing the product or manufacturer's name into a search engine, along with terms like "complaint" or "problem."

Find the Right Price

Find out the *real* cost. Some companies advertise "three easy payments of $49.95." Break out the calculator and figure out what you'll really pay. Don't forget sales tax and shipping or delivery charges. Find out about warranties, and whether shipping or restocking fees apply if you decide to send it back.

Shop around. That one-of-a-kind fitness product may be available at a better price from a local store, or you might get a better deal online. Factor in delivery costs.

Part Four

Exercise Basics

Chapter 23

Exercise and Physical Fitness

Get Physical: Do What You Love

Physical activity helps control weight, builds lean muscle, reduces fat, promotes strong bone, muscle and joint development, and decreases the risk of obesity.

Physical activity is an essential component of a healthy lifestyle. Combined with healthy eating, it can help prevent a range of chronic diseases, including heart disease, cancer, and stroke, which are the three leading causes of death. Physical activity helps control weight, builds lean muscle, reduces fat, promotes strong bone, muscle and joint development, and decreases the risk of obesity.

The U.S. Department of Health and Human Services (HHS) physical activity guidelines for Americans recommends that adults get at least 2½ hours of moderate to vigorous physical activity each week. You don't have to do it all at once; you can spread this activity out over easy 30–minute increments, five days a week. Or you can choose from many activities and do them in bouts of 10 minutes. The HHS also advises doing muscle–strengthening exercises 2 or more days a week.

This chapter includes text excerpted from "Get Physical Do What You Love," Federal Occupational Health (FOH), U.S. Department of Health and Human Services (HHS), February 15, 2013.

Do What You Love

The best exercise is one that you will actually do. So find a form of physical activity that you enjoy–walking, biking, gardening, swimming, as long as it's something that really gets you moving–and find time to do it 5 or more days a week. If it's something you love to do, you'll be much more motivated to do it regularly.

People have different likes and dislikes. This is just as true for physical activity as anything else. Here are some ideas for getting more physically active:

- Take a dance or aerobic exercise class to get your body moving and your heart pumping
- Start a walking club in your neighborhood
- Take public transportation and walk from the station or the bus stop to your office
- Take the stairs rather than the elevator
- Ride your bike or walk to do errands, like light grocery shopping, going to the pharmacy, or picking up dry cleaning
- Go for a hike with friends and family
- Join a local intramural team that plays your favorite sport
- Go swimming
- Play with your kids or your grandkids

Set Realistic Short–and Long–Term Goals

You can also motivate yourself by setting short– and long–term goals. Break down your fitness goals into graduated steps that will logically take you from your short–goals to the longterm ones. For example:

1. I will check with my doctor to see if there are any restrictions or cautions I should be aware of, before I start my new activities.

2. I will begin with 2 sessions of brisk walking for at least 10 minutes (for a total of at least 20 minutes each day) for the first two weeks.

3. I will walk briskly for 30 minutes every morning and do 15 minutes of strength training every other day for the next three weeks.

4. I will jog or cycle for 30 minutes every morning and add 10 more minutes to my strength training routine.

Track Your Progress

Having a clear picture of the advances you're making can help keep you motivated to stay with your program and meet your goals. Forms like those in the resources can help you get a better picture of what activities might be working well for you and which ones you find more challenging. By setting and meeting short–term goals, you can claim many "little victories" that spur you on to reaching your ultimate goal. Remember to celebrate these victories.

Another great tool to help you manage and reach your health goals is the Presidential Active Lifestyle Award (PALA+), a program of the President's Challenge. You can sign up for the six–week program to help you maintain or improve your health.

Way to Go!

Giving yourself a simple reward when you reach you short–or long–term goals can be highly motivating. It reinforces the good work that you're doing and inspires you to do more.

Use the Buddy System

Whatever physical activity you choose to engage in can become more enjoyable when a friend or two is doing it alongside you. Having a friend or a group involved helps keep you motivated, and that can give you a boost whenever you're lagging. Knowing that friends are depending on you to meet them for your activity is just the thing to help get you out of the house and keep you going.

Saving Time

When you're back to a higher level of fitness, you can save time by choosing vigorous physical activities along with your moderate physical activities. You can get similar benefits in less time. Check out the sidebar on moderate vs. vigorous activities for more ideas.

Chapter 24

Types of Physical Activity

The four main types of physical activity are aerobic, muscle-strengthening, bone-strengthening, and stretching. Aerobic activity is the type that benefits your heart and lungs the most.

Aerobic Activity

Aerobic activity moves your large muscles, such as those in your arms and legs. Running, swimming, walking, bicycling, dancing, and doing jumping jacks are examples of aerobic activity. Aerobic activity also is called endurance activity.

Aerobic activity makes your heart beat faster than usual. You also breathe harder during this type of activity. Over time, regular aerobic activity makes your heart and lungs stronger and able to work better.

Other Types of Physical Activity

The other types of physical activity—muscle-strengthening, bone strengthening, and stretching—benefit your body in other ways.

Muscle-strengthening activities improve the strength, power, and endurance of your muscles. Doing pushups and situps, lifting weights, climbing stairs, and digging in the garden are examples of muscle-strengthening activities.

This chapter includes text excerpted from "Types of Physical Activity," National Heart, Lung, and Blood Institute (NHLBI), June 22, 2016.

With bone-strengthening activities, your feet, legs, or arms support your body's weight, and your muscles push against your bones. This helps make your bones strong. Running, walking, jumping rope, and lifting weights are examples of bone-strengthening activities.

Muscle-strengthening and bone-strengthening activities also can be aerobic, depending on whether they make your heart and lungs work harder than usual. For example, running is both an aerobic activity and a bone-strengthening activity.

Stretching helps improve your flexibility and your ability to fully move your joints. Touching your toes, doing side stretches, and doing yoga exercises are examples of stretching.

Levels of Intensity in Aerobic Activity

You can do aerobic activity with light, moderate, or vigorous intensity. Moderate- and vigorous-intensity aerobic activities are better for your heart than light-intensity activities. However, even light-intensity activities are better than no activity at all.

The level of intensity depends on how hard you have to work to do the activity. To do the same activity, people who are less fit usually have to work harder than people who are more fit. So, for example, what is light-intensity activity for one person may be moderate-intensity for another.

Light- and Moderate-Intensity Activities

Light-intensity activities are common daily activities that don't require much effort.

Moderate-intensity activities make your heart, lungs, and muscles work harder than light-intensity activities do.

On a scale of 0 to 10, moderate-intensity activity is a 5 or 6 and produces noticeable increases in breathing and heart rate. A person doing moderate-intensity activity can talk but not sing.

Vigorous-Intensity Activities

Vigorous-intensity activities make your heart, lungs, and muscles work hard.

On a scale of 0 to 10, vigorous-intensity activity is a 7 or 8. A person doing vigorous-intensity activity can't say more than a few words without stopping for a breath.

Examples of Aerobic Activities

Below are examples of aerobic activities. Depending on your level of fitness, they can be light, moderate, or vigorous in intensity:

- Pushing a grocery cart around a store
- Gardening, such as digging or hoeing that causes your heart rate to go up
- Walking, hiking, jogging, running
- Water aerobics or swimming laps
- Bicycling, skateboarding, rollerblading, and jumping rope
- Ballroom dancing and aerobic dancing
- Tennis, soccer, hockey, and basketball

Chapter 25

Step Aerobics

What Is Step Aerobics?

Step aerobics is an aerobic exercise—which means it increases heart rate to pump more oxygenated blood to the muscles—that involves stepping up and down rhythmically on a low bench or platform. The movements, often choreographed in time to music, help to work out the upper and lower body, as well as the cardiovascular system. It is cost-effective, since it does not require the purchase of costly workout equipment, and can be done at home, although health clubs and gyms also often have step-aerobics platforms and classes. Because this type of exercise stresses the heart and respiratory system, it's a good idea to consult a doctor before beginning step aerobics.

History of Step Aerobics

Various types of aerobic exercise began gaining widespread popularity in the 1960s. But step aerobics didn't get its start until 1989, when former gymnast Gin Miller injured her knee and, as a part of her recovery process, tried using her porch steps for physical therapy. She started by doing low-impact workouts on the steps, listening to music while working out to make it more interesting, and soon the concept of step aerobics began spreading.

"Step Aerobics," © 2017 Omnigraphics. Reviewed September 2016.

Benefits of Step Aerobics

The benefits of step aerobics can include:

- Exercising the heart and helping to reduce fat, burn calories, and keep cholesterol in check.

- Reducing stress.

- Toning the body and building muscle endurance.

- Strengthening leg muscles with lower-body movements.

- Reducing weight and helping maintain weight balance.

- Improving coordination and agility.

- Maximizing heart efficiency to help avoid problems like heart disease, diabetes, and joint pain.

- Improving mood and helping reduce depression, tension, mental fatigue, and emotional imbalances.

- Increasing the ability to perform daily tasks.

- Improving overall health.

Getting Ready for Step Aerobics

Step aerobics is done by stepping on and off a raised platform, such as a step, bench, or any other sturdy platform strong enough to hold a person's body weight. The height of the step should be chosen based on the individual's height. To prevent injuries, it is vital to do a ten-minute warm-up before starting the exercise, followed by a cooldown period after the workout. There are basic and advanced levels of step aerobics. For a beginner, it may take some time to get used to the various steps involved in the exercises.

A few of common moves are listed below:

- **The Basic Step.** Step up with right foot, followed by the left; then step down in reverse.

- **The Split Basic Step.** Step up with right foot, then the left; tap the ground with the right foot, then step back up; repeat with the left foot; step down with the right foot, then the left.

- **The Tap Up.** Similar to the Basic Step, but with a tap on the bench by the left foot, then the right.

- **The Repeater.** Step up with the right foot, followed by a knee lift with the left, then tap the ground with the left foot; repeat in reverse.
- **The "A" Step.** Facing the bench sideways, step up with the right foot, then the left; then step down on the far side of the bench with the right foot, then the left; repeat in reverse.
- **The "V" Step.** Perform a Basic Step, but step over the bench, rather than onto it.
- **The "I" Step.** This is a Basic Step, but with a jumping jack on the bench before stepping down.

There are number of other, more complex, steps and countless variations on each of them. Many people like to combine them into personal routines or invent their own steps as they become more proficient. In addition, the various movements can be performed with weights for an even more strenuous workout.

Preventing Injury

Any exercise that is not done properly can cause an injury, and step aerobics is no exception. Here are some precautions that should help prevent injury:

- **Use a sturdy platform.** The step-aerobics platform should be able to support the body's weight during exercise movements, or the surface could break, causing an injury.
- **Step on and off the platform correctly.** The entire foot needs to be placed on the raised platform. If part of the foot hangs off, or if strides are too long, there will be stress on the Achilles tendon, which could lead to a condition called Achilles tendinitis.
- **Don't hop or pound.** Jumping on the platform or floor too hard can cause stress fractures or other injuries.
- **Be sure to wear the proper shoes.** Using improper footwear, like tennis shoes or rubber street shoes, can cause injuries. The proper aerobics or cross-training shoes will be designed to move in all directions, be cushioned in the front area, and will have a wider area for the balls of the feet and an appropriate lift in the heels.
- **Use a platform of the correct size.** If the step or bench is too high, it can cause stress to the calves and heels. It is important to select a platform suited to the individual's height and ability.

References

1. Collins, Sarah. "The History of Aerobics," LiveStrong.com, November 3, 2015.

2. Ramiccio, Marisa. "What Is Step Aerobics? A Beginner's Guide," Symptomfind.com, May 16, 2012.

3. Rifkin, Beth. "The Best Step Aerobics Shoes," LiveStrong.com, October 13, 2015.

4. Tjfit. "Avoiding Injuries in Step Aerobics," SupplementReviews.com, November 14, 2014.

5. McCarron, Joshua. "The Benefits of Step Aerobics," LiveStrong.com, June 2, 2015.

Chapter 26

Kickboxing

Are you looking for a total-body workout that totally kicks butt? How about a way to increase your stamina, flexibility, and strength while listening to your favorite dance mixes?

If this sounds good to you, keep reading to find out what you need to know before you take the kickboxing challenge.

What Is Kickboxing?

Although the true roots of kickboxing date back to Asia 2,000 years ago, modern competitive kickboxing actually started in the 1970s, when American karate experts arranged competitions that allowed full-contact kicks and punches that had been banned in karate.

Because of health and safety concerns, padding and protective clothing and safety rules were introduced into the sport over the years, which led to the various forms of competitive kickboxing practiced in the United States today. The forms differ in the techniques used and the amount of physical contact that is allowed between the competitors.

Currently, one popular form of kickboxing is known as **aerobic** or **cardiovascular** (cardio) **kickboxing**, which combines elements of boxing, martial arts, and aerobics to provide overall physical conditioning and toning. Unlike other types of kickboxing, cardio kickboxing does not involve physical contact between competitors—it's a cardiovascular workout that's done because of its many benefits to the body.

Text in this chapter is excerpted from "Kickboxing," © 1995–2016. The Nemours Foundation/KidsHealth®. Reprinted with permission.

Cardio kickboxing classes usually start with warm-ups and gradually increase in intensity. Kickboxing is a full-body workout that includes movements such as knee strikes, kicks, and punches. Some time at the end of class is usually devoted to cooling down, which usually includes exercises like push-ups and crunches for strength and stretching for flexibility.

Instructional videos and DVDs are also available if you're interested in trying a cardio kickboxing routine at home.

The Basics

Before you decide to jump in and sign up for a class, you should keep a few basic guidelines in mind:

- **Know your current fitness level.** Kickboxing is a high-intensity, high-impact form of exercise, so it's probably not a good idea to plunge in after a long stint as a couch potato. You might try preparing yourself by first taking a low-impact aerobics course or less physical form of exercise and working up to a higher level of endurance. When you do begin kickboxing, allow yourself to be a beginner by working at your own pace and not overexerting yourself to the point of exhaustion.

- **Check it out before you sign up.** If possible, observe or try a class beforehand to see whether it's right for you and to make sure the instructor is willing to modify the routine a bit to accommodate people's different skill levels. Try to avoid classes that seem to move too fast, are too complicated, or don't provide the chance for any individual instruction during or after the class.

- **Find a class act.** Look for an instructor who has both a high-level belt in martial arts and is certified as a fitness instructor by an organization such as the American Council on Exercise (ACE). Also, try to start at a level that suits you and slowly progress to a more intense, fast-paced kickboxing class. Many classes call for intermediate levels of fitness and meet two to three times a week.

- **Comfort is key.** Wear comfortable clothing that allows your arms and legs to move easily in all directions. The best shoes are cross-trainers—not tennis shoes—because cross-trainers allow for side-to-side movements. Gloves or hand wraps are sometimes used during classes—you may be able to buy these where your class is held. Give your instructor a call beforehand so you can be fully prepared.

- **Start slowly and don't overdo it.** The key to a good kickboxing workout is controlled movement. Overextending yourself by kicking too high or locking your arms and legs during movements can cause pulled muscles and tendons and sprained knee or ankle joints. Start with low kicks as you slowly learn proper kickboxing technique. This is **very** important for beginners, who are more prone to developing injuries while attempting quick, complicated kickboxing moves.

- **Drink up.** Drink plenty of fluids before, during, and after your class to quench your thirst and keep yourself hydrated.

- **Talk to your doctor.** It's always a good idea to see your doctor and have a complete physical exam before you begin any type of exercise program—especially one with a lot of aerobic activity like kickboxing. This is extremely important if you have any chronic medical conditions such as asthma or diabetes or are very overweight.

Moves You Can Use

Here are a few moves that you can try at home:

- **Roundhouse kick:** Stand with the right side of your body facing an imaginary target with your knees bent and your feet shoulders' width apart. Lift your right knee, pointing it just to the right of the target and pivoting your body toward the same direction. Kick with your right leg, as though you are hitting the target. Repeat with your other leg.

- **Front kick:** Stand with feet shoulders' width apart. Bend your knees slightly, and pull your right knee up toward your chest. Point your knee in the direction of an imaginary target. Then, kick out with the ball of your foot. Repeat with your other leg.

- **Side kick:** Start with the right side of your body facing a target. Pull your right knee up toward your left shoulder, and bend your knees slightly as you kick in the direction of your target. The outside of your foot or heel should be the part that would hit the target. Repeat with your other leg.

Why Kickboxing?

Besides keeping your body fit, kickboxing has other benefits. According to a study by the ACE, you can burn anywhere from 350 to 450 calories an hour with kickboxing!

Kickboxing also reduces and relieves stress. Its rigorous workout—controlled punching and kicking movements carried out with the discipline and skills required for martial arts—can do wonders for feelings of frustration and anger. Practicing kickboxing moves also can help to improve balance, flexibility, coordination, and endurance.

Kickboxing is also a great way to get a total-body workout while learning simple self-defense moves. Kickboxing fans say the sport helps them to feel more empowered and confident.

So get out there and jab, punch, and kick your way to fitness.

Chapter 27

Aquatic Exercise

Chapter Contents

Section 27.1

Water Fitness

This section includes text excerpted from "Health Benefits of Water-Based Exercise," Centers for Disease Control and Prevention (CDC), May 4, 2016.

Water-Based Exercises and Health Benefits

Swimming is the fourth most popular sports activity in the United States and a good way to get regular aerobic physical activity. Just two and a half hours per week of aerobic physical activity, such as swimming, bicycling, or running, can decrease the risk of chronic illnesses. This can also lead to improved health for people with diabetes and heart disease. Swimmers have about half the risk of death compared with inactive people. People report enjoying water-based exercise more than exercising on land. They can also exercise longer in water than on land without increased effort or joint or muscle pain.

Water-Based Exercise and Chronic Illness

Water-based exercise can help people with chronic diseases. For people with arthritis, it improves use of affected joints without worsening symptoms. People with rheumatoid arthritis have more health improvements after participating in hydrotherapy than with other activities. Water-based exercise also improves the use of affected joints and decreases pain from osteoarthritis.

Water-Based Exercise and Mental Health

Water-based exercise improves mental health. Swimming can improve mood in both men and women. For people with fibromyalgia, it can decrease anxiety and exercise therapy in warm water can decrease depression and improve mood. Water-based exercise can improve the health of mothers and their unborn children and has a positive effect on the mothers' mental health. Parents of children with developmental disabilities find that recreational activities, such as swimming, improve family connections.

Water-Based Exercise and Older Adults

Water-based exercise can benefit older adults by improving the quality of life and decreasing disability. It also improves or maintains the bone health of post-menopausal women.

A Good Choice

Exercising in water offers many physical and mental health benefits and is a good choice for people who want to be more active. When in the water, remember to protect yourself and others from illness and injury by practicing healthy and safe swimming behaviors.

Section 27.2

Healthy Swimming

This section contains text excerpted from the following sources: Text under the heading "Steps of Healthy Swimming" is excerpted from "Steps of Healthy Swimming," Centers for Disease Control and Prevention (CDC), May 27, 2016; Text beginning with the heading "Water-based Exercise and Chronic Illness" is excerpted from "Healthy Swimming," Centers for Disease Control and Prevention (CDC), June 9, 2013; Text under the heading "Exercising in Water" is excerpted from "Staying Active at Any Size," National Institute of Diabetes and Digestive and Kidney Diseases (NIDDK), July 2016.

Steps of Healthy Swimming

You can choose to swim healthy!

We all share the water we swim in, and each of us needs to do our part to help keep ourselves, our families, and our friends healthy. To help protect yourself and other swimmers from germs or injury, here are a few easy and effective steps **all swimmers** can take each time we swim in a public pool or hot tub.

Swimming is the fourth most popular sports activity in the United States and a good way to get regular aerobic physical activity. Just two and a half hours per week of aerobic physical activity, such as

231

swimming, bicycling, or running, can decrease the risk of chronic illnesses. This can also lead to improved health for people with diabetes and heart disease. Swimmers have about half the risk of death compared with inactive people. People report enjoying water-based exercise more than exercising on land. They can also exercise longer in water than on land without increased effort or joint or muscle pain.

Water-based Exercise and Chronic Illness

Water-based exercise can help people with chronic diseases. For people with arthritis, it improves use of affected joints without worsening symptoms. People with rheumatoid arthritis have more health improvements after participating in hydrotherapy than with other activities. Water-based exercise also improves the use of affected joints and decreases pain from osteoarthritis.

Water-based Exercise and Mental Health

Water-based exercise improves mental health. Swimming can improve mood in both men and women. For people with fibromyalgia, it can decrease anxiety and exercise therapy in warm water can decrease depression and improve mood. Water-based exercise can improve the health of mothers and their unborn children and has a positive effect on the mothers' mental health. Parents of children with developmental disabilities find that recreational activities, such as swimming, improve family connections.

Water-based Exercise and Older Adults

Water-based exercise can benefit older adults by improving the quality of life and decreasing disability. It also improves or maintains the bone health of post-menopausal women.

Exercising in water

Swimming and water workouts put less stress on your joints than walking, dancing, or biking. If your feet, back, or joints hurt when you stand, water activities may be best for you. If you feel self-conscious about wearing a bathing suit, you can wear shorts and a T-shirt while you swim.

Swimming:

- lets you be more flexible. You can move your body in water in ways you may not be able to on land.

- reduces your risk of hurting yourself. Water provides a natural cushion, which keeps you from pounding or jarring your joints.

- helps prevent sore muscles.

- keeps you cool, even when you are working hard.

You don't need to know how to swim to work out in water. You can do shallow- or deep-water exercises at either end of the pool without swimming. For instance, you can do laps while holding onto a kickboard and kicking your feet. You also can walk or jog across the width of the pool while moving your arms.

For shallow-water workouts, the water level should be between your waist and chest. During deep-water workouts, most of your body is underwater. For safety and comfort, wear a foam belt or life jacket.

Chapter 28

Walking and Hiking

Chapter Contents

Section 28.1

Walking and Its Popularity in United States

This section includes text excerpted from "Americans Are
Walking More to Improve Their Health," Centers for Disease
Control and Prevention (CDC), May 26, 2014.

Walking for Better Health

**Improve your health by increasing your physical activity.
Start with walking more as part of your daily routine.**

Most everyone knows that physical activity is important for good
health, but not enough actually do it. Obstacles abound, not the least of
which is limited time. Fitting regular physical activity into your daily
schedule may seem difficult at first, but the *2008 Physical Activity
Guidelines* for Americans are more flexible than ever, giving you the
freedom to reach your physical activity goals through different kinds
of activities. It's easier than you think!

Adults need two types of physical activity each week—muscle
strengthening and aerobic. Aerobic activities make you breathe harder
and make your heart and blood vessels healthier. Brisk walking is
the most popular aerobic physical activity among adults in America.

Walking briskly for 2 hours and 30 minutes each week— easily broken up into 5, 30-minute walks—helps you meet the *Physical Activity
Guidelines* and gain health benefits. Add in 2 days that include muscle
strengthening activities—things like sit-ups, push-ups or weight lifting—and you are one of the growing number of adults getting healthier
by increasing their physical activity.

Join the Crowd

More and more Americans are choosing walking as their regular
form of physical activity each day. More than 145 million adults now
include walking as part of a physically active lifestyle. So if you're not
as active as you would like, why not consider walking more each day?

Walking is free, requires no special skills or facilities, and can be
done indoors and outdoors—alone or with others.

Every Step Counts

Increasing physical activity is an important step towards a healthier life. People who are physically active can live longer and have a lower risk for heart disease, stroke, type 2 diabetes, depression, and some cancers. Even if you are inactive, you can benefit from becoming active. Doing some physical activity is better than none.

Commit to Walking More Each Day than You Did the Day Before

Here are a few tips for adding more walking into your day.

- Park the car at the shopping center and walk to all your nearby errands.
- Find a walking buddy. Meet at the same time most days to go for a brisk walk.
- Host a walking meeting—walk and talk over problems with your colleagues for the first 20 minutes then hit the conference room to write down ideas and finish up.
- Make a walk-and-talk date with a friend or family member. Skip the latte and do a loop around the neighborhood instead.
- Take a walking lunch break at work. Keep extra shoes and socks in your filing cabinet.
- Walk while you are waiting. Instead of sitting on the bleachers while your child's at practice, walk around the field. Walk outside the restaurant as you wait for your table to be ready.
- Find a convenient walking path near your home, kids' activities, or work.

Why Choose Walking?

Increased walking has the potential to enliven communities by getting more people out on the streets. It allows you to meet and interact with people, making communities stronger.

Section 28.2

Walking Basics and Stretches

This section includes text excerpted from "Walking... A Step in the Right Direction," National Institute of Diabetes and Digestive and Kidney Diseases (NIDDK), February 2014.

What Are the Benefits of Walking?

Walking is the most popular physical activity among adults. Taking a walk is low cost and doesn't require any special clothes or equipment. Walking may:

- lower your risk of health problems like high blood pressure, heart disease, and diabetes

- strengthen your bones and muscles

- help you burn more calories

- lift your mood

Make walking fun by going to places you enjoy, like a park or shopping center. Bring along a friend or family member to chat with, or listen to some of your favorite music as you walk. Keep the volume low so that you can hear noises around you.

Do I Need to See a Doctor First?

Most people do not need to see a doctor before they start a walking program. But if you answer "yes" to any of the questions below, check with your doctor first.

- Has your doctor told you that you have heart trouble, diabetes, or asthma?

- When you are physically active, do you have pains in your chest, neck, shoulder, or arm?

- Do you often feel faint or have dizzy spells?

- Do you feel very breathless after physical activity?

- Do you have bone or joint problems, like arthritis, that make it difficult for you to walk?

- Are you over 40 years old and have you recently been inactive?

- Do you have a health problem that might keep you from starting a walking program?

How Do I Start?

1. Make a plan

The following questions may help you get started:

- Where will you walk?

- How often will you walk?

- Who will walk with you?

- How far or for how long will you walk?

2. Get ready

Make sure you have anything you may need. Here are some examples:

- shoes with proper arch support, a firm heel, and thick flexible soles

- clothes that keep you dry and comfortable

- a hat or visor for the sun, sunscreen, and sunglasses

- a hat and scarf to cover your head and ears when it's cold outside

3. Go

Divide your walk into three parts:

- Warm up by walking slowly.

- Increase your speed to a brisk walk. This means walking fast enough to raise your heart rate while still being able to speak and breathe easily.

- Cool down by slowing down your pace.

When walking, be sure to use proper form:

- Keep your chin up and your shoulders slightly back.

- Let the heel of your foot touch the ground first, and then roll your weight forward.

- Walk with your toes pointed forward.

- Swing your arms naturally.

4. Add more

As walking becomes easier, walk faster and go farther. Keep track of your progress with a walking journal or log. Record date, time, and distance. Set goals and reward yourself with a relaxing shower or 30 minutes of quiet time to yourself.

Review the sample walking plan for suggestions on how to start and slowly increase walking.

What about Safety?

Keep safety in mind as you plan when and where you will walk.

- Walk with others, when possible, and take a phone and ID with you.

- Let your family and friends know your walking time and route.

- If it is dark outside, wear a reflective vest or brightly colored clothing.

How Can I Make Walking a Habit?

The key to building any habit is to stick with the new behavior. Having a regular walking buddy may help keep you going—even on days when you would rather stay home. You can cheer each other on and serve as role models for friends, family members, and others.

When barriers come up, like time demands or bad weather, think of ways to beat them, like walking inside of a shopping center. If you have a setback, start again as soon as you can. With time, walking will become a part of your daily routine and may make it easier to try other types of physical activity.

How Much Do I Need to Walk?

150 Minutes

Amount of time adults need per week of moderate-intensity aerobic activity (activity that speeds up your heart rate and breathing) to stay healthy.

Break It Down

30 minutes per day x **5** days per week = **150** minutes per week

Walking briskly for 30 minutes per day, 5 days a week will help you meet this goal. But any 10-minute bout of physical activity helps.

Split It Up

10 minutes + **10** minutes + **10** minutes = **30** minutes

If you can't walk for 30 minutes at a time, you can take three 10-minute walks instead.

Step It Up

For more health benefits and to control your weight, you may need to walk more. Aim for 300 minutes each week, or about 1 hour a day for 5 days. The more you walk, the more health benefits you may gain!

Should I Stretch before I Walk?

Most experts advise stretching only after you have warmed up. To warm up, walk slowly for a few minutes before picking up the pace.

Stretching gently at the end of your walk may help build flexibility. Do not bounce or hold your breath when you stretch. Do each stretch slowly and move only as far as you feel comfortable.

If you think that stretching before walking may help you, ask your doctor when and how to do so safely. You may want to discuss these exercises as examples.

Side Reach

- Reach one arm over your head and to the side. Keep your hips steady and your shoulders straight to the side. Hold for 10 seconds and repeat on the other side.

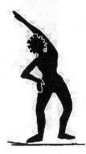

Figure 28.1. *Side Reach*

Wall Push

Lean your hands on a wall and place your feet about 3 to 4 feet away from the wall. Bend one knee and point it toward the wall. Keep your back leg straight with your foot flat and your toes pointed straight ahead. Hold for 10 seconds and repeat with the other leg.

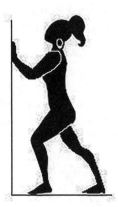

Figure 28.2. *Wall Push*

Knee Pull

Lean your back against a wall. Keep your head, hips, and feet in a straight line. Pull one knee toward your chest, hold for 10 seconds, and then repeat with the other leg.

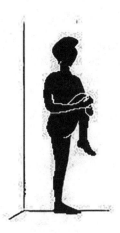

Figure 28.3. *Knee Pull*

Leg Curl

Pull your right foot toward your buttocks with your right hand. Stand straight and keep your bent knee pointing straight down. Hold for 10 seconds and repeat with your other foot and hand.

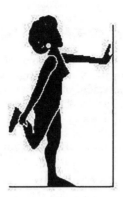

Figure 28.4. *Leg Curl*

Hamstring Stretch

Sit on a sturdy bench or hard surface so that one leg is stretched out on the bench with your toes pointing up. Keep your other foot flat on the surface below. Straighten your back, and if you feel a stretch in the back of your thigh, hold for 10 seconds and then change sides and repeat. If you do not feel a stretch, slowly lean forward from your hips until you feel a stretch.

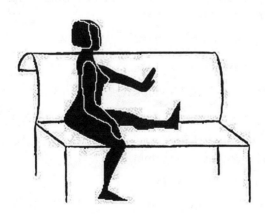

Figure 28.5. *Hamstring Stretch*

Section 28.3

Using a Pedometer

This section contains text excerpted from the following sources: Text
in this section begins with excerpts from "A Guide to Using Your
Pedometer," U.S. Department of Veterans Affairs (VA), August 8,
2012. Reviewed September 2016; Text under the heading "A Sample
Daily Walking Program" is excerpted from "Walking... A Step in the
Right Direction," National Institute of Diabetes and Digestive and
Kidney Diseases (NIDDK), February 2014.

**Walking is a great way to help you lose weight, keep the
weight off, and improve your health.**
Use a Pedometer to:

- Measure how many steps you take.

- Get feedback about your activity.

- Plan, track, and reach your physical activity goals.

How to wear your Pedometer:

- Clip it to your clothing, or place it in a pocket or a bag that you
  carry or wear.

- Use the leash and clip to keep from dropping or losing your
  pedometer.

- Do not get the pedometer wet.

Pedometers do not measure:

- Walking for less than 10 steps or 10 seconds at a time.

- Cycling, swimming, some dancing, basketball, and tennis.

- Distances covered while using a manual wheelchair—this
  requires an odometer/cyclometer.

- Record your steps every day.

- Set goals that you can reach.

- Update your goals every week.

- Start where you are and build up.
- Choose an activity and a setting that you enjoy: outside, at a mall, at a gym, etc.

Ways to add walking to your lifestyle:

- Take a 10-minute walk whenever you can.
- Take the stairs (up or down) instead of the elevator.
- Take 10-minute walks during lunch and breaks at work.
- Park farther away and walk.
- Get off the bus one stop early and walk the rest of the way.
- Step in place while watching television.
- Walk your dog (or borrow a friend's dog).
- Mow your lawn with a push mower or do other yard work.
- For short distances, walk instead of driving your car.

Getting started:

- Wear your pedometer every day for 1 week.
- The pedometer will count your steps in a 24-hour period beginning and ending at midnight.
- Record your steps on your Daily Food and Physical Activity Diary.
- At the end of 1 week, add up your daily steps.
- Determine your daily average by dividing total steps by the number of days.

Increasing your steps:

- Starting with the second week, set a goal to increase your steps. (Example: If you average 3,000 steps per day in first week, then set a goal to increase to 3,500 steps per day.)
- Start at a comfortable level and gradually increase steps.
- Create a weekly walking plan/schedule.
- Take the long way when walking to meetings.
- Find a regular walking partner.

Other important facts:

- For health benefits and weight maintenance, aim for walking or other physical activity for 150 minutes (2½ hours) per week, in periods of at least 10 minutes.

- To help you lose weight, walk or be physically active **more than 2½ hours per week.** Weight loss may be achieved with 300 minutes (5 hours) per week of physical activity.

- Walking and wheeling are easy, inexpensive, and you can do them almost anywhere.

A Sample Daily Walking Program

Your walking sessions may be longer or shorter based on your ability and the advice of your doctor. If you are walking fewer than three times per week, give yourself more than 2 weeks before adding more.

Table 28.1. A Sample Daily Walking Program

Warm-up Time Walk Slowly	Brisk-walk Time	Cool-down Time Walk Slowly and Stretch	Total Time
Weeks 1–2			
5 minutes	5 minutes	5 minutes	15 minutes
Weeks 3–4			
5 minutes	10 minutes	5 minutes	20 minutes
Weeks 5–6			
5 minutes	15 minutes	5 minutes	25 minutes
Weeks 7–8			
5 minutes	20 minutes	5 minutes	30 minutes
Weeks 9–10			
5 minutes	25 minutes	5 minutes	35 minutes
Weeks 11–12			
5 minutes	30 minutes	5 minutes	40 minutes
Weeks 13–14			
5 minutes	35 minutes	5 minutes	45 minutes
Weeks 15–16			
5 minutes	40 minutes	5 minutes	50 minutes
Weeks 17–18			
5 minutes	45 minutes	5 minutes	55 minutes
Weeks 19–20			
5 minutes	50 minutes	5 minutes	60 minutes

Section 28.4

Gearing Up for Hiking

This section includes text excerpted from "Hiking Activity Card," Centers for Disease Control and Prevention (CDC), May 9, 2015.

Gear Up

First, you'll need a good pair of shoes and thick socks designed for this type of activity. You can start with some sturdy sneakers with thick bottoms. When you begin to take on more difficult trails, try a pair of hiking boots, and make sure they fit! Also, get a backpack or fanny pack to carry all of your hiking supplies. Dress in layers and bring along a waterproof jacket with a hood in case you get caught in the rain. And don't forget a hat, sunscreen, and sunglasses because the higher you hike, the more dangerous the sun's rays become.

To keep hiking fun, you always need to be prepared to beat problems that could happen while you're out, like finding the trail if you get lost or stuck in bad weather. Make sure you bring a map of the area you'll be hiking in and a sturdy compass. Don't know how to use a compass? You'll also need to bring plenty of water and extra food, like sports bars or trail mix, in case you have to stay out late and get hungry. The adults on your hike should bring a box of waterproof matches and an Army-style knife. A flashlight and extra batteries will help you find your way if you end up out after dark. Finally, you'll need to bring a first aid kit, in case someone gets hurt during your hike.

Play It Safe

Prep. Get in shape before you head out on your hike. Try walking around your neighborhood with your pack loaded with five pounds more gear than you'll actually carry on your hike. If that goes well, plan a short hike to test your abilities on the trail.

Buddies. Take a friend and an adult along on your hike. That way you can look out for each other and you'll have people to talk to! Also, be sure to let someone who's not going know where you'll be hiking and what time you'll be back.

H2O. Carry lots of water even if you are only planning a short hike. For warm-weather hikes, bring six to eight quarts of water per day. In the cold weather or higher elevations, you can be safe with half that amount. Whenever you are near water, make sure you wet yourself down. Dampen a bandana and wipe your face, neck, and arms or wrap it around your head while you hike.

Blisters and more. To prevent blisters, try spraying your feet with an anti-perspirant before heading out. Bring extra pairs of socks that you can change into if your feet get wet or sweaty—if they aren't made of cotton, they'll keep your feet drier. Once you're on the trail, stop as soon as you feel a "hot spot" on your feet and apply special type of bandage called "moleskin" to the sore area. Also, try using a hiking stick to keep some pressure off of your legs and knees.

Buzz. Don't get bugged by bugs. Protect yourself from bites and stings by using a bug repellant that includes DEET. Repellents that contain DEET are the most effective, but make sure you rub them on according to the directions. A good rule of thumb from the experts is that kids should use repellents with less than 10% DEET. Get your parents to help you put it on your face so you don't get it in your mouth or eyes. And wash your hands after you apply it. Remember that stuff that smells good to you smells good to bugs too, so don't use scented shampoos or lotions before hiking.

Weather watcher. When it's hot, pick trails that are shaded and run near streams. If you need to hike uphill in the sun, first soak yourself down to stay cool. You can also try wearing a wet bandana around your head or neck. Also, try to stay out of cotton clothes. Keep yourself out of bad weather by checking forecasts before you hike and watching the skies once you're out on the trail. During lightening storms, head downhill and away from the direction of the storm, and then squat down and keep your head low.

Keep it yummy. To stay healthy on your hike, you'll need to know how to keep your food and water safe. Remember the four C's: contain, clean, cook, and chill.

How to Play

Take a hike! No, really, take the time to go hiking. Hiking with your friends or family is a great chance to get outdoors, breathe some fresh air, and get active. It's easy to get started. Just look for a trail in a national park near you!

For your first day hike (hiking for a day or less without camping overnight), choose a safe, well-marked trail that doesn't have too many steep climbs. Otherwise, you'll get tired too early and won't make it as far as you want to go. Each time you go hiking, try going a little farther and take a slightly steeper trail. Before you know it you'll be hiking the Appalachian Trail—a 2,167-mile trail that goes all the way from Maine to Georgia!

Chapter 29

Bicycling

Chapter Contents

Section 29.1

Biking Basics

This section includes text excerpted from "Bicycle Activity Card,"
Centers for Disease Control and Prevention (CDC), May 9, 2015.

Just what does it take to become a cyclist?

Gear Up

A Bike. Think of the type of riding you want to do before you buy
one. Mountain bikes are strong and stable and built for gravel roads
and tricky trails. Racing bikes are built to go super fast on pavement,
and sport bikes, a combination of both, are good for many different
purposes.

A Helmet. Your helmet should sit right above your eyebrows and
be tightly buckled so it doesn't slip while you are riding.

Play It Safe

Use your head and wear a helmet! You should always wear a helmet
when you ride—plus, it's the law in many states. It's also important
that your helmet is approved by one of the groups who test helmets to
see which ones are the best: the Consumer Product Safety Commission
(CPSC) or Snell B-95 standards are best for bicycling helmets. Try
not to ride at night or in bad weather, and wear brightly colored, or
reflective clothes whenever you ride so you can be seen. You can even
put reflectors or funky reflective stickers on your bike—who knew
being safe could look so cool? Also, watch out for loose pant legs and
shoe laces that could get caught in your bike chain.

Be street smart. Ride on the right side of the road, moving with
traffic, and obey all traffic signs and signals. Discuss the best riding
routes with your parents—they'll help you determine safe places to
ride near your home.

When you reach an intersection, be sure to stop and look left, right,
and then left again to check for cars—then go. Use hand signals to

show when you're going to turn, and be sure to keep an eye out for rough pavement ahead so you can avoid it. And although you may think you can't go out without your favorite tunes, never wear headphones when you're on your bike.

How to Play

Bicycling can be a great competitive sport, as well as a fun activity to do with your friends. And there are plenty of different types of bicycling depending on your personality. If you love to go fast-n-furious, bicycle racing is probably more your speed. If you like to hit the rocky road, mountain biking sounds more like your taste. And if you just like to pedal for pleasure, any kind of bicycling will do. Try riding to school or to a friend's house!

Section 29.2

Biking-Safety Tips

This section includes text excerpted from "Head Injuries and Bicycle Safety," Centers for Disease Control and Prevention (CDC), January 28, 2015.

What's the Problem?

Millions of Americans ride bicycles, but less than half wear bicycle helmets. For example, a national survey conducted in 2001–2003 found that only 48% of children ages 5–14 years wore bicycle helmets when riding. Further, older children were less likely to wear helmets than younger children.

In 2010 in the United States, 800 bicyclists were killed and an estimated 515,000 sustained bicycle-related injuries that required emergency department care. Roughly half of these cyclists were children and adolescents under the age of 20. Annually, 26,000 of these bicycle-related injuries to children and adolescents are traumatic brain injuries treated in emergency departments.

Who's at Risk?

Any bicyclist who does not wear a bicycle helmet is at increased risk of head injury.

Can It Be Prevented?

Yes. Wearing a properly fitted helmet every time you and your children ride a bicycle is one important prevention method. If children don't want to wear a helmet, find out why. Some children don't like to wear helmets because they fear they will be teased by peers for being "geeky" or because they think helmets are unattractive, uncomfortable, or hot. Talk about these concerns with children and choose a helmet they will want to wear. Other prevention strategies:

- Follow the rules of the road:
  - ride on the right side of the road-with the traffic flow, not against it;
  - obey traffic signs and signals just as if you were driving a car;
  - use correct hand signals;
  - stop at all signs and red lights; and
  - stop and look both ways before entering a street;
- Depending on the laws in your community, children may ride on sidewalks and paths.
- If riding at dawn, at dusk, or at night, wear reflective clothing (not just light-colored clothing) and make sure that the bike has a front headlight and a rear red reflector or flashing red light.

Chapter 30

Running

Running Is a Wonderful Sport

Whether it's as part of a high school track program or cross-country team or just a way of getting in shape, running is a wonderful sport. It's great exercise, virtually anyone can do it, and all you really need to get started is a good pair of sneakers.

But running is not without its risks. Injuries—from sprained ankles and blisters to stress fractures and tendonitis—are common. And runners need to be aware of some hazards (from vehicles to wild animals) when choosing a place to run.

To keep things safe while running, follow these tips:

Avoiding Running Injuries

Up to half of all runners are injured every year, so the odds are good that at some point in your running career you will get injured.

Running, especially on asphalt or other hard surfaces, puts a lot of stress on the legs and back. This can lead to lots of different problems. The most common running injuries include sprained ankles, blisters, tendonitis, chondromalacia (runner's knee), iliotibial band (ITB) syndrome, heel pain, and shinsplints. Teen runners are also at risk of growth plate injuries.

Text in this chapter is excerpted from "Safety Tips: Running," © 1995–2016. The Nemours Foundation/KidsHealth®. Reprinted with permission.

Two steps can help you avoid serious injuries from running:

- **Try to prevent injuries from happening in the first place.**
  Use the right gear, warm up your muscles before you start, and
  take precautions to deal with weather conditions—like staying
  well hydrated in hot weather and keeping muscles warm in the
  cold.

- **Stop running as soon as you notice signs of trouble.**
  Ignoring the warning signs of an injury will only lead to bigger
  problems down the road.

Gear Guidelines

Running might require less gear than other sports, but it is still
vitally important to get the right equipment to minimize the stresses
it puts on your body. Anyone who has ever run in the wrong shoes can
tell you what a painful experience it can be, and anyone who has run
in the wrong socks probably has blisters to prove it.

Here are a few tips to make sure you get the right footwear before
you start running:

Shoes

Before you buy a pair of running sneakers, know what sort of foot
you have. Are your feet wide or narrow? Do you have flat feet? High
arches? Different feet need different sneakers to provide maximum
support and comfort. If you don't know what sort of foot you have or
what kind of sneaker will work best for you, consult a trained professional at a running specialty store.

Minimalist shoes are becoming popular, but there's no evidence
that they reduce injuries. Look for running shoes that provide good
support, starting with a thick, shock-absorbing sole. Runners with flat
feet should choose shoes that advertise "motion control" or "stability."
Runners with high-arched feet should look for shoes that describe
themselves as "flexible" or "cushioned."

Wearing shoes that fit correctly is more important in running than
in virtually any other sport. As you rack up the miles, any hot spots or
discomfort will become magnified and lead to blisters, toenail problems,
and may contribute to leg problems.

If you plan on running on trails or in bad weather, you'll need
trail-running shoes with extra traction, stability, and durability.
Whichever type of shoes you end up purchasing, make sure they are

laced up snugly so they're comfortable but not so tight that they cause discomfort.

Socks

Running socks come in a variety of materials, thicknesses, and sizes. The most important factor is material. Stay away from socks made from 100% cotton. When cotton gets wet, it stays wet, leading to blisters in the summer and cold feet in the winter. Instead, choose socks made from wool or synthetic materials such as polyester and acrylic.

Some runners like thicker socks for extra cushioning while others prefer thin socks, particularly in warm weather. Make sure you wear the socks you plan to wear when running while you try on sneakers to ensure a proper fit.

Choose Where to Run

One of the nice things about running is that you can do it almost anywhere. Running on a track or indoors on a treadmill are options, but lots of runners prefer the variety and challenge of running on roads or trails.

In most cases, it will be possible to simply step out your front door and begin. That being said, there are definitely safer places to run and places that you might want to avoid.

Road Runners

Look for streets that have sidewalks or wide shoulders. If there are no sidewalks or shoulders, and you find yourself having to run in the street, try to find an area with minimal automobile traffic. Always run toward oncoming cars so you can see any potential problems before they reach you.

Avoid running routes that take you through bad neighborhoods. If you're running in an unfamiliar area, be prepared to change your route or turn around if you sense that the area you're headed toward may not be safe. Trust your intuition.

Find someone to run with if you can—there's safety in numbers. Can't find a running partner? Consider joining a running club through your school or the local parks and recreation department. When running in a group, be sure to run single file and keep to the side of the road. Always yield the right-of-way to vehicles at intersections.

Don't assume that cars will stop or alter their paths for you. Obey all traffic rules and signals.

Trail Runners

Choose well-maintained trails. Steer clear of trails that are overgrown or covered with fallen branches—you don't want to trip or encounter ticks or poison ivy! Also, you should avoid trails that travel through deserted areas or take you far away from homes and businesses. Know the location of public phones and the fastest way back to civilization in the event of an emergency.

Watch for dogs or wild animals. If you encounter a mountain lion, bear, or other dangerous animal stop running and face it. Running may trigger the animal's instinct to attack. Make yourself look larger by raising your hands over your head. Give the animal plenty of room to escape. If the animal appears to be acting aggressively, throw rocks, sticks, or whatever is readily available at it. Stay facing the animal.

If you run into an aggressive dog, don't make eye contact—the dog might see this as a threat. The dog may be trying to defend its territory, so stop running and walk to the other side of the street. If the dog approaches, stand still. In a firm, calm voice, say "No" or "Go home." If you keep running into the same dog, choose a new route or file a report with animal control.

Plan for Weather

Rain and Snow

If you intend to run in rain or snow, make sure you dress for the conditions (windproof jacket, hat, gloves, etc.). Wear synthetic fabrics that will help wick away moisture from your body. Consider putting Vaseline or Band-aids on your nipples to keep them from being chafed by a wet shirt.

Wind

If it's windy, run more slowly than you normally would when facing into the wind. This will help you keep from overexerting yourself while still giving you the same amount of exercise. Try to start your run by heading into the wind so that you will have the wind at your back later in the run when you are tired.

Heat

On hot days, drink plenty of water before your run and bring extra water with you. Heat prostration can be a very serious problem for runners. Wear white clothing to reflect the sun's rays and a hat to shade your head from the sun, and stop running if you feel faint or uncomfortable in any way.

Before You Start

Before you begin, warm up. Start with a brisk walk or light jog, or do some jumping jacks to get the blood flowing. Then be sure to stretch well, with a particular focus on your calves, hamstrings, quadriceps, and ankles. Dynamic stretching, where you do slow, controlled movements to improve range of motion is thought to be more effective than static stretching before a run or workout.

Carry a few essentials with you. These include some form of identification, a cell phone or change for a pay phone, and a whistle. Don't wear headphones or earbuds or anything else that might make you less aware of your surroundings while you run.

Tell a friend or family member your running route and when you plan to return. If no one is available, write down your plans so you can be located in the event of an emergency.

While Running

Try to run only during daylight hours, if possible. If you must run at night, avoid dimly lit areas and wear bright and/or reflective clothes so that others can see you clearly.

When you begin, have a definite idea of how far you intend to go. Less experienced runners should start by running short distances until they build up their stamina and get a better idea of how far they can run safely.

Younger teens, are still developing and may be at more risk for injury from over-training and running long distances. As a general guideline, a 10K race is the upper limit of what a 13-year-old should attempt, and no one under 18 should try to run a marathon. (Most marathons limit their entries to people 18 and older.)

Stay alert. The more aware you are of your surroundings and the other people around you, the less vulnerable you will be. Staying safe while running involves the same common sense you use to stay safe anywhere else, like avoiding parked cars and dark areas, and taking note of who is directly behind you and ahead of you.

If a car passes you more than once or seems suspicious, try to note or take a photo of the license plate number. Make it clear that you are aware of the vehicle. Most runners don't get attacked, especially if they take precautions like running in populated areas. You just need to use common sense.

Chapter 31

Strength and Resistance Exercise

Chapter Contents

Section 31.1

Strength / Weight Training Basics

This section includes text excerpted from "Sample Strength
Activity Plan for Beginners," U.S. Department of Veterans
Affairs (VA), December 30, 2014.

About Strength Exercise

To do most of the strength exercises in this plan, you will need to
lift or push weights (or your own body weight), and gradually increase
the amount of weight used. Dumbbells and hand/ ankle weights sold
in sporting goods stores as well as resistance tubing can be purchased.
Get creative and use things in your home like milk or water jugs
filled with sand or water, or socks filled with beans and tied shut at
the ends. You can also use the special strength-training equipment
at a gym or fitness center. There are so many ways to participate in
strength training!

How Much, How Often

- Do strength exercises for all of your major muscle groups at
  least twice a week, but no more than 3 times per week.

- Don't do strength exercises of the same muscle group on any 2
  days in a row.

- Depending on your condition, you might need to start out
  using 1 or 2 pounds of weight or no weight at all. Sometimes,
  the weight of your arms or legs alone is enough to get you
  started.

- Use a minimum weight the first week, and then gradually add
  weight. Starting out with weights that are too heavy can cause
  injuries.

- Gradually add a challenging amount of weight to your strength
  routine. If you don't challenge your muscles, you won't get much
  benefit.

How to Do Strength Exercises

- Do 8–12 repetitions in a row. Wait a minute, and then do another "set" of 8–12 repetitions of the same exercise.

- Take 3 seconds to lift or push a weight into place; hold the position for 1 second, and take another 3 seconds to lower the weight. Don't let the weight drop or let your arms or legs fall in an uncontrolled way. Lowering slowly is very important.

- It should feel somewhere between hard and very hard (15–17 on the Borg Scale) for you to lift or push the weight. It should not feel very, very hard. If you can't lift or push at least 8 times in a row, it's too heavy for you. Reduce the amount of weight. If you can lift more than 12 times in a row without much difficulty, then it's too light for you. Try increasing the amount of weight you are lifting. A little extra weight goes a long way!

- Stretch after strength exercises, as this is when your muscles are warmed up. If you stretch before strength exercises, be sure to warm up your muscles first by light walking and arm pumping.

Safety

- Don't hold your breath or strain during strength exercises. Breathe out as you lift or push, and breathe in as you relax; this may not feel natural at first. Counting out loud helps.

- If you have had your hip or knee joint replaced, check with your doctor to see if there are some lower body exercises that you should skip.

- Avoid jerking or thrusting weights into position or "locking" the joints in your arms and legs. This can cause injuries. Use smooth, steady movements.

- Muscle soreness lasting up to a few days and slight fatigue are normal after muscle-building exercises. Exhaustion, sore joints, and unpleasant muscle pulling are not. These problems mean you are overdoing it.

- None of the exercises should cause pain.

Progressing

- Gradually increasing the amount of weight you use is crucial for building strength.

- When you are able to lift a weight more than 12 times, increase the amount of weight you use at your next session.

- Here is an example of how to progress gradually:

  - Start out with a weight that you can lift only 8 times.

  - Keep using that weight until you become strong enough to lift it 12 to 15 times.

  - Add more weight so that, again, you can lift it only 8 times.

  - Use this weight until you can lift it 12 to 15 times, and then add more weight. Keep repeating.

Sample Schedule

Perform the following exercises, in order, at the recommended frequency. Detailed instructions for each exercise are provided at the end of this handout. Some of this content is adapted from *Exercise: A Guide from the National Institute on Aging.*

Table 31.1. Repetitions, Sets, and Sessions per Exercise

Strength and Balance Exercises	# of repetitions per set	# of sets per session	# of sessions per week
Arm Raise	8–12	2	2–3
Chair Stand	8–12	2	2–3
Biceps Curl	8–12 per side	2 per side	2–3
Plantar Flexion	8–12	2	2–3
Triceps Extension	8–12 per side	2 per side	2–3
Alternative Dip	8–12	2	2–3
Knee Flexion	8–12 per side	2 per side	2–3
Hip Flexion	8–12 per side	2 per side	2–3
Shoulder Flexion	8–12	2	2–3
Knee Extension	8–12 per side	2 per side	2–3
Hip Extension	8–12 per side	2 per side	2–3
Side Leg Raise	8–12 per side	2 per side	2–3

Examples of Strength Exercises

Arm Raise

Strengthens shoulder muscles.

- Sit in armless chair with your back supported by back of chair.

- Keep feet flat on floor even with your shoulders.
- Hold hand weights straight down at your sides, with palms
- facing inward.
- Raise both arms to side, shoulder height.
- Hold the position for 1 second.
- Slowly lower arms to sides. Pause.
- Repeat 8 to 12 times.
- Rest, then do another set of 8 to 12 repetitions.

Chair Stand

Strengthens muscles in abdomen and thighs. Your goal is to do this exercise without using your hands as you become stronger.

- Place pillows on the back of chair.
- Sit toward front of chair, knees bent, feet flat on floor.
- Lean back on pillows in half-reclining position. Keep your back and shoulders straight throughout exercise.
- Raise upper body forward until sitting upright, using hands as little as possible (or not at all, if you can). Your back should no longer lean against pillows.
- Slowly stand up, using hands as little as possible.
- Slowly sit back down. Pause.
- Repeat 8 to 12 times.
- Rest, then do another set of 8 to 12 repetitions.

Biceps Curl

Strengthens upper-arm muscles.

- Sit in armless chair with your back supported by back of chair.
- Keep feet flat on floor even with your shoulders.
- Hold hand weights straight down at your sides, with palms facing inward.
- Slowly bend one elbow, lifting weight toward chest. (Rotate palm to face shoulder while lifting weight.)

- Hold position for 1 second.
- Slowly lower arm to starting position. Pause.
- Repeat with other arm.
- Alternate arms until you have done 8 to 12 repetitions with each arm.
- Rest, then do another set of 8 to 12 alternating repetitions.

Plantar Flexion

Strengthens ankle and calf muscles. Use ankle weights if you are ready.

- Stand straight, feet flat on floor, holding onto a table or chair for balance.
- Slowly stand on tiptoe, as high as possible.
- Hold position for 1 second.
- Slowly lower heels all the way back down. Pause.
- Do the exercise 8 to 12 times.
- Rest, then do another set of 8 to 12 repetitions.

Variation:

As you become stronger, do the exercise standing on one leg only, alternating legs for a total of 8 to 12 times on each leg. Rest, then do another set of 8 to 12 alternating repetitions.

Triceps Extension

Strengthens muscles in back of upper arm. Keep supporting your arm with your hand throughout the exercise. (If your shoulders aren't flexible enough to do this exercise, focus on shoulder stretching exercises. Ask for guidance.)

- Sit in chair with your back supported by back of chair.
- Keep feet flat on floor even with shoulders.
- Hold a weight in one hand. Raise that arm straight toward ceiling, palm facing in.
- Support this arm, below elbow, with other hand.

- Slowly bend raised arm at elbow, bringing hand weight toward same shoulder.
- Slowly straighten arm toward ceiling.
- Hold position for 1 second.
- Slowly bend arm toward shoulder again. Pause.
- Repeat the bending and straightening until you have done the exercise 8 to 12 times.
- Repeat 8 to 12 times with your other arm.
- Rest, then do another set of 8 to 12 alternating repetitions.

Knee Flexion

Strengthens muscles in back of thigh. Use ankle weights if you are ready.

- Stand straight holding onto a table or chair for balance.
- Slowly bend knee as far as possible. Don't move your upper leg at all; bend your knee only.
- Hold position for 1 second.
- Slowly lower foot all the way back down. Pause.
- Repeat with other leg.
- Alternate legs until you have done 8 to 12 repetitions with each leg.
- Rest, then do another set of 8 to 12 alternating repetitions

Hip Flexion

Strengthens thigh and hip muscles. Use ankle weights, if you are ready.

- Stand straight to the side or behind a chair or table, holding on for balance.
- Slowly bend one knee toward chest, without bending waist or hips.
- Hold position for 1 second.
- Slowly lower leg all the way down. Pause.

- Repeat with other leg.

- Alternate legs until you have done 8 to 12 repetitions with each leg.

- Rest, then do another set of 8 to 12 alternating repetitions.

Shoulder Flexion

Strengthens shoulder muscles.

- Sit in armless chair with your back supported by back of chair.

- Keep feet flat on floor even with your shoulders.

- Hold hand weights straight down at your sides, with palms facing inward.

- Raise both arms in front of you (keep them straight and rotate so palms face downward) to shoulder height.

- Hold position for 1 second.

- Slowly lower arms to sides. Pause.

- Repeat 8 to 12 times.

- Rest, then do another set of 8 to 12 repetitions.

Knee Extension

Strengthens muscles in front of thigh and shin. Use ankle weights if you are ready.

- Sit in chair. Only the balls of your feet and your toes should rest on the floor. Put rolled towel under knees, if needed, to lift your feet. Rest your hands on your thighs or on the sides of the chair.

- Slowly extend one leg in front of you as straight as possible.

- Flex ankle so that toes are pulled back towards head.

- Hold position for 1 to 2 seconds.

- Slowly lower leg back down. Pause.

- Repeat with other leg.

- Alternate legs until you have done 8 to 12 repetitions with each leg.

- Rest, then do another set of 8 to 12 alternating repetitions.

Hip Extension

Strengthens buttock and lower-back muscles. Use ankle weights, if you are ready.

- Stand 12 to 18 inches from a table or chair, feet slightly apart.
- Bend forward at hips at about 45-degree angle; hold onto a table or chair for balance.
- Slowly lift one leg straight backwards without bending your knee, pointing your toes, or bending your upper body any farther forward.
- Hold position for 1 second.
- Slowly lower leg. Pause.
- Repeat with other leg.
- Alternate legs until you have done 8 to 12 repetitions with each leg.
- Rest, then do another set of 8 to 12 alternating repetitions.

Side Leg Raise

Strengthens muscles at sides of hips and thighs. Use ankle weights, if you are ready.

- Stand straight, directly behind table or chair, feet slightly apart.
- Hold onto a table or chair for balance.
- Slowly lift one leg 6–12 inches out to side. Keep your back and both legs straight. Don't point your toes outward; keep them facing forward.
- Hold position for 1 second.
- Slowly lower leg. Pause.
- Repeat with other leg.
- Alternate legs until you have done 8 to 12 repetitions with each leg.
- Rest, then do another set of 8 to 12 alternating repetitions.

Examples of Strength/Balance Exercises

Balance exercises can help you stay independent by helping you avoid disability that may result from falling. As you will see, there is a lot of overlap between strength and balance exercises; very often, one exercise serves both purposes.

Any of the lower-body exercises for strength shown in the previous strength section also are balance exercises. They include plantar flexion, hip flexion, hip extension, knee flexion, and side leg raise. Just do your regularly scheduled strength exercises and they will improve your balance at the same time. Also do the knee-extension exercise, which helps you keep your balance

by increasing muscle strength in your upper thighs.

Safety

Don't do more than your regularly scheduled strength exercise sessions to incorporate these balance exercises. Remember that doing strength exercises too often can do more harm than good. Simply do your strength exercises, and incorporate these balance techniques as you progress.

Progressing

These exercises can improve your balance even more if you add the following steps. These exercises instruct you to hold onto a table or chair for balance, so start by holding onto the table with only one hand. As you progress, try holding on with only one fingertip. Next, try these exercises without holding on at all. If you are very

steady on your feet, move on to doing the exercises using no hands, with your eyes closed. Have someone stand close by if you are unsteady.

Plantar Flexion

Do plantar flexion as part of your regularly scheduled strength exercises, and add these modifications as you progress. Hold table with one hand, then one fingertip, then no hands; then do exercise with eyes closed, if steady.

- Stand straight; hold onto a table or chair for balance.
- Slowly stand on tip-toe, as high as possible.
- Hold position for 1 second.
- Slowly lower heels all the way back down. Pause.
- Repeat 8 to 12 times.

270

- Rest, then do another set of 8 to 12 repetitions.

- Add modifications as you progress.

Knee Flexion

Do knee flexion as part of your regularly scheduled strength exercises, and add these modifications as you progress: Hold table with one hand, then one fingertip, then no hands; then do exercise with eyes closed, if steady.

- Stand straight; hold onto a table or chair for balance.

- Slowly bend knee as far as possible, so foot lifts up behind you.

- Hold position for 1 second.

- Slowly lower foot all the way back down. Pause.

- Repeat with other leg.

- Alternate legs until you have done 8 to 12 repetitions with each leg.

- Rest, then do another set of 8 to 12 alternating repetitions.

- Add modifications as you progress.

Hip Flexion

Do hip flexion as part of your regularly scheduled strength exercises, and add these modifications as you progress: Hold table with one hand, then one fingertip, then no hands; then do exercise with eyes closed, if steady.

- Stand straight; hold onto a table or chair for balance.

- Slowly bend one knee toward chest, without bending waist or hips.

- Hold position for 1 second.

- Slowly lower leg all the way down. Pause.

- Repeat with other leg.

- Alternate legs until you have done 8 to 12 repetitions with each leg.

- Rest, then do another set of 8 to 12 alternating repetitions.

- Add modifications as you progress.

Hip Extension

Do hip extension as part of your regularly scheduled strength exercises, and add these modifications as you progress: Hold table with one hand, then one fingertip, then no hands; then do exercise with eyes closed, if steady.

- Stand 12 to 18 inches from a table or chair, feet slightly apart.

- Bend forward at hips at about 45-degree angle; hold onto a table or chair for balance.

- Slowly lift one leg straight backwards without bending your knee, pointing your toes, or bending your upper body any farther forward.

- Hold position for 1 second.

- Slowly lower leg. Pause.

- Repeat with other leg.

- Alternate legs until you have done 8 to 12 repetitions with each leg.

- Rest, then do another set of 8 to 12 alternating repetitions.

- Add modifications as you progress.

Side Leg Raise

Do leg raises as part of your regularly scheduled strength exercises, and add these modifications as you progress: Hold table with one hand, then one fingertip, then no hands; then do exercise with eyes closed, if steady.

- Stand straight, directly behind table or chair, feet slightly apart.

- Hold onto table or chair for balance.

- Slowly lift one leg to side 6–12 inches out to side. Keep your back and both legs straight. Don't point your toes outward; keep them facing forward.

- Hold position for 1 second.

- Slowly lower leg all the way down. Pause.

- Repeat with other leg.

- Alternate legs until you have done 8 to 12 repetitions with each leg.

- Rest, then do another set of 8 to 12 alternating repetitions.

- Add modifications as you progress.

Anytime, Anywhere Balancing Exercises

These types of exercises also improve your balance. You can do them almost anytime, anywhere, and as often as you like, as long as you have something sturdy nearby to hold onto if you become unsteady.

Examples:

- Walk heel-to-toe. Position your heel just in front of the toes of the opposite foot each time you take a step. Your heel and toes should touch or almost touch.

- Stand on one foot (for example, while waiting in line at the grocery store or at the bus stop). Alternate feet.

- Stand up and sit down without using your hands.

Section 31.2

Core-Strengthening Exercises

This section includes text excerpted from "Strengthening Your Core," U.S. Department of Veterans Affairs (VA), March 12, 2014.

Strengthening Your Core

Your body's core is the area around your trunk and pelvis (hips) and is where your center of gravity is located. All body movement involves the core. A weak core can cause poor posture, lower back pain, and increased risk for injury. The benefits of a strong core include:

- Increased protection and support for your back

- Controlled movement

- Improved balance

Strengthening your core requires regular and proper exercise of your body's core muscles. Here are some basic core exercises:

Before you start to exercise your body's core, locate your deepest abdominal muscle—the transversus abdominis—by coughing once. The muscle you feel contracting is your transversus abdominis. We will refer to this muscle as your "abdominals."

Focus on keeping this muscle contracted while doing each of these exercises, and the rest of your core muscles get a workout, too. Once you know how to contract your abdominal muscles, begin the core muscle exercises.

With each exercise, breathe freely and deeply and avoid holding your breath. Coordinate your breathing with the tightening of your abdominals to get the maximum benefit.

Bridge

This exercise works many of your core muscles in combination.

- Lie on your back with your knees bent. Keep your back in a neutral position—not overly arched and not pressed into the floor. Avoid tilting your hips up.

- Cough to tighten your abdominals. Holding the contraction in your abdominals, raise your hips off the floor

- Align your hips with your knees and shoulders. Hold this position and take three deep breaths.

- Return to the start position and repeat. For a challenge, extend one knee while maintaining the bridge position.

Single-Leg Abdominal Press

- Lie on your back with your knees bent and your back in a neutral position.

- Cough and hold to activate your abdominals.

- Raise your right leg off the floor—so that your knee and hip bend at 90-degree angles—and rest your right hand on top of your right knee.

- Push your hand forward while using your abdominal muscles to pull your knee toward your hand. Hold for three deep breaths and return to the start position.

- Repeat this exercise using your left hand and left knee. Keep your arm straight and avoid bending more than 90 degrees at your hip.

Trunk Rotation

- Lie on your back on the floor with your knees bent and your back in a neutral position. Cough and hold to tighten your abdominals.

- Keeping your shoulders on the floor, let your knees fall slowly to the left. Go only as far as is comfortable—you should feel no pain, only a stretch.

- Use your trunk muscles to pull your legs back up to the start position. Repeat the exercise to the right.

Crunch

- Lie on your back and place your feet on a wall with a 90-degree bend at your knees and hips. Cough and hold to activate your abdominals.

- Imagine two dots in a vertical line on your abdomen—one above and one below your bellybutton. Imagine pulling those dots together.

- Use your trunk muscles to raise your head and shoulders off the floor. To avoid straining your neck, cross your arms on your chest, rather than locking them behind your head, and don't raise your head more than shown. Hold for three deep breaths, then return to the start position and repeat.

Quadruped

- Start on your hands and knees with your hands directly below your shoulders and your head and neck aligned with your back.

- Cough and hold your abdominals tight. Raise one arm off the floor and reach ahead. Hold for three deep breaths, return your arm and raise your other arm.

- Repeat the exercise by raising each leg.

- Challenge yourself by raising one arm and the opposite leg together. When raising your leg, avoid rolling your pelvis. Center your hips and tighten your trunk muscles for balance. Do this on both sides.

Chapter 32

Combined Exercise

Chapter Contents

Section 32.1

Cross Training

In order to achieve and maintain a desired level of physical fitness, it is important to make use of a variety of exercises and conditioning techniques. But in the pursuit of fitness, many individuals tend to rely on a single type of exercise or routine and as a result find themselves entrenched in a rut that is difficult to escape. Once a plateau is reached, a creative approach to reinventing your training will help you push through to the next level. Cross training offers a unique approach by drawing on various disciplines and combining them into a powerful and productive fitness routine.

What It Is

Cross training is essentially a program that works muscles and muscle groups from different parts of the body by training in more than one sport, skill, exercise routine, or task. Using this approach, different workout strategies can be combined to create a comprehensive fitness session.

In addition to focusing only on a specific set of muscles, a single, repetitive workout routine also carries the risk of injury by adding stress to the set of muscles and bones involved in the activity. Cross training addresses this by bringing into play a variety of muscle groups, which not only helps avoid injury but also improves overall health.

In sports conditioning, the old thinking was to exercise the set of muscles directly involved in the game in order to maximize proficiency in that particular sport. Experts now believe that cross training—working more muscle groups and adding activities other than the athlete's primary sport—is the best approach, and so cross training has now become standard practice in both professional and amateur sports.

The Benefits of Cross Training

Cross training offers a host of benefits, some of which are listed below:

- It corrects muscle imbalances and improves overall health and mobility.

- The comprehensive workload and variety of exercises lead to increased capability and fitness levels. Cross training supports multiple fitness goals, such as weight loss, muscle gain, and agility.

- Playing sports puts stress on a specific set of muscles, and this can lead to injury from overuse. Cross training, with endurance training and stretches, helps reduce or eliminate such injuries.

- Cross training has been proven effective in rehabilitation. It assists in the healing process and helps athletes maintain fitness levels during recovery. For example, a baseball player with a hamstring injury can swim and work with weights to remain physically fit.

- Cross training improves muscular and cardiovascular fitness. It also relieves stress and boosts productivity at work or while performing daily tasks.

- Cross training relieves the boredom of repeatedly engaging in a single activity by providing variety. This helps people sustain fitness activities in the long run.

Starting a Cross Training Program

A cross training program should entail a variety of activities, including cardio, strength training, flexibility, and balance. Cross training could be as simple as doing different types of exercises in a workout, or it could mean doing one activity in a session but varying it from session to session. For example, one workout could involve just cardio, the next strength training, the next flexibility, and so on.

Since variety is the key to cross training, some people confuse it with circuit training, which involves rotating workouts in which exercises are changed periodically but often still involve only certain parts of the body. Cross training is different from circuit training in that it incorporates cardio, strength training, flexibility, and balance in one coordinated program.

Cross training has been proven to be conducive to overall health and well-being. Its benefits have been recognized by therapists and sports coaches, and its techniques are frequently used in outpatient clinics and sports leagues because of its impressive results. Nevertheless, it is important to consult your doctor before starting a cross-training program, especially if you have chronic conditions like diabetes, high blood pressure, or heart disease.

References

1. Foster, Laeteashai. "Cross Training and the Benefits of Mixing It Up," Bon Secours in Motion, n.d.

2. "The Benefits of Cross Training," Tuvizo.com, n.d.

3. Williard, Jess. "The Benefits of Cross Training," Men's Fitness, n.d.

4. Bouchez, Colette. "Get Stronger and Leaner with Cross Training," WebMD, March 19, 2010.

Section 32.2

Interval Training

"Interval Training," © 2017 Omnigraphics.
Reviewed September 2016.

Interval training is an effective training technique that can help take you to the next level of fitness. Once used only by elite athletes, it has become popular among all types of fitness enthusiasts. With interval training, you can burn more calories in a quick work out and spend less time at the gym. Done properly, interval training can enhance physical performance and transform your physique.

Interval Training Explained

Many fitness programs entail performing exercises in a continuous routine. Interval training, on the other hand, involves short bursts of intense exercise alternated with recovery periods or brief times of low-intensity exercise. The high-intensity and low-intensity periods together form a complete workout cycle. The difficulty level of interval training can be altered by adjusting the intervals. There are two ways of approaching this: The duration and intensity of the individual intervals can be increased; and the total number of intervals in the training session can be changed.

Interval training is comparable to playing sports, which commonly entail periods of high-intensity sprinting and jogging interspersed with brief periods of rest. In this way, it is useful for athletic training, as well as for overall fitness.

Interval training can be practiced easily. There is no need for special equipment, and it only requires a change in the way you perform your exercise routine. For example, if you walk as a form of exercise, you could try jogging for brief periods and alternate with walking for recovery. When swimming, complete a lap at high speed and then rest for the same duration. Repeat this as a cycle. Exercise machines, such as elliptical trainers, treadmills, and stationary cycles often have a built-in interval training function to take you through the alternating stages. If a particular machine lacks this capability, the intervals can be created manually.

The Benefits of Interval Training

Interval training has a number of advantages over some other types of fitness routines:

- Interval training enables you to do the same amount of exercise in less time.

- It is an effective way to lose weight.

- It can help counter the effects of aging.

- You will be burning more calories, even after training.

- Interval training is less tedious than many other kinds of exercise, so you'll have a better chance of sticking to a workout routine.

- It boosts endurance and overall fitness.

- You can switch between a variety of fitness activities and get the same result.

Getting Started

It's best to begin interval training by warming up for at least ten minutes. The workout intervals put a lot of strain on the muscles, so it is important to warm up in order to avoid injuries. And after interval training, be sure to finish with a cool-down period.

You should feel tired—although not completely exhausted—after interval training, otherwise you are not training hard enough. Interval training should generally be done only three times per week, because the body will need 48 hours to recover from the intense bursts. High-performing athletes can train five times each week in an intense training program, but for most people this could be overdoing it.

You can derive significant benefits from as little as 20 minutes of interval training. Once you have reached a certain level of endurance and strength, you can increase the length of your workout to reach the next level.

The high-intensity bursts of interval training exercise many parts of the body and provide a better workout than long durations of moderate exercise. This regimen improves cardiovascular health, aerobic power, speed, and workout threshold levels. It also burns more calories and helps break through fitness plateaus.

Scientists have substantiated the benefits of interval training with a considerable amount of research. In interval training, the body is temporarily unable to supply enough oxygen to the muscles during the intense workout periods. This shortage of oxygen, in turn, increases the metabolism of the body and burns more calories, even for some time after the workout is over. Trainers refer to this mechanism as excess post-exercise oxygen consumption (EPOC), and it has proven to burn fat more effectively than continuous low-intensity workouts.

What Are the Risks?

Interval training is generally safe for healthy individuals and carries little risk unless it is overdone. Nevertheless, before starting a strenuous exercise session be sure to warm up properly, and be careful not to risk injury through overexertion. And always consult a doctor before beginning interval training, especially if you have chronic conditions like diabetes, high blood pressure, or heart disease.

References

1. Bode, Lynn. "Spice Up Your Workouts with Interval Training," Topend Sports, 2003.

2. Herwig. "How to Lose Weight with Interval Training," Runtastic.com, August 5, 2016.

3. "Interval Training for a Stronger Heart," Harvard Health Publications, September, 2015.

4. "Rev up Your Workout with Interval Training," Mayo Clinic, March 24, 2015.

5. "Interval Training," Concept2, Inc., n.d.

6. Duvall, Jeremy. "8 Amazing Fat-Burning Intervals," American Media, Inc., n.d.

7. Shortsleeve, Cassie. "7 Amazing Benefits of Interval Workouts—Backed by Science," American Media, Inc., n.d.

Section 32.3

Boot Camp Workouts

"Boot Camp Workouts," © 2017 Omnigraphics.
Reviewed September 2016.

What It Is

Boot camp workouts are fitness training programs that are modeled on military basic training. Boot camps have become increasingly popular because they exercise every muscle group and require minimal equipment. They generally consist of an hour-long workout that can take place either indoors or outdoors, depending on the trainer or health club.

How It Works

Boot camp workouts are usually conducted in a group and focus on basic exercise activities, such as push-ups, pull-ups, squats, jumping jacks, sit-ups, lunges, crunches, and sprints. The flexibility portions of the workouts may incorporate yoga and Pilates, as well. Boot camp is essentially a type of interval training with bursts of intense workouts alternating with rest periods. It exercises the whole body to build endurance and strength. Anyone can join a boot camp workout provided they have the stamina to complete the session. The exercises are intense, moving rapidly between strength training and cardio, making for a challenging program that builds confidence and self-esteem.

Even though the name is derived from the military, boot camp instructors do not motivate through techniques like yelling and intimidation. Instead, they build camaraderie among participants, relying on the principle that most people tend to push themselves more in a group setting.

Although the group dynamic is a traditional and effective component of boot camps, the workouts can also be done on your own. Popular DVDs are readily available that will help you plan your routine and enable you to work out at home.

The Benefits of Boot Camps

Some of the reasons for the popularity and success of boot camps are listed below:

- They help improve muscle strength and burn fat.

- Completing a strenuous boot camp session boosts confidence and self-esteem, improving both the mind and body.

- An average boot camp workout burns 500 to 600 calories.

- Boot camps are excellent motivators. Participants need to overcome any physical or mental barriers and push themselves with the help of their instructor and fellow trainees.

- Boot camps provide a variety of exercises, making them less repetitious and boring than many other workout programs.

- Special equipment is generally not required for boot camps, since they primarily rely on body weight for strength training, although sometimes hand weights, medicine balls, or other minimal equipment may be used.

- Boot camps create a sense of unity and camaraderie, encouraging the entire group to succeed.

Know the Risks

Boot camp will improve your cardiac health, build muscle, and help you lose weight, but it is a very strenuous workout It is important to consult your doctor before joining a boot camp, especially if you have diabetes, high blood pressure, or high cholesterol. If you have joint pain, arthritis, or other health issues, this type of program may not be for you.

Getting Started

- Boot camps vary, so research different programs in your area to find the best fit. Some camps are tailored for specific groups, such as young adults, older people, or women. Some concentrate on cardio, some stress more weight training, and others incorporate specific kinds of fitness equipment.

- Evaluate the instructor before you commit. Make sure the instructor is experienced and qualified and that his or her motivational style fits your own.

- Make sure the boot camp is appropriate for your level of fitness. Some programs cater to beginners, and others are tailored for more advanced groups. Talk to the instructor ahead of time if you find you are unsure, and let him or her know if you have any injuries that might require special consideration.

- Dress in comfortable workout clothes and wear appropriate shoes. Carry water if you think it won't be available at the site. Snack on fruits, vegetables, and whole grains an hour or two before boot camp to keep your energy level high. And be sure to warm up for at least five minutes before class begins.

- Give 100 percent. Trust your instructor, and push beyond your comfort zone. But listen to your body. Remember, if you are close to injury, no amount of willpower or encouragement will help shake it off. So be smart.

Boot camps are great for people who want to get in shape or maintain their fitness level. They can help you get past a plateau, shed excess weight, and improve your overall health. You only have to be prepared to give your best. If boot camp sounds like your kind of program, check out your local gym, and talk to an instructor about enlisting in one.

References

1. "Boot Camp Workout: Is It Right for You?" Mayo Clinic, March 25, 2016.

2. Sarnataro, Barbara Russi. "Fitness Boot Camps: Should You Enlist?" WebMD, May 27, 2009.

3. Brager, Alana. "The Benefits of Bootcamp," Active.com, n.d.

4. Breene, Sophia. "Know Before You Go: Fitness Boot Camps," Greatist.com, September 3, 2012.

5. Watson, Stephanie. "Boot Camp," WebMD, April 13, 2016.

Chapter 33

Mind-Body Exercise

Chapter Contents

Section 33.1

Introduction to Mind-Body Exercise

This section contains text excerpted from the following sources:
Text under the heading "How Can My Emotions Affect My Health?"
is excerpted from "Mind Body Connection: Strategies to Reduce
Physical and Mental Tension," U.S. Department of Veterans Affairs
(VA), July 2013; Text under the heading "Mind and Body Practices"
is excerpted from "Mind and Body Practices," National Center for
Complementary and Integrative Health (NCCIH), January 27, 2015;
Text beginning with the heading "What the Science Says About
the Safety and Side Effects of Relaxation Techniques" is excerpted
from "Relaxation Techniques for Health," National Center for
Complementary and Integrative Health (NCCIH), May 2016;
Text under the heading "What Is Progressive Muscle Relaxation?"
is excerpted from "Relaxation Techniques for Health," U.S.
Department of Veterans Affairs (VA), May 2016.

How Can My Emotions Affect My Health?

Your body responds to the way you think, feel, and act. This is often called the "mind/body connection." When you are stressed, anxious, or upset, your body tries to tell you that something isn't right. For example, high blood pressure or a stomach ulcer might develop after a particularly stressful event, such as the death of a loved one or friend. Physical signs that your emotional health is out of balance include: change in appetite, headaches, high blood pressure, upset stomach, and many others. Poor emotional health can weaken your body's immune system, making you more likely to get colds and other infections during emotionally difficult times. Also, when you are feeling stressed, anxious, or upset, you may not take care of your health as well as you should. You may not feel like exercising, eating nutritious foods, or taking medicine that your doctor prescribes. Abuse of alcohol, tobacco, or other drugs may also be a sign of poor emotional health.

Mind and Body Practices

Mind and body practices are a large and diverse group of techniques that are administered or taught to others by a trained practitioner or teacher. Examples include acupuncture, massage therapy, meditation, relaxation techniques, spinal manipulation, and yoga.

What Are Relaxation Techniques?

Relaxation techniques include a number of practices such as *progressive relaxation, guided imagery, biofeedback*, self-hypnosis, and deep breathing exercises. The goal is similar in all: to produce the body's natural relaxation response, characterized by slower breathing, lower blood pressure, and a feeling of increased well-being. Meditation and practices that include meditation with movement, such as yoga and tai chi, can also promote relaxation.

- Relaxation techniques are generally considered safe for healthy people. However, occasionally, people report negative experiences such as increased anxiety, intrusive thoughts, or fear of losing control.

- There have been rare reports that certain relaxation techniques might cause or worsen symptoms in people with epilepsy or certain psychiatric conditions, or with a history of abuse or trauma. People with heart disease should talk to their healthcare provider before doing progressive muscle relaxation.

What the Science Says about the Safety and Side Effects of Relaxation Techniques

- Relaxation techniques are generally considered safe for healthy people. However, occasionally, people report negative experiences such as increased anxiety, intrusive thoughts, or fear of losing control.

- There have been rare reports that certain relaxation techniques might cause or worsen symptoms in people with epilepsy or certain psychiatric conditions, or with a history of abuse or trauma. People with heart disease should talk to their healthcare provider before doing progressive muscle relaxation.

Who Teaches Relaxation Techniques?

A variety of professionals, including physicians, psychologists, social workers, nurses, and complementary health practitioners, may teach relaxation techniques. Also, people sometimes learn the simpler relaxation techniques on their own.

The Importance of Practice

Relaxation techniques are skills, and like other skills, they need practice. People who use relaxation techniques frequently are more likely to benefit from them. Regular, frequent practice is particularly important if you're using relaxation techniques to help manage a chronic health problem. Continuing use of relaxation techniques is more effective than short-term use.

Relaxation techniques include the following:

Autogenic Training

In autogenic training, you learn to concentrate on the physical sensations of warmth, heaviness, and relaxation in different parts of your body.

Biofeedback-Assisted Relaxation

Biofeedback techniques measure body functions and give you information about them so that you can learn to control them. Biofeedback-assisted relaxation uses electronic devices to teach you to produce changes in your body that are associated with relaxation, such as reduced muscle tension.

Deep Breathing or Breathing Exercises

This technique involves focusing on taking slow, deep, even breaths.

Guided Imagery

For this technique, people are taught to focus on pleasant images to replace negative or stressful feelings. Guided imagery may be self-directed or led by a practitioner or a recording.

Progressive Relaxation

This technique, also called Jacobson relaxation or progressive muscle relaxation, involves tightening and relaxing various muscle groups. Progressive relaxation is often combined with guided imagery and breathing exercises.

Self-Hypnosis

In self-hypnosis programs, people are taught to produce the relaxation response when prompted by a phrase or nonverbal cue (called a "suggestion").

What Is Progressive Muscle Relaxation?

We all carry tension in different parts of our bodies. This tension may become so habitual that we don't even realize our muscles are tense. Progressive muscle relaxation not only helps release tension from muscles, but it also helps you become more aware of your muscles. This exercise involves sequentially tightening and relaxing various muscle groups.

General Procedure:

- Sit in a chair with eyes closed and your hands loosely in your lap. Take a few slow, deep breaths.

- Extend your right arm in front of you and tense your fist to the point of pressure but not of strain. Hold the tension for 5-7 seconds, and then let your hand relax back into your lap. Let your hand and arm relax for 10-20 seconds.

- Repeat the previous step, tensing and relaxing your right fist for a second time.

- Continue alternating tension with relaxation for each of the remaining muscle groups. Remember to keep breathing as you tense your muscles. After you have tensed and relaxed one muscle group, move on to the next. Below you will find a sample sequence of muscles to tense and relax, but progressive muscle relaxation can be done with a fewer number or greater number of muscle groups as well. For example, you may choose to tense just one fist at a time, both fists at the same time, or perhaps even tense your entire arm along with the fist in the first step. You may also choose to spend more time with an especially tense muscle before moving on to the next muscle. It is not important that you tense your muscles in a certain way. Do this in whatever manner is comfortable for you. You should never tense to the point of pain. Also try to keep any muscles not currently being tensed in a relaxed state. Practice once per day, if possible. It is an acquired skill and you will get better at it with practice.

Possible PMR muscle sequence:

- Hands: Clench each fist

- Upper arms: Bend elbows and tense your upper arms (i.e, 'make a muscle')

- Shoulders: Lift your shoulders towards your ears

- Neck: Let neck drop to your chest
- Forehead and scalp: Raise eyebrows
- Face: Scrunch up face
- Tongue: Press tongue against roof of mouth
- Chest: Tighten chest muscles
- Upper back: Pull shoulders forward
- Lower back: Roll head and upper back down and forward, stretching the lower back (e.g, like touching your toes while sitting in a chair
- Buttocks: Squeeze buttocks
- Abdomen: Tighten stomach muscle
- Thighs: While sitting with knees bent at 90 degree angle, tense thigh muscles / or press upper legs together from knees to hips to create tension
- Calves: Lift toes off ground towards your shins
- Feet: Gently curl toes down so they are pressing into the floor

When you have finished tensing and relaxing each muscle group, sit quietly for another a minute or two. Use your imagination to further relax your muscles. Focus on one muscle group at a time. Going from one to the next, visualize the muscles spreading out; getting long, loose, and more deeply relaxed. Sit quietly for a few more minutes and feel the relaxation.

Section 33.2

Impact of Stress on Body and Mind

This section includes text excerpted from "BAM! Body and Mind,"
Centers for Disease Control and Prevention (CDC), May 9, 2015.

Finding yourself in a hectic situation, whether it's forgetting your homework or missing your ride home, can really stress you out. Are you looking for a safety net for those days that seem to get worse by the second? Could you really use some advice on how to de-stress both your body and your mind? Knowing how to deal can be half the battle!

Check out These 10 Tips to Keep You Cool, Calm, and Collected

Put Your Body in Motion

Moving from the chair to the couch while watching TV is not being physically active! Physical activity is one of the most important ways to keep stress away by clearing your head and lifting your spirits. Physical activity also increases endorphin levels—the natural "feel-good" chemicals in the body which leave you with a naturally happy feeling.

Whether you like full-fledged games of football, tennis, or roller hockey, or you prefer walks with family and friends, it's important to get up, get out, and get moving! Check out the BAM! activity cards and find one that's right for you!

Fuel Up

Start your day off with a full tank—eating breakfast will give you the energy you need to tackle the day. Eating regular meals (this means no skipping dinner) and taking time to enjoy them (nope, eating in the car on the way to practice doesn't count) will make you feel better too.

Make sure to fuel up with fruits, vegetables, proteins (peanut butter, a chicken sandwich, or a tuna salad) and grains (wheat bread, pasta, or some crackers)—these will give you the power you need to make it through those hectic days.

Don't be fooled by the jolt of energy you get from sodas and sugary snacks—this only lasts a short time, and once it wears off, you may feel sluggish and more tired than usual. For that extra boost of energy to sail through history notes, math class, and after school activities, grab a banana, some string cheese, or a granola bar for some power-packed energy!

LOL!

Some say that laughter is the best medicine—well, in many cases, it is! Did you know that it takes 15 facial muscles to laugh? Lots of laughin' can make you feel good—and, that good feeling can stay with you even after the laughter stops. So, head off stress with regular doses of laughter by watching a funny movie or cartoons, reading a joke book (you may even learn some new jokes), or even make up your own riddles...laughter can make you feel like a new person!

Everyone has those days when they do something really silly or stupid—instead of getting upset with yourself, laugh out loud! No one's perfect! Life should be about having fun. So, lighten up!

Have Fun with Friends

Being with people you like is always a good way to ditch your stress. Get a group together to go to the movies, shoot some hoops, or play a board game—or just hang out and talk. Friends can help you work through your problems and let you see the brighter side of things.

Spill to Someone You Trust

Instead of keeping your feelings bottled up inside, talk to someone you trust or respect about what's bothering you. It could be a friend, a parent, someone in your family, or a teacher. Talking out your problems and seeing them from a different view might help you figure out ways to deal with them. Just remember, you don't have to go it alone!

Take Time to Chill

Pick a comfy spot to sit and read, daydream, or even take a snooze. Listen to your favorite music. Work on a relaxing project like putting together a puzzle or making jewelry.

Stress can sometimes make you feel like a tight rubber band—stretched to the limit! If this happens, take a few deep breaths to help yourself unwind. If you're in the middle of an impossible homework problem, take a break! Finding time to relax after (and sometimes during) a hectic day or week can make all the difference.

Catch Some Zzzzz...

Fatigue is a best friend to stress. When you don't get enough sleep, it's hard to deal—you may feel tired, cranky, or you may have trouble thinking clearly. When you're overtired, a problem may seem much bigger than it actually is. You may have a hard time doing a school assignment that usually seems easy, you don't do your best in sports or any physical activity, or you may have an argument with your friends over something really stupid.

Sleep is a big deal! Getting the right amount of sleep is especially important for kids your age. Because your body (and mind) is changing and developing, it requires more sleep to recharge for the next day. So don't resist, hit the hay!

Keep a Journal

If you're having one of those crazy days when nothing goes right, it's a good idea to write things down in a journal to get it off of your chest—like how you feel, what's going on in your life, and things you'd like to accomplish. You could even write down what you do when you're faced with a stressful situation, and then look back and think about how you handled it later. So, find a quiet spot, grab a notebook and pen, and start writing!

Get It Together

Too much to do but not enough time? Forgot your homework? Feeling overwhelmed or discombobulated? Being unprepared for school, practice, or other activities can make for a very stressful day!

Getting everything done can be a challenge, but all you have to do is plan a little and get organized.

Lend a Hand

Get involved in an activity that helps others. It's almost impossible to feel stressed out when you're helping someone else. It's also a great way to find out about yourself and the special qualities you never knew you had! Signing up for a service project is a good idea, but helping others is as easy as saying hello, holding a door, or volunteering to keep a neighbor's pet. If you want to get involved in a more organized volunteer program, try working at a local recreation center, or helping with an after school program. The feeling you will get from helping others is greater than you can imagine!

Most importantly, don't sweat the small stuff! Try to pick a few really important things and let the rest slide—getting worked up over every little thing will only increase your stress. So, toughen up and don't let stressful situations get to you! Remember, you're not alone—everyone has stresses in their lives... it's up to you to choose how to deal with them.

Section 33.3

Yoga

This section includes text excerpted from documents published by three sources. Text under headings marked 1 are excerpted from "Yoga: In Depth," National Center for Complementary and Integrative Health (NCCIH), June 2013; text under heading marked 2 is excerpted from "5 Things You Should Know About Yoga," National Center for Complementary and Integrative Health (NCCIH), September 24, 2015; text under heading marked 3 is excerpted from "Yoga as a Complementary Health Approach," National Center for Complementary and Integrative Health (NCCIH), February 12, 2015.

Yoga is a mind and body practice with historical origins in ancient Indian philosophy. Like other meditative movement practices used for health purposes, various styles of yoga typically combine physical postures, breathing techniques, and meditation or relaxation. This section provides basic information about yoga and summarizes scientific research on effectiveness and safety.

Key Facts[1]

- Recent studies in people with chronic low-back pain suggest that a carefully adapted set of yoga poses may help reduce pain and improve function (the ability to walk and move). Studies also suggest that practicing yoga (as well as other forms of regular exercise) might have other health benefits such as reducing heart rate and blood pressure, and may also help relieve anxiety and depression. Other research suggests yoga is not helpful for asthma, and studies looking at yoga and arthritis have had mixed results.

- People with high blood pressure, glaucoma, or sciatica, and women who are pregnant should modify or avoid some yoga poses.

- Ask a trusted source (such as a healthcare provider or local hospital) to recommend a yoga practitioner. Contact professional organizations for the names of practitioners who have completed an acceptable training program.

- Tell all your healthcare providers about any complementary health approaches you use. Give them a full picture of what you do to manage your health. This will help ensure coordinated and safe care.

5 Things You Should Know About Yoga[2]

Yoga typically combines physical postures, breathing exercises, and meditation or relaxation. Researchers are studying how yoga may be used to help improve health and to learn more about its safe use. If you're thinking about practicing yoga, here are 5 things you should know:

1. Studies suggest that yoga may be beneficial for a number of conditions, including pain. Recent studies in people with chronic low-back pain suggest that a carefully adapted set of yoga poses can help reduce pain and improve function. Other studies also suggest that practicing yoga (as well as other forms of regular exercise) might have other health benefits such as reducing heart rate and blood pressure, and may also help relieve anxiety and depression.

2. Studies show that certain other health conditions may not benefit from yoga. Research suggests that yoga is not helpful for asthma, and studies looking at yoga and arthritis have had mixed results.

3. Yoga is generally considered to be safe in healthy people when practiced appropriately. However, people with high blood pressure, glaucoma, or sciatica, and women who are pregnant should modify or avoid some yoga poses.

4. Practice safely and mindfully. Everyone's body is different, and yoga postures should be modified based on individual abilities. Carefully selecting an instructor who is experienced and is attentive to your needs is an important step toward helping you practice yoga safely. Inform your instructor about any medical issues you have, and ask about the physical demands of yoga.

5. Talk to your healthcare providers about any complementary health practices you use, including yoga. If you're thinking

about practicing yoga, also be sure to talk to your healthcare providers. Give them a full picture of what you do to manage your health. This will help ensure coordinated and safe care.

About Yoga[1]

Yoga in its full form combines physical postures, breathing exercises, meditation, and a distinct philosophy. There are numerous styles of yoga. Hatha yoga, commonly practiced in the United States and Europe, emphasizes postures, breathing exercises, and meditation. Hatha yoga styles include Ananda, Anusara, Ashtanga, Bikram, Iyengar, Kripalu, Kundalini, Viniyoga, and others.

Use of Yoga for Health in the United States[1]

According to the 2007 National Health Interview Survey (NHIS), which included a comprehensive survey on the use of complementary health approaches by Americans, yoga is the sixth most commonly used complementary health practice among adults. More than 13 million adults practiced yoga in the previous year, and between the 2002 and 2007 NHIS, use of yoga among adults increased by 1 percent (or approximately 3 million people). The 2007 survey also found that more than 1.5 million children practiced yoga in the previous year.

Many people who practice yoga do so to maintain their health and well-being, improve physical fitness, relieve stress, and enhance quality of life. In addition, they may be addressing specific health conditions, such as back pain, neck pain, arthritis, and anxiety.

What the Science Says about Yoga[1]

Current research suggests that a carefully adapted set of yoga poses may reduce low-back pain and improve function. Other studies also suggest that practicing yoga (as well as other forms of regular exercise) might improve quality of life; reduce stress; lower heart rate and blood pressure; help relieve anxiety, depression, and insomnia; and improve overall physical fitness, strength, and flexibility. But some research suggests yoga may not improve asthma, and studies looking at yoga and arthritis have had mixed results.

- One National Center for Complementary and Integrative Health (NCCIH)-funded study of 90 people with chronic low-back pain found that participants who practiced Iyengar yoga had significantly less disability, pain, and depression after 6 months.

- In a 2011 study, also funded by NCCIH, researchers compared yoga with conventional stretching exercises or a self-care book in 228 adults with chronic low-back pain. The results showed that both yoga and stretching were more effective than a self-care book for improving function and reducing symptoms due to chronic low-back pain.

- Conclusions from another 2011 study of 313 adults with chronic or recurring low-back pain suggested that 12 weekly yoga classes resulted in better function than usual medical care.

However, studies show that certain health conditions may not benefit from yoga.

- A 2011 systematic review of clinical studies suggests that there is no sound evidence that yoga improves asthma.

- A 2011 review of the literature reports that few published studies have looked at yoga and arthritis, and of those that have, results are inconclusive. The two main types of arthritis—osteoarthritis and rheumatoid arthritis—are different conditions, and the effects of yoga may not be the same for each. In addition, the reviewers suggested that even if a study showed that yoga helped osteoarthritic finger joints, it may not help osteoarthritic knee joints.

Side Effects and Risks[1]

- Yoga is generally low-impact and safe for healthy people **when practiced appropriately under the guidance of a well-trained instructor.**

- Overall, those who practice yoga have a low rate of side effects, and the risk of serious injury from yoga is quite low. However, certain types of stroke as well as pain from nerve damage are among the rare possible side effects of practicing yoga.

- Women who are pregnant and people with certain medical conditions, such as high blood pressure, glaucoma (a condition in which fluid pressure within the eye slowly increases and may damage the eye's optic nerve), and sciatica (pain, weakness, numbing, or tingling that may extend from the lower back to the calf, foot, or even the toes), should modify or avoid some yoga poses.

Yoga as a Complementary Health Approach[3]

Yoga Is One of the Top 10 Complementary Health Approaches

- More than 13 million adults in the U.S. practiced yoga in the previous year.
- Yoga use increased from 5.1% to 6.1% between 2002 and 2007.

Why People Practice Yoga

- 58% do it to maintain health and well-being
- 16% use it to treat specific medical conditions
- 10.5% use it for musculoskeletal conditions
- Of those who used yoga for specific conditions, 22% said their doctor recommended it
- Back pain is the number one reason people use complementary health practices

Yoga's Impact on Low-Back Pain

Back pain is the number one reason people use complementary health practices. Studies found people practicing yoga who experience low-back pain had:

- Significantly less disability, pain, and depression after 6 months than patients in standard care.
- More pain relief than from a self-care book.
- Better function than usual medical care.

Practice Yoga Safely

Follow these tips to minimize your risk of injury:

- Talk to your care provider
- Find a trained and experienced yoga practitioner
- Adapt poses to your individual needs and abilities

Section 33.4

Pilates

Pilates is a body conditioning routine that seeks to build flexibility, strength, endurance, and coordination without adding muscle bulk.

For decades, it's been the exercise of choice for dancers and gymnasts (and now Hollywood actors), but it was originally used to rehabilitate bedridden or immobile patients during World War I.

What Is Pilates?

Pilates improves mental and physical well-being, increases flexibility, and strengthens muscles through controlled movements done as mat exercises or with equipment to tone and strengthen the body.

In addition, pilates increases circulation and helps to sculpt the body and strengthen the body's "core" or "powerhouse" (torso). People who do pilates regularly feel they have better posture, are less prone to injury, and experience better overall health.

Joseph H. Pilates, the founder of the pilates exercise method, was born in Germany. As a child he was frail, living with asthma and other childhood conditions. To build his body and grow stronger, he took up several different sports, eventually becoming an accomplished athlete. As a nurse in Great Britain during World War I, he designed exercise methods and equipment for immobilized patients and soldiers.

In addition to his equipment, Pilates developed a series of mat exercises that focus on the torso. He based these on various exercise methods from around the world, among them the mind-body formats of yoga and Chinese martial arts.

Joseph Pilates believed that our physical and mental health are intertwined. He designed his exercise program around principles that support this philosophy, including concentration, precision, control, breathing, and flowing movements.

There are two ways to exercise in pilates:

1. Today, most people focus on the **mat exercises,** which require only a floor mat and training. These exercises are designed so that your body uses its own weight as resistance.

2. The other method uses a variety of **machines** to tone and strengthen the body, again using the principle of resistance.

Getting Started

The great thing about pilates is that just about everyone—from couch potatoes to fitness buffs—can do it. Because pilates has gained lots of attention recently, classes are usually readily available.

Many fitness centers and YMCAs offer pilates classes, mostly in mat work. Some pilates instructors also offer private classes that can be paid for class by class or in blocks of classes; these may combine mat work with machine work. If your health club makes pilates machines available to members, make sure there's a qualified pilates instructor on duty to teach and supervise you during the exercises.

The fact that pilates is hot and classes are springing up everywhere does have a downside, though: inadequate instruction. As with any form of exercise, it is possible to injure yourself if you have a health condition or don't know exactly how to do the moves. Some gyms send their personal trainers to weekend-long courses and then claim they're qualified to teach pilates (they're not!), and this can lead to injury.

So look for an instructor who is certified by a group that has a rigorous training program. These instructors have completed several hundred hours of training just in pilates and know the different ways to modify the exercises so new students don't get hurt.

The pilates mat program follows a set sequence, with exercises following on from one another in a natural progression, just as Joseph Pilates designed them. Beginners start with basic exercises and build up to include additional exercises and more advanced positioning.

Keep these tips in mind so that you can get the most out of your pilates workout:

- **Stay focused.** Pilates is designed to combine your breathing rhythm with your body movements. Qualified instructors teach ways to keep your breathing working in conjunction with the exercises. You will also be taught to concentrate on your muscles and what you're doing. The goal of pilates is to unite your mind and body, which relieves stress and anxiety.

- **Be comfortable.** Wear comfortable clothes (as you would for yoga—shorts or tights and a T-shirt or tank top are good choices), and keep in mind that pilates is usually done without shoes. If you start feeling uncomfortable, strained, or experience pain, you should stop.

- **Let it flow.** When you perform your exercises, avoid quick, jerky movements. Every movement should be slow, but still strong and flexible. Joseph Pilates worked with dancers and designed his movements to flow like a dance.

- **Don't leave out the heart.** The nice thing about pilates is you don't have to break a sweat if you don't want to—but you can also work the exercises quickly (bearing in mind fluidity, of course!) to get your heart rate going. Or, because pilates is primarily about strength and flexibility, pair your pilates workout with a form of aerobic exercise like swimming or brisk walking.

Most fans of pilates say they stick with the program because it's diverse and interesting. Joseph Pilates designed his program for variety—people do fewer repetitions of a number of exercises rather than lots of repetitions of only a few. He also intended his exercises to be something people could do on their own once they've had proper instruction, cutting down the need to remain dependent on a trainer.

Before you begin any type of exercise program, it's a good idea to talk to your doctor, especially if you have a health problem.

Section 33.5

Tai Chi and Qi Gong

Text in this section is excerpted from "Tai Chi and Qi Gong: In Depth," National Center for Complementary and Integrative Health (NCCIH), August 2015.

What Are Tai Chi and Qi Gong?

Tai chi and qi gong are centuries-old, related mind and body practices. They involve certain postures and gentle movements with mental focus, breathing, and relaxation. The movements can be adapted or practiced while walking, standing, or sitting. In contrast to qi gong, tai chi movements, if practiced quickly, can be a form of combat or self-defense.

How Much Do We Know about Tai Chi and Qi Gong?

Several clinical trials have evaluated the effects of tai chi and qi gong in people with various health conditions.

What Do We Know about the Effectiveness of Tai Chi and Qi Gong?

Practicing tai chi may help to improve balance and stability in older people and in those with Parkinson disease, reduce back pain and pain from knee osteoarthritis, and improve quality of life in people with heart disease, cancer, and other chronic illnesses. Tai chi and qi gong may ease fibromyalgia pain and promote general quality of life. Qi gong may reduce chronic neck pain, but study results are mixed. Tai chi also may improve reasoning ability in older people.

What Do We Know about the Safety of Tai Chi and Qi Gong?

Tai chi and qi gong appear to be safe practices, but it's a good idea to talk with your healthcare providers before beginning any exercise program.

What the Science Says About the Effectiveness of Tai Chi and Qi Gong

Research findings suggest that practicing tai chi may improve balance and stability in older people and those with Parkinson's, reduce pain from knee osteoarthritis, help people cope with fibromyalgia and back pain, and promote quality of life and mood in people with heart failure and cancer. There has been less research on the effects of qi gong, but some studies suggest it may reduce chronic neck pain (although results are mixed) and pain from fibromyalgia. Qi gong also may help to improve general quality of life.

Both also may offer psychological benefits, such as reducing anxiety. However, differences in how the research on anxiety was conducted make it difficult to draw firm conclusions about this.

What the Science Says About Safety of Tai Chi and Qi Gong

Tai chi and qi gong appear to be safe practices. One National Center for Complementary and Integrative Health (NCCIH)-supported review noted that tai chi is unlikely to result in serious injury but it may be associated with minor aches and pains. Women who are pregnant should talk with their healthcare providers before beginning tai chi, qi gong, or any other exercise program.

Training, Licensing, and Certification

Tai chi instructors don't have to be licensed, and the practice is not regulated by the Federal Government or individual states. There's no national standard for qi gong certification. Various tai chi and qi gong organizations offer training and certification programs—with differing criteria and levels of certification for instructors.

NCCIH-Funded Research

NCCIH is supporting studies of tai chi's effects on:

- Symptoms of anxiety and sleep quality in young adults
- Fibromyalgia
- Knee osteoarthritis.
- NCCIH currently is not funding research on qi gong.

More To Consider

Learning tai chi or qi gong from a video or book does not ensure that you're doing the movements correctly or safely.

If you have a health condition, talk with your healthcare provider before starting tai chi or qi gong.

Ask a trusted source (such as your healthcare provider or a nearby hospital) to recommend a tai chi or qi gong instructor. Find out about the training and experience of any instructor you are considering.

Tell all your healthcare providers about any complementary or integrative health approaches you use. Give them a full picture of what you do to manage your health. This will help ensure coordinated and safe care.

Part Five

Fitness Safety

Chapter 34

Safe Physical Activity

Safe and Active

Although physical activity has many health benefits, injuries and other adverse events do sometimes happen. The most common injuries affect the musculoskeletal system (the bones, joints, muscles, ligaments, and tendons). Other adverse events can also occur during activity, such as overheating and dehydration. On rare occasions, people have heart attacks during activity.

The good news is that scientific evidence strongly shows that physical activity is safe for almost everyone. Moreover, the health benefits of physical activity far outweigh the risks.

Still, people may hesitate to become physically active because of concern they'll get hurt. For these people, there is even more good news: They can take steps that are proven to reduce their risk of injury and adverse events.

The Guidelines in this chapter provide advice to help people do physical activity safely. Most advice applies to people of all ages. Specific guidance for particular age groups and people with certain conditions is also provided.

This chapter includes text excerpted from "Chapter 6: Safe and Active," U.S. Department of Health and Human Services (HHS), October 7, 2008. Reviewed September 2016.

Explaining the Guidelines

Physical Activity Is Safe for Almost Everyone

Most people are not likely to be injured when doing moderate-intensity activities in amounts that meet the Physical Activity Guidelines. However, injuries and other adverse events do sometimes happen. The most common problems are musculoskeletal injuries. Even so, studies show that only one such injury occurs for every 1,000 hours of walking for exercise, and fewer than four injuries occur for every 1,000 hours of running.

Both physical fitness and total amount of physical activity affect risk of musculoskeletal injuries. People who are physically fit have a lower risk of injury than people who are not. People who do more activity generally have a higher risk of injury than people who do less activity. So what should people do if they want to be active and safe? The best strategies are to:

- Be regularly physically active to increase physical fitness; and

- Follow the other guidance in this chapter (especially increasing physical activity gradually over time) to minimize the injury risk from doing medium to high amounts of activity.

Following these strategies may reduce overall injury risk. Active people are more likely to have an activity related injury than inactive people. But they appear less likely to have non-activity-related injuries, such as work-related injuries or injuries that occur around the home or from motor vehicle crashes.

Key Guidelines for Safe Physical Activity

To do physical activity safely and reduce risk of injuries and other adverse events, people should:

- Understand the risks and yet be confident that physical activity is safe for almost everyone.

- Choose to do types of physical activity that are appropriate for their current fitness level and health goals, because some activities are safer than others.

- Increase physical activity gradually over time whenever more activity is necessary to meet guidelines or health goals. Inactive people should "start low and go slow" by gradually increasing how often and how long activities are done.

- Protect themselves by using appropriate gear and sports equipment, looking for safe environments, following rules and policies, and making sensible choices about when, where, and how to be active.

- Be under the care of a healthcare provider if they have chronic conditions or symptoms. People with chronic conditions and symptoms should consult their healthcare provider about the types and amounts of activity appropriate for them.

Choose Appropriate Types and Amounts of Activity

People can reduce their risk of injury by choosing appropriate types of activity. As the table shows, the safest activities are moderate intensity and low impact, and don't involve purposeful collision or contact.

Walking for exercise, gardening or yard work, bicycling or exercise cycling, dancing, swimming, and golf are activities with the lowest injury rates. In the amounts commonly done by adults, walking (a moderate–intensity and low-impact activity) has a third or less of the injury risk of running (a vigorous-intensity and higher impact activity).

The risk of injury for a type of physical activity can also differ according to the purpose of the activity. For example, recreational bicycling or bicycling for transportation leads to fewer injuries than training for and competing in bicycle races.

People who have had a past injury are at risk of injuring that body part again. The risk of injury can be reduced by performing appropriate amounts of activity and setting appropriate personal goals. Performing a variety of different physical activities may also reduce the risk of overuse injury.

The risk of injury to bones, muscles, and joints is directly related to the gap between a person's usual level of activity and a new level of activity.

Table 34.1. The Continuum of Injury Risk Associated with Different Types of Activity

The Continuum of Injury Risk Associated with Different Types of Activity		
Injury Risk Level (Risk Level from lower to higher)	**Activity Type**	**Examples**
Lowest Risk	**Commuting**	Walking, bicycling

Table 34.1. Continued

The Continuum of Injury Risk Associated with Different Types of Activity		
Lower Risk	**Lifestyle**	Home repair, gardening/ yard work
Medium Risk	**Recreation/sports No contact**	Walking for exercise, golf, dancing, swimming, running, tennis
Higher Risk	**Recreation/sports Limited contact**	Bicycling, aerobics, skiing, volleyball, baseball, softball
Highest Risk	**Recreation/sports Collision/contact**	Football, hockey, soccer, basketball

Increase Physical Activity Gradually Over Time

Scientific studies indicate that the risk of injury to bones, muscles, and joints is directly related to the gap between a person's usual level of activity and a new level of activity. The size of this gap is called the amount of overload. Creating a small overload and waiting for the body to adapt and recover reduces the risk of injury. When amounts of physical activity need to be increased to meet the Guidelines or personal goals, physical activity should be increased gradually over time, no matter what the person's current level of physical activity.

Scientists have not established a standard for how to gradually increase physical activity over time. The following recommendations give general guidance for inactive people and those with low levels of physical activity on how to increase physical activity:

- Use relative intensity (intensity of the activity relative to a person's fitness) to guide the level of effort for aerobic activity.

- Generally start with relatively moderate-intensity aerobic activity. Avoid relatively vigorous-intensity activity, such as shoveling snow or running. Adults with a low level of fitness may need to start with light activity, or a mix of light- to moderate-intensity activity.

- First, increase the number of minutes per session (duration), and the number of days per week (frequency) of moderate-intensity activity. Later, if desired, increase the intensity.

- Pay attention to the relative size of the increase in physical activity each week, as this is related to injury risk. For example, a 20-minute increase each week is safer for a person who does 200 minutes a week of walking (a 10 percent increase), than for a person who does 40 minutes a week (a 50 percent increase).

The available scientific evidence suggests that adding a small and comfortable amount of light- to moderate–intensity activity, such as 5 to 15 minutes of walking per session, 2 to 3 times a week, to one's usual activities has a low risk of musculoskeletal injury and no known risk of severe cardiac events. Because this range is rather wide, people should consider three factors in individualizing their rate of increase: age, level of fitness, and prior experience.

Age

The amount of time required to adapt to a new level of activity probably depends on age. Youth and young adults probably can safely increase activity by small amounts every week or 2. Older adults appear to require more time to adapt to a new level of activity, in the range of 2 to 4 weeks.

Level of Fitness

Less fit adults are at higher risk of injury when doing a given amount of activity, compared to fitter adults. Slower rates of increase over time may reduce injury risk. This guidance applies to overweight and obese adults, as they are commonly less physically fit.

Prior Experience

People can use their experience to learn to increase physical activity over time in ways that minimize the risk of overuse injury. Generally, if an overuse injury occurred in the past with a certain rate of progression, a person should increase activity more slowly the next time.

Take Appropriate Precautions

Taking appropriate precautions means using the right gear and equipment, choosing safe environments in which to be active, following rules and policies, and making sensible choices about how, when, and where to be active.

Use Protective Gear and Appropriate Equipment

Using personal protective gear can reduce the frequency of injury. Personal protective gear is something worn by a person to protect a specific body part. Examples include helmets, eyewear and goggles, shin guards, elbow and knee pads, and mouth guards.

Using appropriate sports equipment can also reduce risk of injury. Sports equipment refers to sport or activity-specific tools, such as balls, bats, sticks, and shoes.

For the most benefit, protective equipment and gear should be:

- The right equipment for the activity;

- Appropriately fitted;

- Appropriately maintained; and

- Used consistently and correctly.

Be Active in Safe Environments

People can reduce their injury risks by paying attention to the places they choose to be active. To help themselves stay safe, people can look for:

- Physical separation from motor vehicles, such as sidewalks, walking paths, or bike lanes;

- Neighborhoods with traffic-calming measures that slow down traffic;

- Places to be active that are well-lighted, where other people are present, and that are well-maintained (no litter, broken windows);

- Shock-absorbing surfaces on playgrounds;

- Well-maintained playing fields and courts without holes or obstacles;

- Breakaway bases at baseball and softball fields; and

- Padded and anchored goals and goal posts at soccer and football fields.

Follow Rules and Policies That Promote Safety

Rules, policies, legislation, and laws are potentially the most effective and wide-reaching way to reduce activity-related injuries. To get the benefit, individuals should look for and follow these rules, policies, and laws. For example, policies that promote the use of bicycle helmets reduce the risk of head injury among cyclists. Rules against diving into shallow water at swimming pools prevent head and neck injuries.

Make Sensible Choices About How, When, and Where To Be Active

A person's choices can obviously influence the risk of adverse events. By making sensible choices, injuries and adverse events can be prevented. Consider weather conditions, such as extremes of heat and cold. For example, during very hot and humid weather, people lessen the chances of dehydration and heat stress by:

- Exercising in the cool of early morning as opposed to mid-day heat;

- Switching to indoor activities (playing basketball in the gym rather than on the playground);

- Changing the type of activity (swimming rather than playing soccer);

- Lowering the intensity of activity (walking rather than running); and

- Paying close attention to rest, shade, drinking enough fluids, and other ways to minimize effects of heat.

Inactive people who gradually progress over time to relatively moderate-intensity activity have no known risk of sudden cardiac events, and very low risk of bone, muscle, or joint injuries.

Exposure to air pollution is associated with several adverse health outcomes, including asthma attacks and abnormal heart rhythms. People who can modify the location or time of exercise may wish to reduce these risks by exercising away from heavy traffic and industrial sites, especially during rush hour or times when pollution is known to be high. However, current evidence indicates that the benefits of being active, even in polluted air, outweigh the risk of being inactive.

Advice From Healthcare Providers

The protective value of a medical consultation for persons with or without chronic diseases who are interested in increasing their physical activity level is not established. People without diagnosed chronic conditions (such as diabetes, heart disease, or osteoarthritis) and who do not have symptoms (such as chest pain or pressure, dizziness, or joint pain) do not need to consult a healthcare provider about physical activity.

Inactive people who gradually progress over time to relatively moderate-intensity activity have no known risk of sudden cardiac events, and very low risk of bone, muscle, or joint injuries. A person who is habitually active with moderate-intensity activity can gradually increase to vigorous intensity without needing to consult a healthcare provider. People who develop new symptoms when increasing their levels of activity should consult a healthcare provider.

Healthcare providers can provide useful personalized advice on how to reduce risk of injuries. For people who wish to seek the advice of a healthcare provider, it is particularly appropriate to do so when contemplating vigorous-intensity activity, because the risks of this activity are higher than the risks of moderate-intensity activity.

The choice of appropriate types and amounts of physical activity can be affected by chronic conditions. People with symptoms or known chronic conditions should be under the regular care of a healthcare provider. In consultation with their provider, they can develop a physical activity plan that is appropriate for them. People with chronic conditions typically find that moderate-intensity activity is safe and beneficial. However, they may need to take special precautions. For example, people with diabetes need to pay special attention to blood sugar control and proper footwear during activity.

Women who are pregnant and those who've recently had a baby should be under the regular care of a healthcare provider. Moderate-intensity physical activity is generally safe for women with uncomplicated pregnancies, but women should talk with their provider about how to adjust the amounts and types of activity while they are pregnant and right after the baby's birth.

During pregnancy, women should avoid:

- Doing activities that involve lying on their back after the first trimester of pregnancy; and

- Doing activities with high risk of falling or abdominal trauma, including contact or collision sports, such as horseback riding, soccer, basketball, and downhill skiing.

Chapter 35

Workout Safety

Chapter Contents

Section 35.1

Warming Up

This section contains text excerpted from "Why Warm up,
Cool down, and Stretch?" U.S. Department of Veterans
Affairs (VA), March 16, 2014.

Why Warm Up, Cool Down, and Stretch?

You can help prevent injury and reduce muscle soreness if you
warm up before and cool down after physical activity. Warming-up
prepares your muscles and heart for activity. Cooling-down slows your
heart rate gradually and helps prepare your muscles for the next time
you're active.

Warm-ups take 5 to 15 minutes.

1. Do your planned activity, such as walking, but at a lower intensity (slower pace) for a brief time. This may mean walking slowly for
a few minutes before speeding up.

2. Do a few minutes of gentle stretching if you plan to do something
more vigorous than walking.

Cool-downs take 5 to 15 minutes.

1.   To cool down, continue your activity, but slow down the pace
     for a brief time to slow your heart rate.

2.   Stretch all major muscle groups used during the activity.
     Stretching the muscles while they are warm will help increase
     flexibility.

Stretch:

Stretching is important for a good warm-up and cool-down and is
one of the best ways to prevent and avoid muscle soreness, cramps,
and injury. Here are some helpful tips for proper stretching:

• Do a short warm-up before stretching, such as walking or
  marching in place. Stretching is more beneficial when your muscles are warm.

- Stretch in both directions (i.e., if you stretch to the left, don't forget to stretch to the right).

- Avoid fast, jerky movements. Stretch slowly and smoothly.

- Stretches should not be painful. Gentle stretching is best. When you repeat the stretch, you should be able to stretch a little further without pain.

- Hold each stretch for 15–60 seconds. Do not bounce.

- Repeat each stretch 4 or more times.

- Breathe slowly in and out. Do not hold your breath.

- Relax, enjoy, and feel good about yourself.

- Stretch often, if possible every day.

Section 35.2

Basics of Stretching

This section contains text excerpted from the following sources: Text beginning with the heading "What Is Stretching?" is excerpted from "MOVE! Physical Activity Handout," U.S. Department of Veterans Affairs (VA), March 16, 2014; Text under the heading "Ways to Stretch" is excerpted from "Ways to Stretch," Office on Women's Health (OWH), U.S. Department of Health and Human Services (HHS), March 27, 2015.

What Is Stretching?

Stretching prepares your muscles and heart for activity. Cooling-down slows your heart rate gradually and helps prepare your muscles for the next time you're active.

Ways to Stretch

Stretching can help make you more flexible, so you can do activities more easily. It also lengthens and loosens tight muscles.

Not sure how to stretch? Want to learn a great quad stretch, hamstring stretch, and more? Check out the info below:

Stretching Tips

It's a good idea to stretch any time you work out, but try for at least two or three days each week. To stretch well, try these tips:

- **Warm up before you stretch.** Stretching is more helpful when your muscles are warmed up. You can do some light exercises like walking or jogging in place for five to 10 minutes to warm up.

- **Stretch for around 10 minutes.** You can stretch right after you warm up or at the end of your workout—or do both!

- **Go easy on yourself.** You will feel a gentle pull, but if it hurts, stop. And don't forget to breathe.

- **Don't bounce.** A stretch works well if you just hold it. If you are just starting out, try holding a stretch for around 15 seconds. If you are more flexible, you can hold it for a minute.

- **Make sure to repeat each stretch on both sides.** Do each stretch two to four times on each side.

Stretches to Try

Here are some stretches you can practice:

1. Cross Shoulder Stretch

Sit or stand up straight. Keep shoulders even. Extend right arm across chest. Place left hand on the right elbow to gently support your arm. Feel the stretch in your right arm and shoulder. Breathe in through your nose, and breathe out through your mouth. Hold stretch for a count of 15. Repeat this stretch on opposite side, using right hand to stretch left arm and shoulder.

2. Triceps Stretch

Stand up straight, with knees slightly bent, toes facing forward. Place feet hip distance apart. Keep shoulders even. Bend right arm at elbow, with elbow pointing to the sky. Lift arm next to your head. Position right fingers so they touch the shoulder blade area. Place left arm across top of head, and place left hand on the right elbow to gently support the arm during this stretch. You should feel a stretch in the back of your right arm. Breathe in through your nose, and breathe out through your mouth. Hold stretch for a count of 15. Repeat this stretch on the opposite side, using right hand to stretch left triceps.

3. Chest Stretch

Stand up straight, with knees slightly bent, toes facing forward. Place feet hip distance apart. Keep shoulders even. Place arms behind your back. Clasp your hands together, lifting your arms behind your back. Squeeze your shoulder blades together. Feel the stretch in your chest. Breathe in through your nose, and breathe out through your mouth. Hold stretch for count of 15.

4. Quadriceps Stretch

You're going to be standing on one leg, so you may want help staying steady. If so, stand facing a wall or other surface, about 1 foot away from it. Put your right hand against the wall. Raise your left leg behind you and gently grab your foot with your left hand. Relax your left foot in your hand. Press your right hip forward to stretch the muscles in the front of your left thigh. Keep your knees close together. Hold stretch for a count of 15. Repeat the stretch with your right leg.

5. Hamstring Stretch

Lie with your back flat on the floor, with both of your knees bent. Place your feet flat on the floor, about 6 inches apart. Straighten your right knee and put both hands behind your right knee. Slowly lift your right leg, feeling a slight stretching in the back of your thigh. Keep your head relaxed on the floor. If you cannot relax your head on the floor, place a towel around your calf or ankle, holding one side of the towel in each hand. Hold stretch for a count of 15. Repeat the stretch with your left leg.

6. Runner's Stretch

Squat down and put both hands on the floor in front of you. Stretch your right leg straight out behind you and relax your knee on the ground. Keep your left foot flat on the floor and lean forward with your chest on your left knee. Move your weight back to your right leg, keeping it as straight as you can. Do not move your left knee farther forward than your left ankle. Hold stretch for a count of 15. Repeat the stretch with your left leg.

7.Calf Stretch

Stand facing a wall or other surface, about 2 feet away from it, keeping your heels flat and your back straight. Lean forward and press your hands against the wall. Take one step forward with your left leg and bend the knee slightly. Keep your right leg straight and your heel on the ground. Stand up tall with shoulders over hips. Make sure your knee does not move in front of your ankle. You should feel stretching in the muscles in the back of your lower right leg, above your heel. If you need a bigger stretch, move your back farther away from the wall. Hold stretch for a count of 15. Repeat the stretch with your left leg.

Section 35.3

Avoiding Mistakes in the Gym

This section includes text excerpted from "American Council on Exercise (ACE's) Top Ten Mistakes People Make in the Gym," Brookhaven National Laboratory (BNL), U.S. Department of Energy (DOE), August 2, 2004. Reviewed September 2016.

Finding or making time to exercise is the first step toward improving your health, but it's not the only step. Workouts can be challenging and mistakes in the gym are common. At times, these mistakes can cause mild strains or more significant injuries. By changing small parts of your routine, you'll begin to see incredible results.

1. **The all-or-nothing approach.** Not having a full hour to exercise is no reason to skip your workout. Research shows that even 10 minutes of exercise can provide important health benefits

2. **Unbalanced strength-training programs.** Most people tend to focus on certain muscles, such as the abdominals or biceps, because they have a greater impact on appearance or it is where they feel strongest. But to achieve a strong, balanced body, you have to train all the major muscle groups.

3. **Bad form.** The surest way to get injured in a gym is to use bad form. For example, allowing the knee to extend beyond the

toes during a lunge or squat can put undue stress on the knee, and using momentum to lift heavy weights or not exercising through a full range of motion will produce less-than-optimal results.

4. **Not progressing wisely.** Exercising too much, too hard or too often is a common mistake made by many fitness enthusiasts. Rest and gradual progression are important components of a safe and effective exercise program.

5. **Not enough variety.** Too many people find a routine or physical activity they like—and then never change it. Unchanging workouts can lead to boredom, plateaus and, worse case, can lead to injury or burnout.

6. **Not adjusting machines to one's body size.** Most exercise equipment is designed to accommodate a wide range of body types and sizes. But it's up to you to adjust each machine to your body's unique needs. Using improperly adjusted machines will lead to less-than-optimal results and increase your risk of injury.

7. **Focusing on anything but your workout.** The importance of being "mindful" of the task at hand cannot be overstated. Reading or watching TV can adversely affect the quality of your workout because the distraction can literally slow you down.

8. **Not properly cooling down after your workout.** Too many p wrap up their workouts and head straight to the showers. Instead, take a few minutes to lower your heart rate and stretch your muscles. This not only improves flexibility, but also helps prepare the body for your next workout.

9. **Poor gym etiquette.** This can range from simply being rude—lingering on machines long after you are done or chatting loudly on your cell phone—to poor hygiene and not wiping your sweat from machines once you're finished. Always be considerate of other exercisers.

10. **Not setting realistic goals.** Unrealistic and vaguely stated goals are among the leading causes of exercise dropout. The key is to establish a training goal that is specific and appropriate for your fitness and skill levels—something a bit challenging but not overly difficult.

Section 35.4

Safety Equipment

This section contains text excerpted from the following sources: Text beginning with the heading "Safety Equipment," Office on Women's Health (OWH), U.S. Department of Health and Human Services (HHS), March 27, 2015; Text under the heading "Rules of the Road—Bicycling on the Road" is excerpted from "Bicycle Safety," U.S. Department of Transportation (DOT), January 2013.

From helmets to shoes, the right equipment can help keep you safe when playing sports or being active.

Helmets

Helmets help when there's a risk of falling or getting hit in the head, like in baseball, softball, biking, skiing, horseback riding, skateboarding, and inline skating. Make sure you wear a helmet that is made for the activity you are doing. And make sure you know how it is supposed to fit. In some states, the law says you have to wear a helmet while biking. Bike helmets should come with a special sticker from the U.S. Consumer Product Safety Commission (CPSC).

Special Eye Protection

Special eye protection helps prevent many sports-related eye injuries. Sports that have a high risk of eye injury include basketball, baseball, hockey, and racquet sports. Regular glasses or sunglasses will not keep your eyes safe from injury. If you wear regular glasses, the protective eyewear goes over them. If you wear goggles, they should fit snugly and have cushioning for a comfortable fit. Goggles made from a special material called polycarbonate are extremely strong. Ask your coach or eye doctor what type of eye protection you may need.

Mouth Guards

Mouth guards protect your mouth, teeth, and tongue. They offer protection in soccer, lacrosse, basketball, baseball, cheerleading, and other activities in which you could get hit in the mouth. You can get mouth guards at sport stores or from your dentist.

Pads for Your Wrists, Knees, and Elbows

Pads for your wrists, knees, and elbows can help prevent lots of injuries, including broken bones. They are important for activities such as inline skating, snowboarding, and hockey. In some sports, like soccer, your coach may require shin guards, which are pads to protect your lower leg.

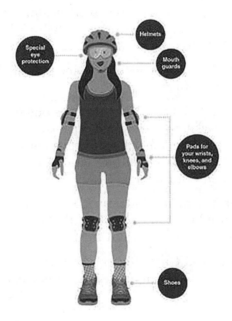

Figure 35.1. *Safety equipment*

Shoes

Shoes need to fit well and be right for your sport. Check with your coach or an athletic shoe salesperson about what shoes to wear. Also ask how often they need to be replaced.

Rules of the Road—Bicycling on the Road

In all States, bicycles on the roadway are considered vehicles, and bicyclists are the drivers, with the same rights and responsibilities as motorists to follow the rules of the road.

When riding, always:

- **Go with the Traffic Flow.** Ride on the right in the same direction as other vehicles. Go with the flow not against it.

- **Obey All Traffic Laws.** A bicycle is a vehicle and you're the driver. When you ride in the street, obey all traffic signs, signals, and lane markings.

- **Yield to Traffic.** Almost always, drivers on a smaller road must yield (wait) for traffic on a major or larger road. If there is no stop sign or traffic signal and you are coming from a smaller roadway (out of a driveway, from a sidewalk, a bike path, etc.), you must slow down and look to see if the way is clear before proceeding. Yield to pedestrians in a crosswalk.

- **Be Predictable.** Ride in a straight line, not in and out of cars. Signal your moves to others.

- **Stay Alert at All Times.** Use your eyes and ears. Watch out for potholes, cracks, wet leaves, storm grates, railroad tracks, or anything that could make you lose control of your bike. Listen for traffic and avoid dangerous situations; don't use personal electronics when you ride.

- **Look Before Turning.** When turning left or right, always look behind you for a break in traffic, and then signal before making the turn. Watch for left- or right-turning traffic.

- **Watch for Parked Cars.** Ride far enough out from the curb to avoid the unexpected from parked cars (like doors opening, or cars pulling out).

Where to Ride Safely

- **Use bike lanes or bike paths, if available.**

- While bicycles are allowed on many roads, riders may feel safer being separated from traffic. A lane or path is a safer choice than riding on a sidewalk.

- Riding on sidewalks puts you in a place where cars do not look for or expect to see moving traffic.

- Sidewalk riding puts you at risk for crashes at driveways and intersections.

- **Children younger than 10 years old are not consistently able to make the decisions necessary to safely ride unsupervised in the street. Therefore, they are safer riding away from traffic.**

- **For anyone riding on a sidewalk:**

- Check the law in your State or jurisdiction to make sure sidewalk riding is allowed.

- Watch for vehicles coming out of or turning into driveways.

- Stop at corners of sidewalks and streets to look for cars and to make sure the drivers see you before crossing.

- Enter a street at a corner and not between parked cars. Alert pedestrians that you are nearby, saying, "Passing on your left," or use a bell or horn.

Chapter 36

Nutrition and Exercise

Chapter Contents

Section 36.1

Healthy Hydration

This section contains text excerpted from the following sources:
Text under the heading "Getting the Basics Right" is excerpted from
"Water and Nutrition," Centers for Disease Control and Prevention
(CDC), June 3, 2014; Text under the heading "Don't Dry out" is
excerpted from "Don't Dry out," NIH News in Health, National
Institutes of Health (NIH), July 2009. Reviewed September 2016.

Getting the Basics Right

Getting enough water every day is important for your health.
Healthy people meet their fluid needs by drinking when thirsty and
drinking with meals. Most of your fluid needs are met through the
water and beverages you drink. However, you can get some fluids
through the foods that you eat. For example, broth soups and foods
with high water content such as celery, tomatoes, or melons can contribute to fluid intake.

Water helps your body:

- Keep your temperature normal

- Lubricate and cushion joints

- Protect your spinal cord and other sensitive tissues

- Get rid of wastes through urination, perspiration, and bowel
  movements

Your body needs more water when you are:

- In hot climates

- More physically active

- Running a fever

- Having diarrhea or vomiting

**If you think you are not getting enough water, these tips
may help:**

- Carry a water bottle for easy access when you are at work of running errands.

- Freeze some freezer safe water bottles. Take one with you for ice-cold water all day long.

- Choose water instead of sugar-sweetened beverages. This can also help with weight management. Substituting water for one 20-ounce sugar sweetened soda will save you about 240 calories. For example, during the school day students should have access to drinking water, giving them a healthy alternative to sugar-sweetened beverages.

- Choose water when eating out. Generally, you will save money and reduce calories.

- Add a wedge of lime or lemon to your water. This can help improve the taste and help you drink more water than you usually do.

Don't Dry Out

You may wonder if you've been drinking enough water, especially when it's hot out. There's a lot of confusing advice out there about how much you really need. The truth is that most healthy bodies are very good at regulating water. Elderly people, young children and some special cases—like people taking certain medications—need to be a little more careful. Here's what you need to know.

"Water is involved in all body processes," says Dr. Jack M. Guralnik of NIH's National Institute on Aging. "You need the proper amount for all those processes to work correctly."

The body regulates how much water it keeps so it can maintain levels of the various minerals it needs to work properly. But every time you breathe out, sweat, urinate or have a bowel movement, you lose some fluid. When you lose fluid, your blood can become more concentrated. Healthy people compensate by releasing stores of water, mostly from muscles. And, of course, you get thirsty. That's your body's way of telling you it needs more water.

At a certain point, however, if you lose enough water, your body can't compensate. Eventually, you can become dehydrated, meaning that your body doesn't have enough fluid to work properly. "Basically, you're drying out," Guralnik says.

Any healthy person can become dehydrated on hot days, when you've been exercising hard or when you have a disease or condition like diarrhea, in which you can lose a lot of fluid very quickly. But dehydration is generally more of a problem in the elderly, who can have a decreased sensitivity to thirst, and very young children who can't yet tell their parents when they're thirsty.

How much water does your body need? Guralnik says you have to consider the circumstances. "If you're active on a hot day, you need more water than if you're sitting in an air-conditioned office," he explains. An average person on an average day needs about 3 quarts of water a day. But if you're out in the hot sun, you'll need a lot more than that.

Signs of dehydration in adults are being thirsty, urinating less often than usual, having dark-colored urine, having dry skin, feeling tired or dizziness and fainting. Signs of dehydration in babies and young children include a dry mouth and tongue, crying without tears, no wet diapers for 3 hours or more, a high fever and being unusually sleepy or drowsy.

If you suspect dehydration, drink small amounts of water over a period of time. Taking too much all at once can overload your stomach and make you throw up. For people exercising in the heat and losing a lot of minerals in sweat, sports drinks can be helpful. But avoid any drinks that have caffeine.

Remember: The best way to deal with dehydration is to prevent it. Make sure to drink enough water in situations where you might become dehydrated. For those caring for small children or older people with conditions that can lead to dehydration, Guralnik advises, "You need to prompt the person to drink fluids and remind them often. It's not just a one-time problem."

Section 36.2

Sports Nutrition

Eat Extra for Excellence

There's a lot more to eating for sports than chowing down on carbs or chugging sports drinks. The good news is that eating to reach your peak performance level likely doesn't require a special diet or supplements. It's all about working the right foods into your fitness plan in the right amounts.

Teen athletes have unique nutrition needs. Because athletes work out more than their less-active peers, they generally need extra calories to fuel both their sports performance and their growth. Depending on how active they are, teen athletes may need anywhere from 2,000 to 5,000 total calories per day to meet their energy needs.

So what happens if teen athletes don't eat enough? Their bodies are less likely to achieve peak performance and may even break down rather than build up muscles. Athletes who don't take in enough calories every day won't be as fast and as strong as they could be and may not be able to maintain their weight. And extreme calorie restriction can lead to growth problems and other serious health risks for both girls and guys, including increased risk for fractures and other injuries.

Athletes and Dieting

Since teen athletes need extra fuel, it's usually a bad idea to diet. Athletes in sports where weight is emphasized—such as wrestling, swimming, dance, or gymnastic—might feel pressure to lose weight, but they need to balance that choice with the possible negative side effects mentioned above.

If a coach, gym teacher, or teammate says that you need to go on a diet, talk to your doctor first or visit a dietitian who specializes in teen athletes. If a health professional you trust agrees that it's safe to diet, then he or she can work with you to develop a plan that allows you get the proper amount of nutrients, and perform your best while also losing weight.

Eat a Variety of Foods

You may have heard about "carb loading" before a game. But when it comes to powering your game for the long haul, it's a bad idea to focus on only one type of food.

Carbohydrates are an important source of fuel, but they're only one of many foods an athlete needs. It also takes vitamins, minerals, protein, and fats to stay in peak playing shape.

Muscular Minerals and Vital Vitamins

Calcium helps build the strong bones that athletes depend on, and iron carries oxygen to muscles. Most teens don't get enough of these minerals, and that's especially true of teen athletes because their needs may be even higher than those of other teens.

To get the iron you need, eat lean (not much fat) meat, fish, and poultry; green, leafy vegetables; and iron-fortified cereals. Calcium—a must for protecting against stress fractures—is found in dairy foods, such as low-fat milk, yogurt, and cheese.

In addition to calcium and iron, you need a whole bunch of other vitamins and minerals that do everything from help you access energy to keep you from getting sick. Eating a balanced diet, including lots of different fruits and veggies, should provide the vitamins and minerals needed for good health and sports performance.

Protein Power

Athletes may need more protein than less-active teens, but most teen athletes get plenty of protein through regular eating. It's a myth that athletes need a huge daily intake of protein to build large, strong muscles. Muscle growth comes from regular training and hard work. And taking in too much protein can actually harm the body, causing dehydration, calcium loss, and even kidney problems.

Good sources of protein are fish, lean meats and poultry, eggs, dairy, nuts, soy, and peanut butter.

Carb Charge

Carbohydrates provide athletes with an excellent source of fuel. Cutting back on carbs or following low-carb diets isn't a good idea for athletes because restricting carbohydrates can cause a person to feel tired and worn out, which ultimately affects performance.

Good sources of carbohydrates include fruits, vegetables, and grains. Choose whole grains (such as brown rice, oatmeal, whole-wheat bread) more often than their more processed counterparts like white rice and white bread. That's because whole grains provide both the energy athletes need to perform and the fiber and other nutrients they need to be healthy.

Sugary carbs such as candy bars or sodas are less healthy for athletes because they don't contain any of the other nutrients you need. In addition, eating candy bars or other sugary snacks just before practice or competition can give athletes a quick burst of energy and then leave them to "crash" or run out of energy before they've finished working out.

Fat Fuel

Everyone needs a certain amount of fat each day, and this is particularly true for athletes. That's because active muscles quickly burn through carbs and need fats for long-lasting energy. Like carbs, not all fats are created equal. Experts advise athletes to concentrate on eating healthier fats, such as the unsaturated fat found in most vegetable oils, some fish, and nuts and seeds. Try to not to eat too much trans fat–like partially hydrogenated oils–and saturated fat, that is found in high fat meat and high fat dairy products, like butter.

Choosing when to eat fats is also important for athletes. Fatty foods can slow digestion, so it's a good idea to avoid eating these foods for a few hours before and after exercising.

Shun Supplements

Protein and energy bars don't do a whole lot of good, but they won't really do you much harm either. Energy drinks have lots of caffeine, though, so no one should drink them before exercising.

Other types of supplements can really do some damage.

Anabolic steroids can seriously mess with a person's hormones, causing side effects like testicular shrinkage and baldness in guys and facial hair growth in girls. Steroids can cause mental health problems, including depression and serious mood swings.

Some supplements contain hormones that are related to testosterone (such as dehydroepiandrosterone, or DHEA for short). These supplements can have similar side effects to anabolic steroids. Other sports supplements (like creatine, for example) have not been tested in people younger than 18. So the risks of taking them are not yet known.

Salt tablets are another supplement to watch out for. People take them to avoid dehydration, but salt tablets can actually lead to dehydration. In large amounts, salt can cause nausea, vomiting, cramps, and diarrhea and may damage the lining of the stomach. In general, you are better off drinking fluids in order to maintain hydration. Any salt you lose in sweat can usually be made up with sports drinks or food eaten after exercise.

Ditch Dehydration

Speaking of dehydration, **water** is just as important to unlocking your game power as food. When you sweat during exercise, it's easy to become overheated, headachy, and worn out—especially in hot or humid weather. Even mild dehydration can affect an athlete's physical and mental performance.

There's no one-size-fits-all formula for how much water to drink. How much fluid each person needs depends on the individual's age, size, level of physical activity, and environmental temperature.

Experts recommend that athletes drink before and after exercise as well as every 15 to 20 minutes during exercise. Don't wait until you feel thirsty, because thirst is a sign that your body has needed liquids for a while. But don't force yourself to drink more fluids than you may need either. It's hard to run when there's a lot of water sloshing around in your stomach!

If you like the taste of sports drinks better than regular water, then it's OK to drink them. But it's important to know that a sports drink is really no better for you than water unless you are exercising for more than 60 to 90 minutes or in really hot weather. The additional carbohydrates and electrolytes may improve performance in these conditions, but otherwise your body will do just as well with water.

Avoid drinking carbonated drinks or juice because they could give you a stomachache while you're competing.

Never drink energy drinks before exercising. Energy drinks contain a large amount of caffeine and other ingredients that have caffeine-like effects.

Caffeine

Caffeine is a diuretic. That means it causes a person to urinate (pee) more. It's not clear whether this causes dehydration or not, but to be safe, it's wise to stay away from too much caffeine. That's especially true if you'll be exercising in hot weather.

When it comes to caffeine and exercise, it's good to weigh any benefits against potential problems. Although some studies find that caffeine may help adults perform better in endurance sports, other studies show too much caffeine may hurt.

Caffeine increases heart rate and blood pressure. Too much caffeine can leave an athlete feeling anxious or jittery. Caffeine can also cause trouble sleeping. All of these can drag down a person's sports performance. Plus, taking certain medications—including supplements—can make caffeine's side effects seem even worse.

Never drink energy drinks before exercising. These products contain a large amount of caffeine and other ingredients that have caffeine-like effects.

Game-Day Eats

Your performance on game day will depend on the foods you've eaten over the past several days and weeks. But you can boost your performance even more by paying attention to the food you eat on game day. Strive for a game-day diet rich in carbohydrates, moderate in protein, and low in fat.

Here are some guidelines on what to eat and when:

- **Eat a meal 2 to 4 hours before the game or event:** Choose a protein and carbohydrate meal (like a turkey or chicken sandwich, cereal and milk, chicken noodle soup and yogurt, or pasta with tomato sauce).

- **Eat a snack less than 2 hours before the game:** If you haven't had time to have a pre-game meal, be sure to have a light snack such as low-fiber fruits or vegetables (like plums, melons, cherries, carrots), crackers, a bagel, or low-fat yogurt.

Consider not eating anything for the hour before you compete or have practice because digestion requires energy—energy that you want to use to win. Also, eating too soon before any kind of activity can leave food in the stomach, making you feel full, bloated, crampy, and sick.

Everyone is different, so get to know what works best for you. You may want to experiment with meal timing and how much to eat on practice days so that you're better prepared for game day.

Section 36.3

Using Dietary Supplements Wisely

This section includes text excerpted from "Dietary
Supplements: What You Need to Know," U.S. Food and
Drug Administration (FDA), January 6, 2016.

Dietary Supplements can be beneficial to your health — but taking supplements can also involve health risks. The U.S. Food and Drug Administration (FDA) does not have the authority to review dietary supplement products for safety and effectiveness before they are marketed.

Dietary Supplements:

You've heard about them, may have used them, and may have even recommended them to friends or family. While some dietary supplements are well understood and established, others need further study. Read on for important information for you and your family about dietary supplements.

Before making decisions about whether to take a supplement, talk to your healthcare provider. They can help you achieve a balance between the foods and nutrients you personally need.

What Are Dietary Supplements?

Dietary supplements include such ingredients as vitamins, minerals, herbs, amino acids, and enzymes. Dietary supplements are marketed in forms such as tablets, capsules, softgels, gelcaps, powders, and liquids.

What Are the Benefits of Dietary Supplements?

Some supplements can help assure that you get enough of the vital substances the body needs to function; others may help reduce the risk of disease. But supplements should not replace complete meals which are necessary for a healthful diet – so, be sure you eat a variety of foods as well.

Unlike drugs, supplements are not intended to treat, diagnose, prevent, or cure diseases. That means supplements should not make claims, such as "reduces pain" or "treats heart disease." Claims like these can only legitimately be made for drugs, not dietary supplements.

Are There Any Risks in Taking Supplements?

Yes. Many supplements contain active ingredients that have strong biological effects in the body. This could make them unsafe in some situations and hurt or complicate your health. For example, the following actions could lead to harmful – even life-threatening – consequences.

- Combining supplements
- Using supplements with medicines (whether prescription or over-the-counter)
- Substituting supplements for prescription medicines
- Taking too much of some supplements, such as vitamin A, vitamin D, or iron

Some supplements can also have unwanted effects before, during, and after surgery. So, be sure to inform your healthcare provider, including your pharmacist about any supplements you are taking.

Some Common Dietary Supplements

- Calcium
- Echinacea
- Fish Oil
- Ginseng
- Glucosamine and/or
- Chondroitin Sulphate
- Garlic
- Vitamin D
- St. John's Wort
- Saw Palmetto
- Ginkgo
- Green Tea

Note: These examples do not represent either an endorsement or approval by FDA.

How Can I Find out More about the Dietary Supplement I'm Taking?

Dietary supplement labels must include name and location information for the manufacturer or distributor.

If you want to know more about the product that you are taking, check with the manufacturer or distributor about:

- Information to support the claims of the product

- Information on the safety and effectiveness of the ingredients in the product.

How Can I Be a Smart Supplement Shopper?

Be a savvy supplement user. Here's how:

- When searching for supplements on the internet, use noncommercial sites (e.g, NIH, FDA, USDA) rather than doing blind searches.

- Watch out for false statements like "works better than [a prescription drug]," "totally safe," or has "no side effects."

- Be aware that the term natural doesn't always means safe.

- Ask your healthcare provider for help in distinguishing between reliable and questionable information.

- Always remember – safety first!

Report Problems to FDA

Notify FDA if the use of a dietary supplement caused you or a family member to have a serious reaction or illness (even if you are not certain that the product was the cause or you did not visit a doctor or clinic).

Follow these steps:

- Stop using the product.

- Contact your healthcare provider to find out how to take care of the problem.

- Report problems to FDA in either of these ways:

  - Contact the Consumer Complaint Coordinator in your area.

  - File a safety report online through the Safety Reporting Portal.

Section 36.4

Anabolic Steroids

This section includes text excerpted from "DrugFacts: Anabolic Steroids," National Institute on Drug Abuse (NIDA), March 2016.

What Are Anabolic Steroids?

Anabolic steroids are synthetic variations of the male sex hormone testosterone. The proper term for these compounds is anabolic-androgenic steroids. "Anabolic" refers to muscle building, and "androgenic" refers to increased male sex characteristics. Some common names for anabolic steroids are Gear, Juice, Roids, and Stackers.

Healthcare providers can prescribe steroids to treat hormonal issues, such as delayed puberty. Steroids can also treat diseases that cause muscle loss, such as cancer and AIDS. But some athletes and bodybuilders abuse these drugs to boost performance or improve their physical appearance.

How Do People Abuse Anabolic Steroids?

People who abuse anabolic steroids usually take them orally or inject them into the muscles. These doses may be 10 to 100 times higher than doses prescribed to treat medical conditions. Steroids are also applied to the skin as a cream, gel, or patch.

Some athletes and others who abuse steroids believe that they can avoid unwanted side effects or maximize the drugs' effects by taking them in ways that include:

- cycling—taking doses for a period of time, stopping for a time, and then restarting

- stacking—combining two or more different types of steroids

- pyramiding—slowly increasing the dose or frequency of abuse, reaching a peak amount, and then gradually tapering off

There is no scientific evidence that any of these practices reduce the harmful medical consequences of these drugs.

How Do Anabolic Steroids Affect the Brain?

Anabolic steroids work differently from other drugs of abuse; they do not have the same short-term effects on the brain. The most important difference is that steroids do not trigger rapid increases in the brain chemical dopamine, which causes the "high" that drives people to abuse other substances. However, long-term steroid abuse can act on some of the same brain pathways and chemicals—including dopamine, serotonin, and opioid systems—that are affected by other drugs. This may result in a significant effect on mood and behavior.

Short-Term Effects

Abuse of anabolic steroids may lead to mental problems, such as:

- paranoid (extreme, unreasonable) jealousy

- extreme irritability

- delusions—false beliefs or ideas

- impaired judgment

Extreme mood swings can also occur, including "roid rage"—angry feelings and behavior that may lead to violence.

What Are the Other Health Effects of Anabolic Steroids?

Aside from mental problems, steroid use commonly causes severe acne. It also causes the body to swell, especially in the hands and feet.

Long-Term Effects

Anabolic steroid abuse may lead to serious, even permanent, health problems such as:

- kidney problems or failure

- liver damage

- enlarged heart, high blood pressure, and changes in blood cholesterol, all of which increase the risk of stroke and heart attack, even in young people

Several other effects are gender- and age-specific:

In men:

- shrinking testicles

- decreased sperm count

- baldness
- development of breasts
- increased risk for prostate cancer

In women:

- growth of facial hair or excess body hair
- male-pattern baldness
- changes in or stop in the
- menstrual cycle
- enlarged clitoris
- deepened voice

In teens:

- stunted growth (when high hormone levels from steroids signal to the body to stop bone growth too early)
- stunted height (if teens use steroids before their growth spurt)
- Some of these physical changes, such as shrinking sex organs in men, can add to mental side effects such as mood disorders.

Are Anabolic Steroids Addictive?

Even though anabolic steroids do not cause the same high as other drugs, they can lead to addiction. Studies have shown that animals will self-administer steroids when they have the chance, just as they do with other addictive drugs. People may continue to abuse steroids despite physical problems, high costs to buy the drugs, and negative effects on their relationships. These behaviors reflect steroids' addictive potential. Research has further found that some steroid users turn to other drugs, such as opioids, to reduce sleep problems and irritability caused by steroids.

People who abuse steroids may experience withdrawal symptoms when they stop use, including:

- mood swings
- fatigue
- restlessness
- loss of appetite

- sleep problems

- decreased sex drive

- steroid cravings

One of the more serious withdrawal symptoms is depression, which can sometimes lead to suicide attempts.

How Can People Get Treatment for Anabolic Steroid Addiction?

Some people seeking treatment for anabolic steroid addiction have found behavioral therapy to be helpful. More research is needed to identify the most effective treatment options.

In certain cases of severe addiction, patients have taken medicines to help treat symptoms of withdrawal. For example, healthcare providers have prescribed anti-depressants to treat depression and pain medicines for headaches and muscle and joint pain. Other medicines have been used to help restore the patient's hormonal system.

Points to Remember

- Anabolic steroids are synthetic variations of the male sex hormone testosterone.

- Healthcare providers can prescribe steroids to treat various medical conditions. But some athletes and bodybuilders abuse these drugs to boost performance or improve their physical appearance.

- People who abuse anabolic steroids usually take them orally or inject them into the muscles. They are also applied to the skin as a cream, gel, or patch.

- Some athletes and other people abuse steroids by cycling, stacking, and pyramiding them.

- Abuse of anabolic steroids may lead to short-term effects such as mental problems. Extreme mood swings can also occur, including "roid rage"—angry feelings and behavior that may lead to violence.

- Continued steroid abuse can act on some of the same brain pathways and chemicals—including dopamine, serotonin, and opioid systems—that are affected by other drugs.

- Anabolic steroid abuse may lead to serious long-term, even permanent, health problems. Several other effects are gender- and age-specific.

- People who inject steroids increase their risk of contracting or transmitting HIV/AIDS or hepatitis.

- Even though anabolic steroids do not cause the same high as other drugs, they can lead to addiction.

- Some people seeking treatment for anabolic steroid addiction have found behavioral therapy to be helpful. In certain cases of severe addiction, patients have received medicines to help treat symptoms of withdrawal.

Chapter 37

Preventing Sports Injuries

Chapter Contents

Section 37.1

Understanding Sports Injuries

This section includes text excerpted from "Handout on Health: Sports Injuries," National Institute of Arthritis and Musculoskeletal and Skin Diseases (NIAMS), February 2016.

In recent years, increasing numbers of people of all ages have been heeding their health professionals' advice to get active for all of the health benefits exercise has to offer. But for some people—particularly those who overdo or who don't properly train or warm up—these benefits can come at a price: **sports injuries**.

What Are Sports Injuries?

The term "sports injury," in the broadest sense, refers to the kinds of injuries that most commonly occur during sports or exercise. Some sports injuries result from accidents; others are due to poor training practices, improper equipment, lack of conditioning, or insufficient warm-up and stretching.

Following are some of the most common sports injuries.

- Muscle sprains and strains

- Tears of the ligaments that hold joints together

- Tears of the tendons that support joints and allow them to move

- Dislocated joints

- Fractured bones, including vertebrae.

Sprains and Strains

A *sprain* is a stretch or tear of a ligament, the band of connective tissues that joins the end of one bone with another. Sprains are caused by trauma such as a fall or blow to the body that knocks a joint out of position and, in the worst case, ruptures the supporting ligaments. Sprains can range from first degree (minimally stretched ligament) to third degree (a complete tear). Areas of the body most vulnerable to sprains are ankles, knees, and wrists. Signs of a sprain include varying degrees of tenderness or pain; bruising; inflammation; swelling; inability to move a limb or joint; or joint looseness, laxity, or instability.

A *strain* is a twist, pull, or tear of a muscle or tendon, a cord of tissue connecting muscle to bone. It is an acute, noncontact injury that results from overstretching or overcontraction. Symptoms of a strain include pain, muscle spasm, and loss of strength. Although it's hard to tell the difference between mild and moderate strains, severe strains not treated professionally can cause damage and loss of function.

Knee Injuries

Because of its complex structure and weight-bearing capacity, the knee is a commonly injured joint.

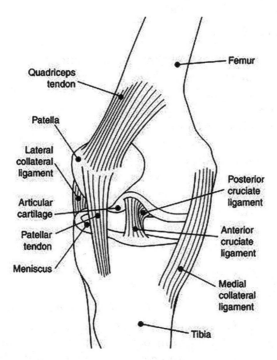

Figure 37.1. *Lateral View of the Knee*

Knee injuries can range from mild to severe. Some of the less severe, yet still painful and functionally limiting, knee problems are runner's knee (pain or tenderness close to or under the knee cap at the front or side of the knee), iliotibial band syndrome (pain on the outer side of the knee), and tendinitis, also called tendinosis (marked by degeneration within a tendon, usually where it joins the bone).

More severe injuries include bone bruises or damage to the cartilage or ligaments. There are two types of cartilage in the knee. One is the meniscus, a crescent-shaped disc that absorbs shock between the thigh (femur) and lower leg bones (tibia and fibula). The other is a surface-coating (or articular) cartilage. It covers the ends of the bones where they meet, allowing them to glide against one another. The four major ligaments that support the knee are the anterior cruciate ligament (ACL), the posterior cruciate ligament (PCL), the medial collateral ligament (MCL), and the lateral collateral ligament (LCL).

Knee injuries can result from a blow to or twist of the knee; from improper landing after a jump; or from running too hard, too much, or without proper warm-up.

Compartment Syndrome

In many parts of the body, muscles (along with the nerves and blood vessels that run alongside and through them) are enclosed in a "compartment" formed of a tough membrane called fascia. When muscles become swollen, they can fill the compartment to capacity, causing interference with nerves and blood vessels as well as damage to the muscles themselves. The resulting painful condition is referred to as compartment syndrome.

Compartment syndrome may be caused by a one-time traumatic injury (acute compartment syndrome), such as a fractured bone or a hard blow to the thigh, by repeated hard blows (depending upon the sport), or by ongoing overuse (chronic exertional compartment syndrome), which may occur, for example, in long-distance running.

Shin Splints

Although the term "shin splints" has been widely used to describe any sort of leg pain associated with exercise, the term actually refers to pain along the tibia or shin bone, the large bone in the front of the lower leg. This pain can occur at the front outside part of the lower leg, including the foot and ankle (anterior shin splints) or at the inner edge of the bone where it meets the calf muscles (medial shin splints).

Shin splints are primarily seen in runners, particularly those just starting a running program. Risk factors for shin splints include overuse or incorrect use of the lower leg; improper stretching, warm-up, or exercise technique; overtraining; running or jumping on hard surfaces; and running in shoes that don't have enough support. These injuries are often associated with flat (overpronated) feet.

Achilles Tendon Injuries

An Achilles tendon injury results from a stretch, tear, or irritation to the tendon connecting the calf muscle to the back of the heel. These injuries can be so sudden and agonizing that they have been known to bring down charging professional football players in shocking fashion.

The most common cause of Achilles tendon tears is a problem called tendinitis, a degenerative condition caused by aging or overuse. When a tendon is weakened, trauma can cause it to rupture.

Achilles tendon injuries are common in middle-aged "weekend warriors" who may not exercise regularly or take time to stretch properly before an activity. Among professional athletes, most Achilles injuries seem to occur in quick-acceleration, jumping sports like football and basketball, and almost always end the season's competition for the athlete.

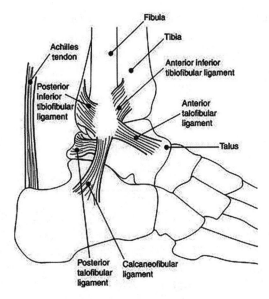

Figure 37.2. *Lateral View of the Ankle*

Fractures

A fracture is a break in the bone that can occur from either a quick, one-time injury to the bone (acute fracture) or from repeated stress to the bone over time (stress fracture).

Acute fractures: Acute fractures can be simple (a clean break with little damage to the surrounding tissue) or compound (a break

351

in which the bone pierces the skin with little damage to the surrounding tissue). Most acute fractures are emergencies. One that breaks the skin is especially dangerous because there is a high risk of infection.

Stress fractures: Stress fractures occur largely in the feet and legs and are common in sports that require repetitive impact, primarily running/jumping sports such as gymnastics or track and field. Running creates forces two to three times a person's body weight on the lower limbs.

The most common symptom of a stress fracture is pain at the site that worsens with weight-bearing activity. Tenderness and swelling often accompany the pain.

Dislocations

When the two bones that come together to form a joint become separated, the joint is described as being dislocated. Contact sports such as football and basketball, as well as high-impact sports and sports that can result in excessive stretching or falling, cause the majority of dislocations. A dislocated joint is an emergency situation that requires medical treatment.

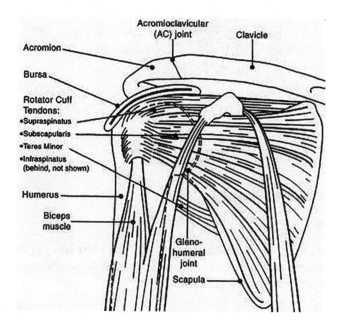

Figure 37.3. *The Shoulder Joint*

The joints most likely to be dislocated are some of the hand joints. Aside from these joints, the joint most frequently dislocated is the shoulder. Dislocations of the knees, hips, and elbows are uncommon.

What Should I Do If I Suffer an Injury?

Whether an injury is acute or chronic, there is never a good reason to try to "work through" the pain of an injury. When you have pain from a particular movement or activity, STOP! Continuing the activity only causes further harm.

Some injuries require prompt medical attention, while others can be self-treated. Here's what you need to know about both types:

When to Seek Medical Treatment

You should call a health professional if:

- The injury causes severe pain, swelling, or numbness.

- You can't tolerate any weight on the area.

- The pain or dull ache of an old injury is accompanied by increased swelling or joint abnormality or instability.

When and How to Treat at Home

If you don't have any of the above symptoms, it's probably safe to treat the injury at home—at least at first. If pain or other symptoms worsen, it's best to check with your healthcare provider. Use the RICE method to relieve pain and inflammation and speed healing. Follow these four steps immediately after injury and continue for at least 48 hours.

- *Rest.* Reduce regular exercise or activities of daily living as needed. If you cannot put weight on an ankle or knee, crutches may help. If you use a cane or one crutch for an ankle injury, use it on the uninjured side to help you lean away and relieve weight on the injured ankle.

- *Ice.* Apply an ice pack to the injured area for 20 minutes at a time, four to eight times a day. A cold pack, ice bag, or plastic bag filled with crushed ice and wrapped in a towel can be used. To avoid cold injury and frostbite, do not apply the ice for more than 20 minutes. (Note: Do not use heat immediately after an injury. This tends to increase internal bleeding or swelling.

Heat can be used later on to relieve muscle tension and promote relaxation.)

- *Compression.* Compression of the injured area may help reduce swelling. Compression can be achieved with elastic wraps, special boots, air casts, and splints. Ask your healthcare provider for advice on which one to use.

- *Elevation.* If possible, keep the injured ankle, knee, elbow, or wrist elevated on a pillow, above the level of the heart, to help decrease swelling.

Who Should I See for My Injury?

Although severe injuries will need to be seen immediately in an emergency room, particularly if they occur on the weekend or after office hours, most musculoskeletal sports injuries can be evaluated and, in many cases, treated by your primary healthcare provider.

Depending on your preference and the severity of your injury or the likelihood that your injury may cause ongoing, long-term problems, you may want to see, or have your primary healthcare professional refer you to, one of the following:

- An **orthopaedic surgeon** is a doctor specializing in the diagnosis and treatment of the musculoskeletal system, which includes bones, joints, ligaments, tendons, muscles, and nerves.

- A **physical therapist/physiotherapist** is a healthcare professional who can develop a rehabilitation program. Your primary care physician may refer you to a physical therapist after you begin to recover from your injury to help strengthen muscles and joints and prevent further injury.

Section 37.2

Common Sports Injuries and Their Prevention

This section includes text excerpted from "Fast Facts about Sports Injuries," National Institute of Arthritis and Musculoskeletal and Skin Diseases (NIAMS), November 2014.

List of Common Sports Injuries

"Sports injuries" are injuries that happen when playing sports or exercising. Some are from accidents. Others can result from poor training practices or improper gear. Some people get injured when they are not in proper condition. Not warming up or stretching enough before you play or exercise can also lead to injuries. The most common sports injuries are:

- Sprains and strains
- Knee injuries
- Swollen muscles
- Achilles tendon injuries
- Pain along the shin bone
- Fractures
- Dislocations

What Can People Do to Prevent Sports Injuries?

These tips can help you avoid sports injuries.

- Don't bend your knees more than half way when doing knee bends.
- Don't twist your knees when you stretch. Keep your feet as flat as you can.
- When jumping, land with your knees bent.
- Do warm up exercises before you play any sport.
- Always stretch before you play or exercise.
- Don't overdo it.
- Cool down after hard sports or workouts.

- Wear shoes that fit properly, are stable, and absorb shock.
- Use the softest exercise surface you can find; don't run on asphalt or concrete.
- Run on flat surfaces.

For adults:

- Don't be a "weekend warrior." Don't try to do a week's worth of activity in a day or two.
- Learn to do your sport right. Use proper form to reduce your risk of "overuse" injuries.
- Use safety gear.
- Know your body's limits.
- Build up your exercise level gradually.
- Strive for a total body workout of cardiovascular, strength-training, and flexibility exercises.

For parents and coaches:

- Group children by their skill level and body size, not by their age, especially for contact sports.
- Match the child to the sport. Don't push the child too hard to play a sport that she or he may not like or be able to do.
- Try to find sports programs that have certified athletic trainers.
- See that all children get a physical exam before playing.
- Don't play a child who is injured.
- Get the child to a doctor, if needed.
- Provide a safe environment for sports.

For children:

- Be in proper condition to play the sport.
- Get a physical exam before you start playing sports.
- Follow the rules of the game.
- Wear gear that protects, fits well, and is right for the sport.
- Know how to use athletic gear.

- Don't play when you are very tired or in pain.

- Always warm up before you play.

- Always cool down after you play.

Section 37.3

Sports-Related Concussions: What Youngsters Need to Know

This section contains text excerpted from the following sources: Text beginning with the heading "What Is a Concussion?" is excerpted from "Concussion Information Sheet," Centers for Disease Control and Prevention (CDC), May 3, 2016; Text under the heading "What Should I Do If I Think I Have a Concussion?" is excerpted from "Fact Sheet for Athletes," Centers for Disease Control and Prevention (CDC), December 27, 2015; Text under the heading "Concussion Treatment" is excerpted from "Mild Traumatic Brain Injury-Concussion," U.S. Department of Veterans Affairs (VA), October 2010. Reviewed September 2016.

What Is a Concussion?

A concussion is a type of traumatic brain injury—or TBI—caused by a bump, blow, or jolt to the head or by a hit to the body that causes the head and brain to move quickly back and forth. This fast movement can cause the brain to bounce around or twist in the skull, creating chemical changes in the brain and sometimes stretching and damaging the brain cells.

What Should I Do If I Think I Have a Concussion?

Report It

Tell your coach and parent if you think you or one of your teammates may have a concussion. You won't play your best if you are not feeling well, and playing with a concussion is dangerous. Encourage your teammates to also report their symptoms.

Get Checked out by a Doctor

If you think you have a concussion, do not return to play on the day of the injury. Only a doctor or other healthcare provider can tell if you have a concussion and when it's OK to return to school and play.

Give Your Brain Time to Heal

Most athletes with a concussion get better within a couple of weeks. For some, a concussion can make everyday activities, such as going to school, harder. You may need extra help getting back to your normal activities. Be sure to update your parents and doctor about how you are feeling.

How Can I Tell If I Have a Concussion?

You may have a concussion if you have any of these symptoms after a bump, blow, or jolt to the head or body:

- Get a headache
- Feel dizzy, sluggish, or foggy
- Are bothered by light or noise
- Have double or blurry vision
- Vomit or feel sick to your stomach
- Have trouble focusing or problems remembering
- Feel more emotional or "down"
- Feel confused
- Have problems with sleep

A concussion feels different to each person, so it's important to tell your parents and doctor how you feel. You might notice concussion symptoms right away, but sometimes it takes hours or days until you notice that something isn't right.

How Can I Help My Team?

Protect Your Brain

All your teammates should avoid hits to the head and follow the rules for safe play to lower chances of getting a concussion.

Be a Team Player

If one of your teammates has a concussion, tell them that they're an important part of the team, and they should take the time they need to get better.

Concussion Treatment

- Moderate to severe TBI are medical conditions that require specialty care from providers such as neurologists, physiatrists, and rehabilitative therapy services.

- Currently there are neither biomarkers nor objective tests to routinely diagnose concussion. A good, thorough patient history and physical examination are essential.

- TBI is often treated in a multidisciplinary fashion through clinical care practice; patient care coordination; provider, patient and family education; and emerging medical technologies that enhance TBI care.

- Care strategies are based on the severity of brain injury. More severe brain injuries may require comprehensive, multidisciplinary approaches to care. Physical therapy, occupational therapy and speech language therapy are all examples of the type of services that may need to be included

- in a rehabilitative care program.

- Clinical care practice may include treatment of symptoms, rest/recovery strategies, and educational intervention and rehabilitation to optimize function. Providers should emphasize a positive prognosis for mild TBI, as a vast majority of patients will be symptom free within 3-6 months.

- The brain has a remarkable ability to adjust after injury. Each brain injury and its recovery are different. Brain injury rehabilitation assists patients in reaching maximum levels of independence.

- Symptoms following concussion may overlap with the clinical presentation of other diagnoses, such as PTSD and depression, as well as co-morbid physical injuries in the context of polytrauma. It is important to evaluate all associated symptoms to include physical, cognitive, and emotional sequelae. The strategy relies on a target-symptom approach in the context of an individualized treatment plan, facilitated by the primary care provider.

- When recovering from mild TBI, tips and advice to the patient include: getting plenty of sleep; keeping a daily journal of activities, feelings, and symptoms; returning to normal activities gradually; avoiding high-risk activities that could lead to another brain injury; following doctors' directions; not drinking alcoholic beverages; and being patient.

- Advice should be simple and provided in writing.

- For memory problems, advise your patient to get into the habit of writing down important information. If important items are frequently lost or misplaced, putting those items in the same place each time is helpful. One strategy is to use a personal planner to record where important documents, phone numbers, etc. can be found.

Section 37.4

Sports-Related Concussions: What Parents Need to Know

This section contains text excerpted from the following sources: Text beginning with the heading "What Is a Concussion?" is excerpted from "Fact Sheet for Athletes," Centers for Disease Control and Prevention (CDC), December 27, 2015; Text under the heading "What Should I Do If I Think I Have a Concussion?" is excerpted from "Concussion Information Sheet," Centers for Disease Control and Prevention (CDC), May 3, 2016.

What Is a Concussion?

A concussion is a brain injury that affects how your brain works. It can happen when your brain gets bounced around in your skull after a fall or hit to the head.

How Can I Help Keep My Children or Teens Safe?

Sports are a great way for children and teens to stay healthy and can help them do well in school. To help lower your children's or teens' chances of getting a concussion or other serious brain injury, you should:

- Help create a culture of safety for the team.

- Work with their coach to teach ways to lower the chances of getting a concussion.

- Talk with your children or teens about concussion and ask if they have concerns about reporting a concussion. Talk with them about their concerns; emphasize the importance of reporting concussions and taking time to recover from one.

- Ensure that they follow their coach's rules for safety and the rules of the sport.

- Tell your children or teens that you expect them to practice good sportsmanship at all times.

- When appropriate for the sport or activity, teach your children or teens that they must wear a helmet to lower the chances of the most serious types of brain or head injury. However, there is no "concussion-proof" helmet. So, even with a helmet, it is important for children and teens to avoid hits to the head.

Talk with Your Children and Teens about Concussion

Tell them to report their concussion symptoms to you and their coach right away. Some children and teens think concussions aren't serious or worry that if they report a concussion they will lose their position on the team or look weak. Be sure to remind them that it's better to miss one game than the whole season.

Concussions Affect Each Child and Teen Differently

While most children and teens with a concussion feel better within a couple of weeks, some will have symptoms for months or longer. Talk with your children's or teens' healthcare provider if their concussion symptoms do not go away or if they get worse after they return to their regular activities.

How Can I Spot a Possible Concussion?

Children and teens who show or report one or more of the signs and symptoms listed below—or simply say they just "don't feel right" after a bump, blow, or jolt to the head or body—may have a concussion or other serious brain injury.

Signs Observed by Parents or Coaches

• Appears dazed or stunned.

• Forgets an instruction, is confused about an assignment or position, or is unsure of the game, score, or opponent.

• Moves clumsily.

• Answers questions slowly.

• Loses consciousness (even briefly).

• Shows mood, behavior, or personality changes.

• Can't recall events prior to or after a hit or fall.

Symptoms Reported by Children and Teens

• Headache or "pressure" in head.

• Nausea or vomiting.

• Balance problems or dizziness, or double or blurry vision.

• Bothered by light or noise.

• Feeling sluggish, hazy, foggy, or groggy.

• Confusion, or concentration or memory problems.

• Just not "feeling right," or "feeling down."

What Are Some More Serious Danger Signs to Look out For?

In rare cases, a dangerous collection of blood (hematoma) may form on the brain after a bump, blow, or jolt to the head or body and can squeeze the brain against the skull. Call 9-1-1 or take your child or teen to the emergency department right away if, after a bump, blow, or jolt to the head or body, he or she has one or more of these danger signs:

• One pupil larger than the other.

• Drowsiness or inability to wake up.

- A headache that gets worse and does not go away. Slurred speech, weakness, numbness, or decreased coordination.
- Repeated vomiting or nausea, convulsions or seizures (shaking or twitching).
- Unusual behavior, increased confusion, restlessness, or agitation.
- Loss of consciousness (passed out/knocked out).
- Even a brief loss of consciousness should be taken seriously.

What Should I Do If My Child or Teen Has a Possible Concussion?

As a parent, if you think your child or teen may have a concussion, you should:

1. Remove your child or teen from play.

2. Keep your child or teen out of play the day of the injury. Your child or teen should be seen by a healthcare provider and only return to play with permission from a healthcare provider who is experienced in evaluating for concussion.

3. Ask your child's or teen's healthcare provider for written instructions on helping your child or teen return to school. You can give the instructions to your child's or teen's school nurse and teacher(s) and return-to-play instructions to the coach and/or athletic trainer.

Do not try to judge the severity of the injury yourself. Only a healthcare provider should assess a child or teen for a possible concussion. Concussion signs and symptoms often show up soon after the injury. But you may not know how serious the concussion is at first, and some symptoms may not show up for hours or days.

The brain needs time to heal after a concussion. A child's or teen's return to school and sports should be a gradual process that is carefully managed and monitored by a healthcare provider.

Chapter 38

Safety Information to Help Prevent Sports Injuries

Childhood Sports Injuries: A Common and Serious Problem

Like Raoul, more than 38 million children and adolescents participate in organized sports in the United States each year. Still more participate in informal recreational activities. Although sports participation provides numerous physical and social benefits, it also has a downside: the risk of sports-related injuries. According to the Centers for Disease Control and Prevention (CDC), more than 2.6 million children 0 to 19 years old are treated in the emergency department each year for sports and recreation-related injuries.

These injuries are by far the most common cause of musculoskeletal injuries in children treated in emergency departments. They are also the single most common cause of injury-related primary care office visits.

The Most Common Sports-Related Injuries in Kids

Although sports injuries can range from scrapes and bruises to serious brain and spinal cord injuries, most fall somewhere between

This chapter includes text excerpted from "Childhood Sports Injuries and Their Prevention: A Guide for Parents with Ideas for Kids," National Institute of Arthritis and Musculoskeletal and Skin Diseases (NIAMS), June 2013.

the two extremes. Here are some of the more common types of injuries.

Sprains and Strains

A sprain is an injury to a ligament, one of the bands of tough, fibrous tissue that connects two or more bones at a joint and prevents excessive movement of the joint. An ankle sprain is the most common athletic injury.

A strain is an injury to either a muscle or a tendon. A muscle is a tissue composed of bundles of specialized cells that, when stimulated by nerve messages, contract and produce movement. A tendon is a tough, fibrous cord of tissue that connects muscle to bone. Muscles in any part of the body can be injured.

Growth Plate Injuries

In some sports accidents and injuries, the growth plate may be injured. The growth plate is the area of developing tissues at the end of the long bones in growing children and adolescents. When growth is complete, sometime during adolescence, the growth plate is replaced by solid bone. The long bones in the body include:

- the long bones of the hand and fingers (metacarpals and phalanges)
- both bones of the forearm (radius and ulna)
- the bone of the upper leg (femur)
- the lower leg bones (tibia and fibula)
- the foot bones (metatarsals and phalanges)

If any of these areas become injured, it's important to seek professional help from an orthopaedic surgeon, a doctor who specializes in bone injuries.

Repetitive Motion Injuries

Painful injuries such as stress fractures (a hairline fracture of the bone that has been subjected to repeated stress) and tendinitis (inflammation of a tendon) can occur from overuse of muscles and tendons. Some of these injuries don't always show up on X-rays, but they do cause pain and discomfort. The injured area usually responds to rest, ice, compression, and elevation (RICE). Other treatments can include crutches, cast immobilization, and physical therapy.

Heat-Related Illnesses

Heat-related illnesses include:

- dehydration (deficit in body fluids)

- heat exhaustion (nausea, dizziness, weakness, headache, pale and moist skin, heavy perspiration, normal or low body temperature, weak pulse, dilated pupils, disorientation, and fainting spells)

- heat stroke (headache, dizziness, confusion, and hot dry skin, possibly leading to vascular collapse, coma, and death).

Heat injuries are always dangerous and can be fatal. Heat-related injuries are a particular problem for children because children perspire less than adults and require a higher core body temperature to trigger sweating. Playing rigorous sports in the heat requires close monitoring of both body and weather conditions. Fortunately, heat-related illnesses can be prevented.

Preventing and Treating Injuries

Injuries can happen to any child who plays sports, but there are some things that can help prevent and treat injuries.

Prevention

- Enroll your child in organized sports through schools, community clubs, and recreation areas that are properly maintained. Any organized team activity should demonstrate a commitment to injury prevention. Coaches should be trained in first aid and CPR, and should have a plan for responding to emergencies. Coaches should be well versed in the proper use of equipment, and should enforce rules on equipment use.

- Organized sports programs may have adults on staff who are certified athletic trainers. These individuals are trained to prevent, recognize, and provide immediate care for athletic injuries.

- Make sure your child has—and consistently uses—proper gear for a particular sport. This may reduce the chances of being injured.

- Make warm-ups and cool-downs part of your child's routine before and after sports participation. Warm-up exercises make the body's tissues warmer and more flexible. Cool-down exercises loosen muscles that have tightened during exercise.

- Make sure your child has access to water or a sports drink while playing. Encourage him or her to drink frequently and stay properly hydrated. Remember to include sunscreen and a hat (when possible) to reduce the chance of sunburn, which is a type of injury to the skin. Sun protection may also decrease the chances of malignant melanoma—a potentially deadly skin cancer—or other skin cancers that can occur later in life.

- Learn and follow safety rules and suggestions for your child's particular sport. You'll find some more sport-specific safety suggestions below.

Treatment

- Treatment for sports-related injuries will vary by injury. But if your child suffers a soft tissue injury (such as a sprain or strain) or a bone injury, the best immediate treatment is easy to remember: RICE (rest, ice, compression, elevation) the injury. Get professional treatment if any injury is severe. A severe injury means having an obvious fracture or dislocation of a joint, prolonged swelling, or prolonged or severe pain.

Keep Kids Exercising

Luckily for Raoul, his injury wasn't serious. In a few weeks, he will be fully recovered and able to play again. Even though Raoul got hurt, it's important that he continue some type of regular exercise and sports involvement after the injury heals. Exercise may reduce his chances of obesity, which is becoming more common in children. It may also reduce his risk of diabetes, a disease that can be associated with a lack of exercise and poor eating habits. Exercise also helps him build social skills and provides him with a general sense of well-being. Sports participation is an important part of learning how to build team skills.

As a parent, it is important for you to encourage your children to be physically active. It's also important to match your child to the sport, and not push him or her too hard into an activity that he or she may not like or be capable of doing. Teach your children to follow the rules and to play it safe when they get involved in sports, so they'll spend more time having fun in the game and be less likely to be sidelined with an injury. You should be mindful of the risks associated with different sports and take important measures to reduce the chance of injury. For sport-specific suggestions, see the information below.

Sport-Specific Safety Information

Here are some winning ways to help prevent an injury from occurring, so you are less likely to get that alarming phone call like Raoul's mom did.

Basketball

- **Common injuries and locations:** sprains, strains, bruises, fractures, scrapes, dislocations, cuts, injuries to teeth, ankles, and knees. (Injury rates are higher in girls, especially for the anterior cruciate ligament or ACL, the wide ligament that limits rotation and forward movement of the shin bone.)

- **Safest playing with:** eye protection, elbow and knee pads, mouth guard, athletic supporters for males, proper shoes, water. If playing outdoors, wear sunscreen and, when possible, a hat.

- **Injury prevention:** strength training (particularly knees and shoulders), aerobics (exercises that develop the strength and endurance of heart and lungs), warm-up exercises, proper coaching, and use of safety equipment.

Track and Field

- **Common injuries:** strains, sprains, scrapes from falls.

- **Safest playing with:** proper shoes, athletic supporters for males, sunscreen, water.

- **Injury prevention:** proper conditioning and coaching.

Football

- **Common injuries and locations:** bruises, sprains, strains, pulled muscles, tears to soft tissues such as ligaments, broken bones, internal injuries (bruised or damaged organs), concussions, back injuries, sunburn. Knees and ankles are the most common injury sites.

- **Safest playing with:** helmet, mouth guard, shoulder pads, athletic supporters for males, chest/rib pads, forearm, elbow, and thigh pads, shin guards, proper shoes, sunscreen, water.

- **Injury prevention:** proper use of safety equipment, warm-up exercises, proper coaching techniques and conditioning.

Baseball and Softball

- **Common injuries:** soft tissue strains, impact injuries that include fractures caused by sliding and being hit by a ball, sunburn.

- **Safest playing with:** batting helmet, shin guards, elbow guards, athletic supporters for males, mouth guard, sunscreen, cleats, hat, detachable, "breakaway bases" rather than traditional, stationary ones.

- **Injury prevention:** proper conditioning and warm-ups.

Soccer

- **Common injuries:** bruises, cuts and scrapes, headaches, sunburn.

- **Safest playing with:** shin guards, athletic supporters for males, cleats, sunscreen, water.

- **Injury prevention:** aerobic conditioning and warm-ups, and proper training in "heading" (that is, using the head to strike or make a play with the ball).

Gymnastics

- **Common injuries:** sprains and strains of soft tissues.

- **Safest playing with:** athletic supporters for males, safety harness, joint supports (such as neoprene wraps), water.

- **Injury prevention:** proper conditioning and warm-ups.

Treat Injuries with "RICE"

Rest: Reduce or stop using the injured area for at least 48 hours. If you have a leg injury, you may need to stay off of it completely.

Ice: Put an ice pack on the injured area for 20 minutes at a time, four to eight times per day. Use a cold pack, ice bag, or a plastic bag filled with crushed ice that has been wrapped in a towel.

Compression: Ask your child's doctor about elastics wraps, air casts, special boots, or splints that can be used to compress an injured ankle, knee, or wrist to reduce swelling.

Elevation: Keep the injured area elevated above the level of the heart to help decrease swelling. Use a pillow to help elevate an injured limb.

Chapter 39

Overtraining and Compulsive Exercise

Chapter Contents

Section 39.1

Overtraining in Women and the Risk to Bone Health

This section includes text excerpted from "Exercise and Bone Health for Women: The Skeletal Risk of Overtraining," National Institute of Arthritis and Musculoskeletal and Skin Diseases (NIAMS), May 15, 2016.

Are you exercising too much? Eating too little? Have your menstrual periods stopped or become irregular? If so, you may be putting yourself at high risk for several serious problems that could affect your health, your ability to remain active, and your risk for injuries. You also may be putting yourself at risk for developing osteoporosis, a disease in which bone density is decreased, leaving your bones vulnerable to fracture (breaking).

Why Is Missing My Period Such a Big Deal?

Some athletes see amenorrhea (the absence of menstrual periods) as a sign of successful training. Others see it as a great answer to a monthly inconvenience. And some young women accept it blindly, not stopping to think of the consequences. But missing your periods is often a sign of decreased estrogen levels. And lower estrogen levels can lead to osteoporosis, a disease in which your bones become brittle and more likely to break.

Usually, bones don't become brittle and break until women are much older. But some young women, especially those who exercise so much that their periods stop, develop brittle bones, and may start to have fractures at a very early age. Some 20-year-old female athletes have been said to have the bones of an 80- year-old woman. Even if bones don't break when you're young, low estrogen levels during the peak years of bone-building, the preteen and teen years, can affect bone density for the rest of your life. And studies show that bone growth lost during these years may never be regained.

Broken bones don't just hurt—they can cause lasting physical malformations. Have you noticed that some older women and men have stooped postures? This is not a normal sign of aging. Fractures from osteoporosis have left their spines permanently altered.

Overtraining can cause other problems besides missed periods. If you don't take in enough calcium and vitamin D (among other nutrients), bone loss may result. This may lead to decreased athletic performance, decreased ability to exercise or train at desired levels of intensity or duration, and increased risk of injury.

Who Is at Risk for These Problems?

Girls and women who engage in rigorous exercise regimens or who try to lose weight by restricting their eating are at risk for these health problems. They may include serious athletes, "gym rats" (who spend considerable time and energy working out), and girls and women who believe "you can never be too thin."

How Can I Tell If Someone I Know, Train with, or Coach May Be at Risk for Bone Loss, Fracture, and Other Health Problems?

Here are some signs to look for:

- missed or irregular menstrual periods

- extreme or "unhealthy-looking" thinness

- extreme or rapid weight loss

- behaviors that reflect frequent dieting, such as eating very little, not eating in front of others, trips to the bathroom following meals, preoccupation with thinness or weight, focus on low-calorie and diet foods, possible increase in the consumption of water and other no- and low-calorie foods and beverages, possible increase in gum chewing, limiting diet to one food group, or eliminating a food group

- frequent intense bouts of exercise (e.g., taking an aerobics class, then running 5 miles, then swimming for an hour, followed by weight-lifting)

- an "I can't miss a day of exercise/practice" attitude

- an overly anxious preoccupation with an injury

- exercising despite illness, inclement weather, injury, and other conditions that might lead someone else to take the day off

- an unusual amount of self-criticism or self dissatisfaction

- indications of significant psychological or physical stress, including: depression, anxiety or nervousness, inability to concentrate, low levels of self-esteem, feeling cold all the time, problems sleeping, fatigue, injuries, and constantly talking about weight

How Can I Make Needed Changes to Improve My Bone Health?

If you recognize some of these signs in yourself, the best thing you can do is to make your diet more healthful. That includes consuming enough calories to support your activity level. If you've missed periods, it's best to check with a doctor to make sure it's not a sign of some other problem and to get his or her help as you work toward a more healthy balance of food and exercise. Also, a doctor can help you take steps to protect your bones from further damage.

What Can I Do If I Suspect a Friend May Have Some of These Signs?

First, be supportive. Approach your friend or teammate carefully, and be sensitive. She probably won't appreciate a lecture about how she should be taking better care of herself. But maybe you could share this information with her or suggest that she talk to a trainer, coach, or doctor about the symptoms she's experiencing.

My Friend Drinks a Lot of Diet Sodas. She Says This Helps Keep Her Trim

Girls and women who may be dieting often drink diet sodas rather than milk. Yet, milk and other dairy products are a good source of calcium, an essential ingredient for healthy bones. Drinking sodas instead of milk can be a problem, especially during the teen years when rapid bone growth occurs. If you (or your friend) find yourself drinking a lot of sodas, try drinking half as many sodas each day, and gradually add more milk and dairy products to your diet. A frozen yogurt shake can be an occasional low-fat, tasty treat. Or try a fruit smoothie made with frozen yogurt, fruit, or calcium-enriched orange juice.

My Coach and I Think I Should Lose Just a Little More Weight. I Want to Be Able to Excel at My Sport!

Years ago, it was not unusual for coaches to encourage athletes to be as thin as possible for many sports (e.g., dancing, gymnastics, figure skating, swimming, diving, and running). However, many coaches now realize that being too thin is unhealthy and can negatively affect performance. It's important to exercise and watch what you eat. However, it's also important to develop and maintain healthy bones and bodies. Without these, it will not matter how fast you can run, how thin you are, or how long you exercise each day. Balance is the key!

I'm Still Not Convinced. If My Bones Become Brittle, so What? What's the Worst Thing That Could Happen to Me?

Brittle bones may not sound as scary as a fatal or rare disease. The fact is that osteoporosis can lead to fractures. It can cause disability.

Imagine having so many spine fractures that you've lost inches in height and walk bent over. Imagine looking down at the ground everywhere you go because you can't straighten your back. Imagine not being able to find clothes that fit you. Imagine having difficulty breathing and eating because your lungs and stomach are compressed into a smaller space. Imagine having difficulty walking, let alone exercising, because of pain and misshapen bones. Imagine constantly having to be aware of what you are doing and having to do things so slowly and carefully because of a very real fear and dread of a fracture—a fracture that could lead to a drastic change in your life, including pain, loss of independence, loss of mobility, loss of freedom, and more. Osteoporosis isn't just an "older person's" disease. Young women also experience fractures. Imagine being sidelined because of a broken bone and not being able to get those good feelings you get from regular activity.

Eating for Healthy Bones

How much calcium do I need? It's very important to your bone health that you receive adequate daily amounts of calcium, vitamin D, phosphorus, and magnesium. These vitamins and minerals are the most influential in building bones and teeth. The chart on the next page will help you decide how much calcium you need.

Where can I get calcium and vitamin D? Dairy products are the primary food sources of calcium. Choose low-fat milk, yogurt, cheeses, ice cream, or products made or served with these choices to fulfill your daily requirement. Three servings of dairy products per day should give you at least 900 mg (milligrams) of calcium. Green vegetables are another source. A cup of broccoli, for example, has about 136 mg of calcium.

Milk and dairy products. Many great snack and meal items contain calcium. With a little planning and "know-how," you can make meals and snacks calcium-rich!

- **Milk.** Wouldn't a tall, cold glass of this refreshing thirst quencher be great right now? If you're concerned about fat and calories, choose reduced-fat or fat-free milk. You can drink it plain or with a low- or no-fat syrup or flavoring, such as chocolate syrup, vanilla extract, hazelnut flavoring, or cinnamon.

- **Cheese.** Again, you can choose the low- or no-fat varieties. Use all different types of cheese for sandwiches, bagels, omelets, vegetable dishes, pasta creations, or as a snack by itself!

- **Pudding (prepared with milk).** You can now purchase (or make from a mix) pudding in a variety of flavors with little or no fat, such as chocolate fudge, lemon, butterscotch, vanilla, and pistachio. Try them all!

- **Yogurt.** Add fruit. Eat it plain. Add a low- or no-fat sauce or syrup. No matter how you choose to eat this calcium-rich food, yogurt remains a quick, easy, and convenient choice. It's also available in a variety of flavors. Try mocha-fudge-peppermint swirl if you're more adventurous at heart and vanilla if you're a more traditional yogurt snacker!

- **Frozen yogurt (or fat-free ice cream).** Everybody loves ice cream. And now, without the unnecessary fat, you can enjoy it more often! Mix yogurt, milk, and fruit to create a breakfast shake. Have a cone at lunchtime or as a snack. A scoop or two after dinner can be cool and refreshing.

What are other sources of calcium? Many foods you already buy and eat may be "calcium-fortified." Try calcium-fortified orange juice or calcium-fortified cereal. Check food labels to see if some of your other favorite foods may be good sources of calcium. You also can take calcium supplements if you think you may not be getting enough from your diet.

Section 39.2

Compulsive Exercise

About Compulsive Exercise

Compulsive exercise (also called **obligatory exercise and anorexia athletica**) is best defined by an exercise addict's frame of mind: He or she no longer chooses to exercise but feels compelled to do so and struggles with guilt and anxiety if he or she doesn't work out. Injury, illness, an outing with friends, bad weather—none of these will deter those who compulsively exercise. In a sense, exercising takes over a compulsive exerciser's life because he or she plans life around it.

Of course, it's nearly impossible to draw a clear line dividing a healthy amount of exercise from too much. The government's 2005 dietary guidelines, published by the U.S. Department of Agriculture (USDA) and the U.S. Department of Health and Human Services (HHS), recommend at least 60 minutes of physical activity for kids and teens on most—if not all—days of the week.

Experts say that repeatedly exercising beyond the requirements for good health is an indicator of compulsive behavior, but because different amounts of exercise are appropriate for different people, this definition covers a range of activity levels. However, several workouts a day, every day, is overdoing it for almost anyone.

Much like with eating disorders, many people who engage in compulsive exercise do so to feel more in control of their lives, and the majority of them are female. They often define their self-worth through their athletic performance and try to deal with emotions like anger or depression by pushing their bodies to the limit. In sticking to a rigorous workout schedule, they seek a sense of power to help them cope with low self-esteem.

Although compulsive exercising doesn't have to accompany an eating disorder, the two often go hand in hand. In anorexia nervosa, the excessive workouts usually begin as a means to control weight and become more and more extreme. As the rate of activity increases, the amount the person eats might decrease. Someone with bulimia also may use exercise as a way to compensate for binge eating.

Compulsive exercise behavior can grow out of student athletes' demanding practice schedules and their quest to excel. Pressure, both external (from coaches, peers, or parents) and internal, can drive an athlete to go too far to be the best. He or she ends up believing that just one more workout will make the difference between first and second place . . . then keeps adding more workouts.

Eventually, compulsive exercising can breed other compulsive behavior, from strict dieting to obsessive thoughts about perceived flaws. Exercise addicts may keep detailed journals about their exercise schedules and obsess about improving themselves. Unfortunately, these behaviors often compound each other, trapping the person in a downward spiral of negative thinking and low self-esteem.

Why Is Exercising Too Much a Bad Thing?

We all know that regular exercise is an important part of a healthy lifestyle. But few people realize that too much can cause physical and psychological harm:

- Excessive exercise can damage tendons, ligaments, bones, cartilage, and joints, and when minor injuries aren't allowed to heal, they often result in long-term damage. Instead of building muscle, too much exercise actually destroys muscle mass, especially if the body isn't getting enough nutrition, forcing it to break down muscle for energy.

- Girls who exercise compulsively may disrupt the balance of hormones in their bodies. This can change their menstrual cycles (some girls lose their periods altogether, a condition known as **amenorrhea**) and increase the risk of premature bone loss (**osteoporosis**). And of course, working their bodies so hard leads to exhaustion and constant fatigue.

- An even more serious risk is the stress that excessive exercise can place on the heart, particularly when someone is also engaging in unhealthy weight loss behaviors such as restricting intake, vomiting, and using diet pills or supplements. In extreme cases, the combination of anorexia and compulsive exercise can be fatal.

- Psychologically, exercise addicts are often plagued by anxiety and depression. They may have a negative image of themselves and feel worthless. Their social and academic lives may suffer as they withdraw from friends and family to fixate on exercise. Even if they want to succeed in school or in relationships, working out always comes first, so they end up skipping homework or missing out on time spent with friends.

Warning Signs

Someone may be exercising compulsively if he or she:

- won't skip a workout, even if tired, sick, or injured
- doesn't enjoy exercise sessions, but feels obligated to do them
- seems anxious or guilty when missing even one workout
- does miss one workout and exercises twice as long the next time
- is constantly preoccupied with his or her weight and exercise routine
- doesn't like to sit still or relax because of worry that not enough calories are being burnt
- has lost a significant amount of weight
- exercises more after eating more
- skips seeing friends, gives up activities, and abandons responsibilities to make more time for exercise
- seems to base self-worth on the number of workouts completed and the effort put into training
- is never satisfied with his or her own physical achievements

It's important, too, to recognize the types of athletes who are more prone to compulsive exercise because their sports place a particular emphasis on being thin. Ice skaters, gymnasts, wrestlers, and dancers can feel even more pressure than most athletes to keep their weight down and their body toned. Runners also frequently fall into a cycle of obsessive workouts.

Getting Professional Help

If you recognize some of the warning signs of compulsive exercise in your child, call your doctor to discuss your concerns. After evaluating your child, the doctor may recommend medical treatment and/or other therapy.

Because compulsive exercise is so often linked to an eating disorder, a community agency that focuses on treating these disorders might be able to offer advice or referrals. Extreme cases may require hospitalization to get a child's weight back up to a safe range.

Treating a compulsion to exercise is never a quick-fix process—it may take several months or even years. But with time and effort, kids can get back on the road to good health. Therapy can help improve self-esteem and body image, as well as teach them how to deal with emotions. Sessions with a nutritionist can help develop healthy eating habits. Once they know what to watch out for, kids will be better equipped to steer clear of unsafe exercise and eating patterns.

Ways to Help at Home

Parents can do a lot to help a child overcome a compulsion to exercise:

- Involve kids in preparing nutritious meals.

- Combine activity and fun by going for a hike or a bike ride together as a family.

- Be a good body-image role model. In other words, don't fixate on your own physical flaws, as that just teaches kids that it's normal to dislike what they see in the mirror.

- Never criticize another family member's weight or body shape, even if you're just kidding around. Such remarks might seem harmless, but they can leave a lasting impression on kids or teens struggling to define and accept themselves.

- Examine whether you're putting too much pressure on your kids to excel, particularly in a sport (because some teens turn to exercise to cope with pressure). Take a look at where kids might be feeling too much pressure. Help them put it in perspective and find other ways to cope.

Most important, just be there with constant support. Point out all of your child's great qualities that have nothing to do with working out—small daily doses of encouragement and praise can help improve self-esteem.

If you teach kids to be proud of the challenges they've faced and not just the first-place ribbons they've won, they will likely be much happier and healthier kids now and in the long run.

Chapter 40

Exercising Safely Outdoors

Chapter Contents

Section 40.1

Exercising in Hot Weather

This section includes text excerpted from "Exercising in Hot Weather," Division of Commissioned Corps Personnel and Readiness (DCCPR), August 5, 2007. Reviewed September 2016.

It Is Hot Outside!

Understanding warm and/or hot weather definitions is very important for an athlete or just an exerciser for fitness so that they may better comprehend heat illness, preventative measures, and treatment options if necessary. Of the many relevant heat related definitions, the heat index is one of the most important.

Steadman or Heat Index: The combination of air temperature and humidity that gives a description of how the temperature feels. This is not the actual air temperature. When the heat index is at or over 90 degrees Fahrenheit, extreme caution should be considered before exercising outdoors.

Heat Illness: What Is It and How Do You Manage It?

Heat illness or exertional heat illness progresses along a continuum from the mild (heat rash and/or heat cramps and/or heat syncope) through the moderate (heat exhaustion) to the life-threatening (heatstroke). Anyone is susceptible to a heat-related exertional illness. It is very important that the athlete or exerciser understand that the presentation of signs and symptoms associated with heat exertional illness does not necessarily follow this continuum. A dehydrated, non-acclimated or deconditioned individual may right away present with signs and symptoms consistent with heat stroke and not the milder symptoms first.

Heat Cramps are associated with excessive sweating during exercise and are usually caused by dehydration, electrolyte (primarily salt) loss, and inadequate blood flow to the peripheral muscles. They usually occur in the quadriceps, hamstrings, and calves.

Treatment for heat cramps is rehydration with an electrolyte (salt) solution and muscle stretch.

Heat Syncope results from physical exertion in a hot environment. In an effort to increase heat loss, the skin blood vessels dilate to such an extent that blood flow to the brain is reduced causing symptoms of headache, dizziness, faintness, increased heart rate, nausea, vomiting, restlessness, and possibly even a brief loss of consciousness.

Treatment for heat syncope is to sit or lie down in a cool environment with elevation of the feet. Hydration is very important so there is not a possible progression to heat exhaustion or heat stroke.

Heat Exhaustion is a shock-like condition that occurs when excessive sweating causes dehydration and electrolyte loss. A person with heat exhaustion may have headache, nausea, dizziness, chills, fatigue, and extreme thirst. Signs of heat exhaustion are pale and clammy skin, rapid and weak pulse, loss of coordination, decreased performance, dilated pupils, and profuse sweating.

Treatment for heat exhaustion is to immediately stop the activity and properly hydrate with chilled water and/or an electrolyte replacement sport beverage. The exerciser should be cleared by his/her physician before resuming sport or other strenuous outdoor activities.

Exertional Heat Stoke (Hyperthermia) is a life-threatening condition in which the body's thermal regulatory mechanism is overwhelmed. There are two types heat stroke—fluid depleted (slow onset) and fluid intact (fast onset). Fluid depleted means that the individual is not hydrating at a rate sufficient to function in a heat challenge situation. Fluid intact means that the extreme heat overwhelms the individual even though the fluid level is sufficient. Key signs of heat stroke are hot skin (not necessarily dry skin), peripheral vasoconstriction (pale or ashen colored skin), high pulse rate, high respiratory rate, decreased urine output, and a core temperature (taken rectally) over 104 or 105 degrees Fahrenheit, and pupils may be dilated and unresponsive to light.

Treatment for heat stroke is to move the person to a cool shaded area and reduce the body temperature immediately. If immediate medical attention is not available, immerse the person in a cool bath while covering the extremities with cool wet cloths and massaging the extremities to propel the cooled blood back into the core.

Exercise Induced Hyponatremia (water intoxication) is most commonly associated with prolonged exertion during sustained, high-intensity endurance activities such as marathons or triathlons. In most cases, it is attributable to excess free water intake, which fails to replenish the sometimes massive sodium losses that result from sweating. Symptoms of hyponatremia can vary from light-headedness, malaise, nausea, to altered mental status. Risk factors include hot weather, female athletes/exercisers, poor performance, and possibly the use of nonsteroidal anti-inflammatory medications.

As a treatment for hyponatremia, new guidelines advise runners to drink only as much fluid as they lose due to sweating during a race. The International Marathon Medical Directors Association recommends that, during extended exercise, athletes drink no more than 31 ounces (or about 800 milliliters) of water per hour. Individuals involved in strenuous exercise in warm or hot weather should consider the sodium (salt) concentration of the beverage being consumed.

How Can You Prevent Exertional Heat Related Illnesses?

Some recommendations on how to prevent exertional heat related illness include:

- When exercising in high heat and humidity, rest 10 minutes for every hour and change wet clothing frequently.

- Avoid the midday sun by exercising before 10 a.m. or after 6 p.m., if possible.

- Use a sunscreen with a rating of SPF-15 or lower dependent upon skin type. Ratings above SPF-15 can interfere with the skin's thermal regulation.

- Wear light-weight and breathable clothing.

- Weigh yourself pre and post exercise. If there is a less than a 2 percent weight loss after exercise, you are considered mildly dehydrated. With a 2 percent and greater weight loss, you are considered dehydrated.

During hot weather training, dehydration occurs more frequently and has more severe consequences. Drink early and at regular intervals according to the American College of Sports Medicine. The perception of thirst is a poor index of the magnitude of fluid deficit. Monitoring your weight loss and ingesting chilled volumes of fluid during exercise at a rate equal to that lost from sweating is a better method to preventing dehydration.

- Rapid fluid replacement is not recommended for rehydration. Rapid replacement of fluid stimulates increased urine production, which reduces the body water retention.

- Individuals involved in a short bout of exercise are generally fine with water fluid replacement of an extra 8-16 ounces. A sports drink (with salt and potassium) is suggested for exercise lasting longer than an hour, such as a marathon, and at a rate of about 16 to 24 ounces an hour depending upon the amount you sweat and the heat index.

- Replace fluids after long bouts of exercise (greater than an hour) at a rate of 16 ounces of fluid per pound of body weight lost during exercise.

- Avoid caffeinated, protein, and alcoholic drinks, e.g., colored soda, coffee, tea.

- Acclimate to exercising outdoors, altitude, and physical condition. General rule of thumb is 10-14 days for adults and 14-21 days for children (prepubescent) and older adults (> 60 years). Children and older adults are less heat tolerant and have a less effective thermoregulatory system.

- Educate and prepare yourself for outdoor activities. Many Web sites offer heat index calculations for your local weather conditions.

Summer weather does not have to sideline your outdoor exercise regimen. The above suggestions can help you plan and find ways to modify your routine to exercise safely in warm, hot, and humid weather.

Section 40.2

Exercising In Cold Weather

This section includes text excerpted from "Exercising in Cold Weather," Division of Commissioned Corps Personnel and Readiness (DCCPR), February 19, 2007. Reviewed September 2016.

Dangers of Exposure

Cold temperature can cause life and limb threatening cold-related disorders. Cold-related disorders can be systemic or local.

Systemic Response to Cold Exposure

Hypothermia is a systemic response to cold and occurs when the core body temperature drops below 95 degrees F. It can begin even when air temperatures are at 50 degrees F. Hypothermia requires immediate medical attention.

Signs and symptoms of hypothermia include: chills, fatigue or drowsiness, pain in the extremities, euphoria, slurred speech, slow and weak pulse, shivering, and collapse and/or unconsciousness.

Local Responses to Cold Exposure

Frostbite is freezing of local tissues that can occur if ambient temperature is less than 30 degrees F. Frostbite must be treated as a burn and requires medical treatment. Frost nip and trench foot are skin disorders resulting from extreme cooling of the skin and underlying tissue, but without actual freezing of the tissues. Damp clothing accelerates heat loss, which causes frost nip and trench foot. Frost nip can also occur when the wind chill is –22 degrees F.

How to Protect Yourself and Prevent Cold Related Injuries When Exercising

- Environmental conditions that must be considered in the management of cold stress along with exercise demands are air temperature and air speed. Personal protective practices are recommended for exercise at air temperatures below 50 degrees F. Proper clothing is the primary protection against cold-related disorders. Layering of clothing is always the recommended choice with physical activity outdoors. The amount of layering depends on the intensity of the activity and the temperature. Generally, each quarter-inch of clothing adds one layer of insulation. Any exposed skin, however, is still at risk for excessive local cooling and can lead to frostbite.

- The following are examples of how much layering of clothing is needed if the air temperature is 20 degrees F. If you are going to do a high intensity activity like running or speed biking, you will need approximately one layer (a quarter-inch thick total) of clothing. If you are going to do a light intensity activity like walking you will need at least three layers (three quarters of an inch thick total) of clothing.

Other Tips to Reduce the Risk of Cold Exposure during Exercise

The following practices are recommended for exercise at air temperatures below 50 degrees F:

- Plan your activity to avoid fatigue at a location removed from a warm recovery station. For example, if you run outdoors on an off-road (e.g., trail) setting, you may want to consider an alternative, pedestrian-friendly route through a neighborhood that offers potential shelter (e.g., coffee shop) along the way should it be needed.

- Anticipate, wear, and adjust as necessary proper clothing. Key word here is layers!

- Seek relief from cold stress exposure when you experience sensation(s) of extreme discomfort, especially at the extremities; fatigue or weakness; or loss of coordination.

- Frequently drink warm, caffeine-free fluids containing carbohydrates. Not only will this help keep your core temperature above 95 degrees F, but this will also keep you hydrated and with ready energy. For example, pour your lukewarm sports drink in an insulated container when doing outdoor exercise.

- Change wet clothing immediately, especially if the air temperature is less than 36 degrees F.

- Seek medical advice for repeated or unusual intolerance to cold, such as repeated episodes of frost nip, appearances of welts, or severe shivering. It is recommended to have medical approval for exercising at wind chills of less than 11 degrees F. Winter weather does not have to sideline your outdoor exercise regimen. The above suggestions can help you find ways to modify your routine to safely exercise in cold weather conditions. And, no matter what the season of the year is, you should maintain a healthy lifestyle through a balanced diet, regular exercise, adequate sleep, and avoiding drug abuse.

Winter weather does not have to sideline your outdoor exercise regimen. The above suggestions can help you find ways to modify your routine to safely exercise in cold weather conditions. And, no matter what the season of the year is, you should maintain a healthy lifestyle through a balanced diet, regular exercise, adequate sleep, and avoiding drug abuse.

Section 40.3

Air Pollution and Exercise

This section includes text excerpted from "Physical Activity and Air Pollution Exposure," U.S. Environmental Protection Agency (EPA), February 10, 2014.

Outdoor Activity and Air Pollution

- Exposure to air pollution is associated with several adverse health outcomes, including asthma attacks and abnormal heart rhythms.

- People who can modify the location or time of exercise may wish to reduce these risks by exercising away from heavy traffic and industrial sites, especially during rush hour or times when pollution is known to be high.

- However, current evidence indicates that the benefits of being active, even in polluted air, outweigh the risk of being inactive.

Air Pollution Exposure While Being Active

How Physical Activity Affects Air Pollution Dose

- Concentration varies across microenvironments
- When and where activity occurs
- Time spent in microenvironment
- Duration of activity (e.g., active travel vs. driving)
- Ventilation rate correlates with intensity of activity
- Increased ventilation rate: more breaths/minute
- Increased velocity of breaths: forces air deeper into lungs and increases deposition fraction
- More mouth breathing: bypasses nasal filtration
- Dose is dependent on age, sex, and body size

Air Pollution and Physical Activity Joint Health Effects

- Mortality risks vs. benefits
- Studies on increasing active travel consistently show that benefits (physical activity) > risks (air pollution and injury)
- Modeled predictions of hypothetical scenarios using relative risk data from literature
- Built environment plays an important role in determining air pollution and physical activity levels

Short-term Exposure and Lung Function

- 60 adults with asthma walk for 2 hours along two different routes
- Larger decline in lung function after walking more polluted route

Long-term Exposure and Asthma Incidence

- Playing ≥3 sports increased risk of asthma in high ozone communities, but not in low ozone communities

Air Quality and Outdoor Activity Guidance for Schools

- Goal: Keep kids active
- Take into consideration that air pollution exposures during school day are of short duration
- 15 minute recess
- 30 minute PE class

Part Six

Physical Fitness for People with Health Conditions

Chapter 41

Introduction to Exercise with a Health Condition

Regular exercise and physical activity are important to the physical and mental health of almost everyone, including older adults. Being physically active can help you continue to do the things you enjoy and stay independent as you age. Regular physical activity over long periods of time can produce long-term health benefits. In addition, regular exercise and physical activity can reduce the risk of developing some diseases and disabilities that develop as people grow older. In some cases, exercise is an effective treatment for many chronic conditions. For example, studies show that people with arthritis, heart disease, or diabetes benefit from regular exercise.

Exercise also helps people with high blood pressure, balance problems, or difficulty walking. One of the great things about physical

This chapter contains text excerpted from the following sources: Text in this chapter begins with excerpts from "Exercise and Physical Activity: Your Everyday Guide from the National Institute on Aging," National Institute on Aging (NIA), February 16, 2016; Text beginning with the heading "Talking with Your Doctor about Exercise and Physical Activity" is excerpted from "Exercise and Physical Activity: Your Everyday Guide from the National Institute on Aging," National Institute on Aging (NIA), February 16, 2016; Text under the heading "Physical Activity for People with Chronic Medical Conditions" is excerpted from "Chapter 7: Additional Considerations for Some Adults," Office of Disease Prevention and Health Promotion (ODPHP), U.S. Department of Health and Human Services (HHS), July 21, 2016.

activity is that there are so many ways to be active. For example, you can be active in short spurts throughout the day, or you can set aside specific times of the day on specific days of the week to exercise. Many physical activities—such as brisk walking, raking leaves, or taking the stairs whenever you can—are free or low cost and do not require special equipment.

Talking with Your Doctor about Exercise and Physical Activity

You may want to talk with your doctor, if you aren't used to energetic activity and you want to start a vigorous exercise program or significantly increase your physical activity. You also should talk with your doctor if you have any health problems. This does not mean that exercise is dangerous. Doctors rarely tell people not to exercise, but they may have certain safety tips for those who have recently had hip or back surgery, those with uncontrolled health problems, or those with chronic conditions such as diabetes, heart disease, or arthritis.

Your activity level is an important topic to discuss with your doctor as part of your ongoing preventive healthcare. Talk about exercise at least once a year if your health is stable, and more often if your health is getting better or worse over time so that you can adjust your exercise program. Your doctor can help you choose activities that are best for you and reduce any risks. Here are a few things you may want to discuss:

- Ask whether there are exercises or activities you should avoid. An illness or surgery may affect how you exercise. For example, if you've had hip or back surgery, you may need to modify or avoid some exercises, or if you develop blood clots in your legs, you will have to restrict your activity for a time. Your doctor can tell you how to increase your physical activity gradually as you recover.

- Talk about any unexplained symptoms, such as chest pain or pressure, pain in your joints, dizziness, or shortness of breath. Postpone exercise until the problem is diagnosed and treated.

- Make sure your preventive care is up to date. For example, women age 65 and older should have regular tests for osteoporosis. Weight-bearing exercises—such as walking and lifting weight—are especially helpful for those with osteoporosis.

- Understand how any ongoing health conditions affect exercise and physical activity. For example, people with arthritis may need to avoid some types of activity, especially when joints are swollen or inflamed. Those with diabetes may need to adjust their daily schedule, meal plan, or medications when planning their activities.

- Talk to your doctor if you think you might have an uncontrolled medical condition that might affect the type of exercise you should be doing. For example, it is important to know how to exercise safely if your blood pressure or diabetes is not under control.

Safety First: When to Check with Your Doctor

Almost anyone, at any age, can do some type of exercise and physical activity. You can still be active even if you have a long-term condition like heart disease or diabetes. In fact, exercise and physical activity may help. But, talk with your doctor if you aren't used to energetic activity. Other reasons to check with your doctor before you exercise include:

- Any new symptom you haven't yet discussed
- Dizziness or shortness of breath
- Chest pain or pressure
- The feeling that your heart is skipping, racing, or fluttering
- Blood clots
- An infection or fever with muscle aches
- Unplanned weight loss
- Foot or ankle sores that won't heal
- Joint swelling
- A bleeding or detached retina, eye surgery, or laser treatment
- A hernia
- Recent hip or back surgery

Physical Activity for People with Chronic Medical Conditions

Adults with chronic conditions should engage in regular physical activity because it can help promote their quality of life and reduce the risk of developing new conditions. The type and amount of physical activity should be determined by a person's abilities and the severity of the chronic condition. Three examples are provided below to illustrate the benefits of physical activity for persons with chronic conditions.

Physical Activity for Adults with Osteoarthritis

Osteoarthritis is a common condition in older adults, and people can live many years with osteoarthritis. People with osteoarthritis are commonly concerned that physical activity can make their condition worse. Osteoarthritis can be painful and cause fatigue, making it hard to begin or maintain regular physical activity. Yet people with this condition should get regular physical activity to lower their risk of getting other chronic diseases, such as heart disease or type 2 diabetes, and to help maintain a healthy body weight.

Strong scientific evidence indicates that both aerobic activity and muscle-strengthening activity provide therapeutic benefits for persons with osteoarthritis. When done safely, physical activity does not make the disease or the pain worse. Studies show that adults with osteoarthritis can expect improvements in pain, physical function, quality of life, and mental health with regular physical activity.

Physical Activity for Adults with Type 2 Diabetes

Physical activity in adults with type 2 diabetes shows how important it can be for people with a chronic disease to be active. Physical activity has important therapeutic effects in people with diabetes, but it is also routinely recommended to reduce risk of other diseases and help promote a healthy body weight.

For example, strong scientific evidence shows that physical activity protects against heart disease in people with diabetes. Moderate-intensity activity for about 150 minutes a week helps to substantially lower the risk of heart disease. A person who moves toward 300 minutes (5 hours) or more of moderate-intensity activity a week gets even greater benefit.

Physical Activity for Cancer Survivors

With modern treatments, many people with cancer can either be cured or survive for many years, living long enough to be at risk of other chronic conditions, such as high blood pressure or type 2 diabetes. Some cancer survivors are at risk of recurrence of the original cancer. Some have experienced side effects of the cancer treatment.

Like other adults, cancer survivors should engage in regular physical activity for its preventive benefits. Physical activity in cancer survivors can reduce risk of new chronic diseases. Further, studies suggest physically active adults with breast or colon cancer are less like to die prematurely or have a recurrence of the cancer. Physical activity may also play a role in reducing adverse effects of cancer treatment.

Chapter 42

Physical Activity for People with Disabilities

Chapter Contents

Section 42.1

Healthy Living for People with Disabilities

This section includes text excerpted from "Healthy Living," Centers
for Disease Control and Prevention (CDC), March 30, 2016.

People with Disabilities Can Live a Healthy Life

People with disabilities need healthcare and health programs for
the same reasons anyone else does—to stay well, active, and a part of
the community.

Having a disability does not mean a person is not healthy or that he
or she cannot be healthy. Being healthy means the same thing for all
of us—getting and staying well so we can lead full, active lives. That
means having the tools and information to make healthy choices and
knowing how to prevent illness.

For people with disabilities, it also means knowing that health
problems related to a disability can be treated. These problems, also
called secondary conditions, can include pain, depression, and a greater
risk for certain illnesses.

To be healthy, people with disabilities require healthcare that meets
their needs as a whole person, not just as a person with a disability.
Most people with or without disabilities can stay healthy by learning
about and living healthy lifestyles.

Leading a Long and Healthy Life

Although people with disabilities sometimes have a harder time
getting and staying healthy than people without disabilities, there
are things we can all do to get and stay healthy.

Tips for leading a long and healthy life:

- Be physically active every day.

- Eat healthy foods in healthy portions.

- Don't get too much sun.

- Get regular checkups.

- Don't smoke.

- Use medicines wisely.

- If you drink alcoholic beverages, drink in moderation.

- Get help for substance abuse.

- Stay in touch with family and friends.

- If you need help, talk with your healthcare professional.

Getting the Best Possible Healthcare

People with disabilities must get the care and services they need to help them be healthy.

If you have a disability, there are many things you can do to make sure you are getting the best possible healthcare:

- Know your body, how you feel when you are well and when you're not.

- Talk openly with your healthcare professional about your concerns.

- Find healthcare professionals that you are comfortable with in your area.

- Check to be sure you can physically get into your healthcare professional's office, such as having access to ramps or elevators if you use an assistive device like a wheelchair or scooter.

- Check to see if your healthcare professional's office has the equipment you need, such as an accessible scale or examining table.

- Ask for help from your healthcare professional's office staff if you need it.

- Think about your questions and health concerns before you visit your healthcare professional so that you're prepared.

- Bring your health records with you.

- Take a friend with you if you are concerned you might not remember all your questions or what is said by the healthcare professional.

- Get it in writing. Write down, or have someone write down for you, what is said by the healthcare professional.

Physical Activity

Adults of all shapes, sizes, and abilities can benefit from being physically active, including those with disabilities. For important health benefits, all adults should do both aerobic and muscle-strengthening physical activities. Regular aerobic physical activity increases heart and lung functions; improves daily living activities and independence; decreases chances of developing chronic diseases; and improves mental health.

Adults with disabilities should try to get at least 2 hours and 30 minutes (150 minutes) a week of moderate-intensity aerobic physical activity (i.e., brisk walking; wheeling oneself in a wheelchair) or at least 1 hour and 15 minutes (75 minutes) a week of vigorous-intensity aerobic physical activity (i.e., jogging, wheelchair basketball) or a mix of both moderate- and vigorous-intensity aerobic physical activities each week. A rule of thumb is that 1 minute of vigorous-intensity activity is about the same as 2 minutes of moderate-intensity activity. They should avoid inactivity as some physical activity is better than none.

Muscle-strengthening activities should include moderate and high intensity, and involve all major muscle groups on two or more days a week (i.e., working with resistance-band, adapted yoga) as these activities provide additional health benefits. All children and adolescents should do 1 hour (60 minutes) or more of physical activity each day.

If a person with a disability is not able to meet the physical activity guidelines, they should engage in regular physical activity based on their abilities and should avoid inactivity. Adults with disabilities should talk to their healthcare provider about the amounts and types of physical activity that are appropriate for their abilities.

Tips for getting fit:

- Talk to your doctor about how much and what kind of physical activity is right for you.

- Find opportunities to increase physical activity regularly in ways that meet your needs and abilities.

- Start slowly, based on your abilities and fitness level (e.g., be active for at least 10 minutes at a time, slowly increase activity over several weeks, if necessary).

- Avoid inactivity. Some activity is better than none!

Section 42.2

Working with Your Doctor to Increase Physical Activity

This section includes text excerpted from "Increasing Physical Activity among Adults with Disabilities," Centers for Disease Control and Prevention (CDC), April 11, 2016.

More than 21 million US adults 18–64 years of age have a disability. These are adults with serious difficulty walking or climbing stairs; hearing; seeing; or concentrating, remembering, or making decisions. Adults with disabilities are three times more likely to have heart disease, stroke, diabetes, or cancer than adults without disabilities. Aerobic physical activity can help reduce the impact of these chronic diseases, yet nearly half of all adults with disabilities get no leisure time aerobic physical activity.

Doctors and Other Health Professionals Can Play a Role

Doctors and other health professionals can play a role in promoting physical activity among their adult patients with disabilities. Adults with disabilities were 82% more likely to be physically active if their doctor recommended it, than if they did not get a doctor recommendation. However, only 44% of adults with disabilities who visited a doctor in the past year received a physical activity recommendation from their doctor.

Doctors and other health professionals can use these four steps to increase physical activity among adults with disabilities:

1. Remember that physical activity guidelines are for everybody

2. Ask about physical activity

3. Discuss barriers to physical activity

4. Recommend physical activity options

1. Remember the Physical Activity Guidelines Are for Everybody

Doctors and other health professionals should recommend physical activity, based on the 2008 Physical Activity Guidelines, to their patients with disabilities. Adults of all shapes, sizes, and abilities can benefit from being physically active, including those with disabilities.

2. Ask about Physical Activity

Doctors should recommend to their adult patients with disabilities to get physical activity on a regular basis that is consistent with their abilities. Doctors can ask about physical activity levels of their patients with disabilities by asking questions such as:

- How much physical activity are you currently doing each week?
  - How often?
  - How long?
  - At what intensity level?
- What types of physical activity do you enjoy, now or in the past?
- How can you add more physical activity to your life?

3. Discuss Barriers with Patients

Adults with disabilities face barriers to getting aerobic physical activity. Discuss the following barriers with your patients with disabilities to help them find ways to get physical activity in the built and natural environment, including:

- Knowing about and getting to programs, places, and spaces where they can be physically active;
- Having social support (e.g., setting up a buddy system, making contracts with others to complete specified levels of physical activity, or setting up walking groups or other groups to provide friendship and support) for physical activity;
- Having limited information about accessible facilities and programs; and
- Finding fitness and health professionals who can provide physical activity options that match their specific abilities.

4. Recommend Physical Activity Options

Recommend physical activity to your patients with disabilities, but remember they need to:

- Engage in the amount and types of physical activity that are right for them;

- Find opportunities to increase regular physical activity in ways that meet their needs and abilities;

- Start slowly based on their abilities and fitness level (e.g, active for at least 10 minutes at a time, slowly increase activity over several weeks, if necessary);

- Include aerobic physical activities that make them breathe harder and their heart beat faster for important health benefits, such as reducing the risk of heart disease, stroke, diabetes, and some cancers;

- Know that most aerobic physical activity may need to be modified, adapted, or may need additional assistance or equipment; and

- Avoid being physically inactive. Some physical activity is better none.

Aerobic physical activities may include:

- Aquatic therapy
- Ballroom dancing
- Brisk walking
- Cross-country and downhill skiing
- Hand-crank bicycling
- Hiking
- Horseback riding
- Nordic Walking
- Rowing
- Seated volleyball
- Swimming laps

- Water aerobics

- Wheeling oneself in wheelchair

- Wheelchair basketball, tennis, football, or softball

Section 42.3

Stay Active with a Disability: Quick Tips

This section includes text excerpted from "Stay Active with
a Disability: Quick Tips," Office of Disease Prevention and
Health Promotion (ODPHP), U.S. Department of Health and
Human Services (HHS), March 23, 2016.

Regular physical activity is good for everyone's health, including
people with disabilities.

Getting active can help you:

- Strengthen your heart

- Build strong muscles and bones

- Improve coordination

- Relieve stress, improve your mood, and feel better about yourself

Before you start...

- Talk to your doctor about the types and amounts of physical
  activity that are right for you. If you are taking medicine, be
  sure to find out how it will affect your physical activity.

- It's also a good idea to talk to a trained exercise professional.
  Find a fitness center near you that is comfortable and accessible.
  Ask if they have experience working with people with similar
  disabilities.

**Aim for 2 hours and 30 minutes a week of moderate aerobic
activities.**

- Choose aerobic activities—activities that make your heart beat
  faster—like walking fast or wheeling yourself in a wheelchair,
  swimming, or raking leaves.

- Start slowly. Be active for at least 10 minutes at a time and gradually build up to doing 30 minutes at a time.

- Aim for 30 minutes of aerobic activity on most days of the week.

Do strengthening activities 2 days a week.

- These include activities like crunches (sit-ups), push-ups, or lifting weights.

- Try working on the muscles that you use less often because of your disability.

Find support and stick with it.

- Take along a friend, especially if you are trying out a new activity.

- If you don't meet your physical activity goal, don't give up. Start again tomorrow.

- Be active according to your abilities. Remember, some physical activity is better than none!

Chapter 43

Physical Fitness for People Who Are Overweight

Chapter Contents

Section 43.1

Understanding Obesity

This section includes text excerpted from "Defining
Childhood Obesity," Centers for Disease Control and
Prevention (CDC), June 16, 2015.

Defining Childhood Obesity

Body mass index (BMI) is a measure used to determine childhood overweight and obesity. Overweight is defined as a BMI at or above the 85th percentile and below the 95th percentile for children and teens of the same age and sex. Obesity is defined as a BMI at or above the 95th percentile for children and teens of the same age and sex.

BMI is calculated by dividing a person's weight in kilograms by the square of height in meters. For children and teens, BMI is age- and sex-specific and is often referred to as BMI-for-age. A child's weight status is determined using an age- and sex-specific percentile for BMI rather than the BMI categories used for adults. This is because children's body composition varies as they age and varies between boys and girls. Therefore, BMI levels among children and teens need to be expressed relative to other children of the same age and sex.

For example, a 10-year-old boy of average height (56 inches) who weighs 102 pounds would have a BMI of 22.9 kg/m2. This would place the boy in the 95th percentile for BMI, and he would be considered as obese. This means that the child's BMI is greater than the BMI of 95% of 10-year-old boys in the reference population.

The Centers for Disease Control and Prevention (CDC) Growth Charts are the most commonly used indicator to measure the size and growth patterns of children and teens in the United States. BMI-for-age weight status categories and the corresponding percentiles were based on expert committee recommendations and are shown in the following table.

BMI does not measure body fat directly, but research has shown that BMI is correlated with more direct measures of body fat, such as

Table 43.1. Growth Charts

Weight Status Category	Percentile Range
Underweight	Less than the 5th percentile
Normal or Healthy Weight	5th percentile to less than the 85th percentile
Overweight	85th to less than the 95th percentile
Obese	95th percentile or greater

skinfold thickness measurements, bioelectrical impedance, densitometry (underwater weighing), dual energy X-ray absorptiometry (DXA) and other methods. BMI can be considered an alternative to direct measures of body fat. A trained healthcare provider should perform appropriate health assessments in order to evaluate an individual's health status and risks.

Childhood Obesity Causes

Childhood obesity is a complex health issue. It occurs when a child is well above the normal or healthy weight for his or her age and height. The main causes of excess weight in youth are similar to those in adults, including individual causes such as behavior and genetics. Behaviors can include dietary patterns, physical activity, inactivity, medication use, and other exposures. Additional contributing factors in our society include the food and physical activity environment, education and skills, and food marketing and promotion.

Behavior

Healthy behaviors include a healthy diet pattern and regular physical activity. Energy balance of the number of calories consumed from foods and beverages with the number of calories the body uses for activity plays a role in preventing excess weight gain. A healthy diet pattern follows the *Dietary Guidelines for Americans* which emphasizes eating whole grains, fruits, vegetables, lean protein, low-fat and fat-free dairy products and drinking water. The *Physical Activity Guidelines for Americans* recommends children do at least 60 minutes of physical activity every day.

Having a healthy diet pattern and regular physical activity is also important for long term health benefits and prevention of chronic diseases such as Type 2 diabetes and heart disease.

411

Community Environment

American society has become characterized by environments that promote increased consumption of less healthy food and physical inactivity. It can be difficult for children to make healthy food choices and get enough physical activity when they are exposed to environments in their home, child care center, school, or community that are influenced by:

- Advertising of less healthy foods.

- Variation in licensure regulations among child care centers.

- No safe and appealing place, in many communities, to play or be active.

- Limited access to healthy affordable foods.

- Greater availability of high-energy-dense foods and sugar sweetened beverages.

- Increasing portion sizes.

- Lack of breastfeeding support.

Consequences of Obesity

Health Risks Now

- Obesity during childhood can have a harmful effect on the body in a variety of ways. Children who are obese have a greater risk of:

- High blood pressure and high cholesterol, which are risk factors for cardiovascular disease (CVD). In one study, 70% of obese children had at least one CVD risk factor, and 39% had two or more.

- Increased risk of impaired glucose tolerance, insulin resistance and type 2 diabetes.

- Breathing problems, such as sleep apnea, and asthma.

- Joint problems and musculoskeletal discomfort.

- Fatty liver disease, gallstones, and gastro-esophageal reflux (i.e., heartburn).

- Psychological stress such as depression, behavioral problems, and issues in school.

- Low self-esteem and low self-reported quality of life.

- Impaired social, physical, and emotional functioning.

Health Risks Later

- Children who are obese are more likely to become obese adults. Adult obesity is associated with a number of serious health conditions including heart disease, diabetes, metabolic syndrome, and cancer.

- If children are obese, obesity, and disease risk factors in adulthood are likely to be more severe.

Defining Adult Overweight and Obesity

Weight that is higher than what is considered as a healthy weight for a given height is described as overweight or obese. Body Mass Index, or BMI, is used as a screening tool for overweight or obesity.

Adult Body Mass Index (BMI)

Body mass index (BMI) is a person's weight in kilograms divided by the square of height in meters. A high BMI can be an indicator of high body fatness.

- If your BMI is less than 18.5, it falls within the underweight range.

- If your BMI is 18.5 to <25, it falls within the normal.

- If your BMI is 25.0 to <30, it falls within the overweight range.

- If your BMI is 30.0 or higher, it falls within the obese range.

Obesity is frequently subdivided into categories:

- Class 1: BMI of 30 to < 35

- Class 2: BMI of 35 to < 40

- Class 3: BMI of 40 or higher. Class 3 obesity is sometimes categorized as "extreme" or "severe" obesity.

Note: At an individual level, BMI can be used as a screening tool but is not diagnostic of the body fatness or the health of an individual. A trained healthcare provider should perform appropriate health assessments in order to evaluate an individual's health status and risks.

See the following table for an example.

Table 43.2. Weight Range and BMI

Height	Weight Range	BMI	Considered
5' 9"	124 lbs or less	Below 18.5	Underweight
	125 lbs to 168 lbs	18.5 to 24.9	Healthy weight
	169 lbs to 202 lbs	25.0 to 29.9	Overweight
	203 lbs or more	30 or higher	Obese
	271 lbs or more	40 or higher	Class 3 Obese

BMI does not measure body fat directly, but research has shown that BMI is moderately correlated with more direct measures of body fat obtained from skinfold thickness measurements, bioelectrical impedance, underwater weighing, dual energy X-ray absorptiometry (DXA) and other methods.

Furthermore, BMI appears to be strongly correlated with various adverse health outcomes consistent with these more direct measures of body fatness.

Adult Obesity Causes

Obesity is a complex health issue to address. Obesity results from a combination of causes and contributing factors, including individual factors such as behavior and genetics. Behaviors can include dietary patterns, physical activity, inactivity, medication use, and other exposures. Additional contributing factors in our society include the food and physical activity environment, education and skills, and food marketing and promotion.

Obesity is a serious concern because it is associated with poorer mental health outcomes, reduced quality of life, and the leading causes of death in the U.S. and worldwide, including diabetes, heart disease, stroke, and some types of cancer.

Behavior

Healthy behaviors include a healthy diet pattern and regular physical activity. Energy balance of the number of calories consumed from foods and beverages with the number of calories the body uses for activity plays a role in preventing excess weight gain.[1,2] A healthy diet pattern follows the *Dietary Guidelines for Americans* which emphasizes eating whole grains, fruits, vegetables, lean protein, low-fat and fat-free dairy products and drinking water. The *Physical Activity Guidelines for Americans* recommends adults do at least 150 minutes of moderate intensity activity or 75 minutes of vigorous intensity activity, or a combination of both, along with 2 days of strength training per week.

Having a healthy diet pattern and regular physical activity is also important for long term health benefits and prevention of chronic diseases such as Type 2 diabetes and heart disease.

Community Environment

People and families may make decisions based on their environment or community. For example, a person may choose not to walk or bike to the store or to work because of a lack of sidewalks or safe bike trails. Community, home, child care, school, healthcare, and workplace settings can all influence people's daily behaviors. Therefore, it is important to create environments in these locations that make it easier to engage in physical activity and eat a healthy diet.

Genetics

Do Genes Have a Role in Obesity?

Genetic changes in human populations occur too slowly to be responsible for the obesity epidemic. Nevertheless, the variation in how people respond to the environment that promotes physical inactivity and intake of high-calorie foods suggests that genes do play a role in the development of obesity.

How Could Genes Influence Obesity?

Genes give the body instructions for responding to changes in its environment. Studies have identified variants in several genes that may contribute to obesity by increasing hunger and food intake.

Rarely, a clear pattern of inherited obesity within a family is caused by a specific variant of a single gene (monogenic obesity). Most obesity, however, probably results from complex interactions among multiple genes and environmental factors that remain poorly understood (multifactorial obesity).

What about Family History?

Healthcare practitioners routinely collect family health history to help identify people at high risk of obesity-related diseases such as diabetes, cardiovascular diseases, and some forms of cancer. Family health history reflects the effects of shared genetics and environment among close relatives. Families can't change their genes but they can change the family environment to encourage healthy eating habits and physical activity. Those changes can improve the health of family members—and improve the family health history of the next generation.

Other Factors: Diseases and Drugs

Some illnesses may lead to obesity or weight gain. These may include Cushing's disease, and polycystic ovary syndrome. Drugs such as steroids and some antidepressants may also cause weight gain. The science continues to emerge on the role of other factors in energy balance and weight gain such as chemical exposures and the role of the microbiome.

A healthcare provider can help you learn more about your health habits and history in order to tell you whether behaviors, illnesses, medications, and/or psychological factors are contributing to weight gain or making weight loss hard.

Consequences of Obesity

Health Consequences

People who are obese, compared to those with a normal or healthy weight, are at increased risk for many serious diseases and health conditions, including the following:

- Body pain and difficulty with physical functioning
- Osteoarthritis (a breakdown of cartilage and bone within a joint)
- High blood pressure (Hypertension)
- High LDL cholesterol, low HDL cholesterol, or high levels of triglycerides (Dyslipidemia)
- Type 2 diabetes
- Coronary heart disease
- Stroke
- Gallbladder disease
- Sleep apnea and breathing problems
- Some cancers (endometrial, breast, colon, kidney, gallbladder, and liver)

- Low quality of life

- Mental illness such as clinical depression, anxiety, and other mental disorders

- All-causes of death (mortality)

Economic and Societal Consequences

Obesity and its associated health problems have a significant economic impact on the U.S. healthcare system. Medical costs associated with overweight and obesity may involve direct and indirect costs. Direct medical costs may include preventive, diagnostic, and treatment services related to obesity. Indirect costs relate to morbidity and mortality costs including productivity. Productivity measures include 'absenteeism' (costs due to employees being absent from work for obesity-related health reasons) and 'presenteeism' (decreased productivity of employees while at work) as well as premature mortality and disability.

Section 43.2

Physical Fitness at Any Size

This section includes text excerpted from "Staying Active at Any Size," National Institute of Diabetes and Digestive and Kidney Diseases (NIDDK), July 30, 2016.

Physical activity may seem hard if you're overweight. You may get short of breath or tired quickly. Finding or affording the right clothes and equipment may be frustrating. Or, perhaps you may not feel comfortable working out in front of others.

The good news is you can overcome these challenges. Not only can you be active at any size, you can have fun and feel good at the same time.

Can Anyone Be Active?

Research strongly shows that physical activity is safe for almost everyone. The health benefits of physical activity far outweigh the risks.

The activities discussed here are safe for most people. If you have problems moving or staying steady on your feet, or if you get out of breath easily, talk with a healthcare professional before you start. You also should talk with a healthcare professional if you are unsure of your health, have any concerns that physical activity may be unsafe for you, or have:

- a chronic disease such as diabetes, high blood pressure, or heart disease

- a bone or joint problem—for example, in your back, knee, or hip—that could get worse if you change your physical activity level

Why Should I Be Active?

Being active may help you live longer and protect you from developing serious health problems, such as type 2 diabetes, heart disease, stroke, and certain types of cancer. Regular physical activity is linked to many health benefits, such as:

- lower blood pressure and blood glucose, or blood sugar

- healthy bones, muscles, and joints

- a strong heart and lungs

- better sleep at night and improved mood

The *Physical Activity Guidelines for Americans* define regular physical activity as at least 2½ hours a week of moderate-intensity activity, such as brisk walking. Brisk walking is a pace of 3 miles per hour or faster. A moderate-intensity activity makes you breathe harder but does not overwork or overheat you.

You may reach this goal by starting with 10 minutes of activity 3 days per week, and working up to 30 minutes a day 5 days a week. If you do even more activity, you may gain even more health benefits.

When combined with healthy eating, regular physical activity may also help you control your weight. However, research shows that even if you can't lose weight or maintain your weight loss, you still can enjoy important health benefits from regular physical activity.

Physical activity also can be a lot of fun if you do activities you enjoy and are active with other people. Being active with others may give you a chance to meet new people or spend more time with family and friends. You also may inspire and motivate one another to get and stay active.

What Do I Need to Know about Becoming Active?

Choosing physical activities that match your fitness level and health goals can help you stay motivated and keep you from getting hurt. You may feel some minor discomfort or muscle soreness when you first become active. These feelings should go away as you get used to your activity. However, if you feel sick to your stomach or have pain, you may have done too much. Go easier and then slowly build up your activity level. Some activities, such as walking or water workouts, are less likely to cause injuries.

If you have been inactive, start slowly and see how you feel. Gradually increase how long and how often you are active. If you need guidance, check with a healthcare or certified fitness professional.

Here are some tips for staying safe during physical activity:

- Wear the proper safety gear, such as a bike helmet if you are bicycling.

- Make sure any sports equipment you use works and fits properly.

- Look for safe places to be active. For instance, walk in well-lit areas where other people are around. Be active with a friend or group.

- Stay hydrated to replace the body fluids you lose through sweating and to prevent you from getting overheated.

- If you are active outdoors, protect yourself from the sun with sunscreen and a hat or protective visor and clothing.

- Wear enough clothing to keep warm in cold or windy weather. Layers are best.

If you don't feel right, stop your activity. If you have any of the following warning signs, stop and seek help right away:

- pain, tightness, or pressure in your chest or neck, shoulder, or arm

- extreme shortness of breath

- dizziness or sickness

Check with a healthcare professional about what to do if you have any of these warning signs. If your activity is causing pain in your joints, feet, ankles, or legs, you also should consult a healthcare professional to see if you may need to change the type or amount of activity you are doing.

419

What Kinds of Activities Can I Do?

You don't need to be an athlete or have special skills or equipment to make physical activity part of your life. Many types of activities you do every day, such as walking your dog or going up and down steps at home or at work, may help improve your health.

Try different activities you enjoy. If you like an activity, you're more likely to stick with it. Anything that gets you moving around, even for a few minutes at a time, is a healthy start to getting fit.

Walking

Walking is free and easy to do—and you can do it almost anywhere. Walking will help you:

- burn calories

- improve your fitness

- lift your mood

- strengthen your bones and muscles

If you are concerned about safety, try walking in a shopping mall or park where it is well lit and other people are around. Many malls and parks have benches where you can take a quick break. Walking with a friend or family member is safer than walking alone and may provide the social support you need to meet your activity goals.

If you don't have time for a long walk, take several short walks instead. For example, instead of a 30-minute walk, add three 10-minute walks to your day. Shorter spurts of activity are easier to fit into a busy schedule.

Walking tips

- Wear comfortable, well-fitting walking shoes with a lot of support, and socks that absorb sweat.

- Dress for the weather if you are walking outdoors. In cold weather, wear layers of clothing you can remove if you start getting too warm. In hot weather, protect yourself against the sun and heat.

- Warm up by walking more slowly for the first few minutes. Cool down by slowing your pace.

Dancing

Dancing can be a lot of fun while it tones your muscles, strengthens your heart and lungs, and boosts your mood. You can dance at a health club, dance studio, or even at home. Just turn on some lively music and start moving. You also can dance to a video on your TV or computer.

If you have trouble standing on your feet for a long time, try dancing while sitting down. Chair dancing lets you move your arms and legs to music while taking the weight off your feet.

Bicycling

Riding a bicycle spreads your weight among your arms, back, and hips. For outdoor biking, you may want to try a mountain bike. Mountain bikes have wider tires and are sturdier than bikes with thinner tires. You can buy a larger seat to make biking more comfortable.

For indoor biking, you may want to try a recumbent bike. On this type of bike, you sit lower to the ground with your legs reaching forward to the pedals. Your body is in more of a reclining position, which may feel better than sitting straight up. The seat on a recumbent bike is also wider than the seat on a regular bike.

If you decide to buy a bike, check how much weight it can support to make sure it is safe for you.

Workout clothing tips

- Clothes made of fabrics that absorb sweat are best for working out.

- Comfortable, lightweight clothes allow you to move more easily.

- Tights or spandex shorts are the best bottoms to wear to prevent inner-thigh chafing.

- Women should wear a bra that provides extra support during physical activity.

Water Workouts

Swimming and water workouts put less stress on your joints than walking, dancing, or biking. If your feet, back, or joints hurt when you stand, water activities may be best for you. If you feel self-conscious about wearing a bathing suit, you can wear shorts and a T-shirt while you swim.

Exercising in water

- lets you be more flexible. You can move your body in water in ways you may not be able to on land.

- reduces your risk of hurting yourself. Water provides a natural cushion, which keeps you from pounding or jarring your joints.

- helps prevent sore muscles.

- keeps you cool, even when you are working hard.

You don't need to know how to swim to work out in water. You can do shallow- or deep-water exercises at either end of the pool without swimming. For instance, you can do laps while holding onto a kickboard and kicking your feet. You also can walk or jog across the width of the pool while moving your arms.

For shallow-water workouts, the water level should be between your waist and chest. During deep-water workouts, most of your body is underwater. For safety and comfort, wear a foam belt or life jacket.

Tips for protecting your hair

If you're worried that pool water will damage or mess up your hair, try these tips:

- Use a swim cap to help protect your hair from pool chemicals and getting wet.

- Wear a natural hairstyle, short braids, locs, or twists, which may be easier to style after a water workout.

- Buy a shampoo to remove chlorine buildup, available at most drug stores, if your hair feels dry or damaged after a pool workout.

Strength Training

Strength training involves using free weights, weightlifting machines, resistance bands, or your own body weight to make your muscles stronger. Lower-body strength training will improve your balance and prevent falls.

Strength training may help you:

- build and maintain strong muscles as you get older

- continue to perform activities of daily living, such as carrying groceries or moving furniture

- keep your bones strong, which may help prevent osteoporosis and fractures

If you are just starting out, using a weightlifting machine may be safer than dumbbells. As you get fit, you may want to add free-weight exercises with dumbbells.

You do not need a weight bench or large dumbbells to do strength training at home. You can use a pair of hand weights to do bicep curls. You can also use your own body weight: for example, get up and down from a chair.

Proper form is very important when lifting weights. You may hurt yourself if you don't lift weights properly. You may want to schedule a session with a certified fitness professional to learn which exercises to do and how to do them safely. Check with your health insurer about whether your health plan covers these services.

If you decide to buy a home gym, check how much weight it can support to make sure it is safe for you.

Strength-training tips

If you're worried that pool water will damage or mess up your hair, try these tips:

- Aim for 2 to 3 days per week of strength-training activities.

- Try to perform each exercise 8 to 12 times. If that's too hard, the weight you are lifting is too heavy. If it's too easy, your weight is too light.

- Try to exercise all the major muscle groups. These groups include the muscles of the legs, hips, chest, back, abdomen, shoulders, and arms.

- Don't work the same muscles 2 days in a row. Your muscles need time to recover.

Mind and Body Exercise

Your local hospital or fitness, recreation, or community center may offer classes such as yoga, tai chi, or Pilates. You also may find some of these workouts online and can download them to a computer, smartphone, or other device. These types of activities may help you:

- become stronger and more flexible

- feel more relaxed

- improve balance and posture

These classes also can be a lot of fun and add variety to your workout routine. If some movements are hard to do or you have injuries you are concerned about, talk with the instructor about how to adapt the exercises and poses to meet your needs—or start with a beginner's class.

Daily Life Activities

Daily life activities, such as cleaning out the attic or washing the car, are great ways to get moving. Small changes can add more physical activity to your day and improve your health. Try these:

- Take 2- to 3-minute walking breaks at work several times a day, if possible.

- Stand, walk, or stretch in place during TV commercials.

- Take the stairs instead of the elevator or escalator whenever you can.

- Park farther from where you are going and walk the rest of the way.

Even a shopping trip can be exercise because it provides a chance to walk and carry your bags. Chores such as mowing the lawn, raking leaves, and gardening also count.

Where Can I Be Active?

You can find many fun places to be active. Having more than one place may keep you from getting bored. Here are some options:

- Join or take a class at a local fitness, recreation, or community center.

- Enjoy the outdoors by taking a hike or going for a walk in a safe local park, neighborhood, or mall.

- Work out in the comfort of your own home with a workout video or by finding a fitness channel on your TV, tablet, or other mobile device.

Tips for choosing a fitness center

If you're worried that pool water will damage or mess up your hair, try these tips:

- Make sure the center has exercise equipment for people who weigh more and staff to show you how to use it.

- Ask if the center has any special classes for people just starting out, older adults, or people with mobility or health issues.

- See if you can try out the center or take a class before you join.

- Try to find a center close to work or home. The quicker and easier the center is to get to, the better your chances of using it often.

- Make sure you understand the rules for joining and ending your membership, what your membership fee covers, any related costs, and the days and hours of operation.

How Can I Get past My Roadblocks?

You most likely will face roadblocks that keep you from meeting your physical activity goals. Think about what keeps you from being active, then try to come up with creative ways to address those roadblocks. Here are a few examples to help you get started:

Table 43.3. Barrier and Solution

Barrier	Solution
I don't have enough time.	Instead of doing one long workout session, build in three 10-minute bursts of activity during your day, such as a brisk walk. Even standing up instead of sitting at your desk has benefits.
I just don't like exercise.	Good news! You don't have to run a marathon or go to the gym all the time to benefit from being active. To make physical activity more fun, try something you enjoy doing, such as dancing to the radio or taking a yoga class with friends. Many people find they start to like exercise better the more they do it.
I'm worried about my health or getting hurt.	If you have a hard time being active because of your health, talk with a healthcare professional first. A certified fitness professional can also guide you on how to be active safely.
I feel self-conscious working out in front of others.	Start being active at home until you feel more confident. Be active with friends who will support and encourage you.

How Can I Stick with My Physical Activity Plan?

Sticking with a plan to be physically active can be a challenge. Online tools such as the SuperTracker and the NIH Bodyweight Planner can help. The SuperTracker is a free, online physical activity-, food-, and weight-tracking tool. The NIH Bodyweight Planner, part of the SuperTracker, lets you make personalized calorie and physical activity plans to reach specific goals within a specific time period.

You also can download fitness apps that let you enter information to track your progress using a computer or smart phone or other mobile device.

Devices you can wear, such as pedometers and fitness trackers, may help you count steps, calories, and minutes of physical activity. Trackers can help you set goals and monitor progress. You wear most of these devices on your wrist like a watch, or clipped to your clothing.

Keeping an activity journal is another good way to help you stay motivated and on track to reach your fitness goals.

Set goals. As you track your activity, try to set specific short- and long-term goals. For example, instead of "I will be more active," set a goal such as "I will take a walk after lunch at least 2 days a week." Getting started with a doable goal is a good way to form a new habit. A short-term goal may be to walk 5 to 10 minutes, 5 days a week. A long-term goal may be to do at least 30 minutes of moderate-intensity physical activity on most days of the week.

Get support. Ask a family member or friend to be active with you. Your workout buddy can help make your activities more fun and can cheer you on and help you meet your goals.

Track progress. You may not feel as though you are making progress, but when you look back at where you started, you may be pleasantly surprised. Making regular activity part of your life is a big step. Start slowly and praise yourself for every goal you set and achieve.

Review your goals. Did you meet your goals? If not, why? Are they doable? Did you hit a roadblock trying to meet your goal? What will you do differently next week? Brainstorm some options to overcome future roadblocks. Ask a friend or family member to help support your goals.

Pick nonfood rewards. Whether your goal is to be active 15 minutes a day, to walk farther than you did last week, or simply to stay positive, recognizing your efforts is an important part of staying on track. Decide how you will reward yourself. Some ideas for rewards include getting new music to charge you up or buying new workout gear.

Be patient with yourself. Don't get discouraged if you have setbacks from time to time. If you can't achieve your goal the first time or can only stick to your goals for part of the week, remind yourself that this is all part of establishing new habits.

Look ahead. Try to focus on what you will do differently moving forward, rather than on what went wrong. Pat yourself on the back for trying.

Most importantly, don't give up. Any movement, even for a short time, is a good thing. Each activity you add to your life is another step toward a healthier you.

Section 43.3

Weight-Loss and Weight Training Myths

This section includes text excerpted from "Weight-Loss and Nutrition Myths," National Institute of Diabetes and Digestive and Kidney Diseases (NIDDK), October 2014.

Weight-Loss and Diet Myths

Myth: Fad diets will help me lose weight and keep it off.

Fact: Fad diets are not the best way to lose weight and keep it off. These diets often promise quick weight loss if you strictly reduce what you eat or avoid some types of foods. Some of these diets may help you lose weight at first. But these diets are hard to follow. Most people quickly get tired of them and regain any lost weight.

Fad diets may be unhealthy. They may not provide all of the nutrients your body needs. Also, losing more than 3 pounds a week after the first few weeks may increase your chances of developing gallstones (solid matter in the gallbladder that can cause pain). Being on a diet of fewer than 800 calories a day for a long time may lead to serious heart problems.

TIP: Research suggests that safe weight loss involves combining a reduced-calorie diet with physical activity to lose 1/2 to 2 pounds a week (after the first few weeks of weight loss). Make healthy food choices. Eat small portions. Build exercise into your daily life. Combined, these habits may be a healthy way to lose weight and keep it off. These habits may also lower your chances of developing heart disease, high blood pressure, and type 2 diabetes.

Myth: Grain products such as bread, pasta, and rice are fattening. I should avoid them when trying to lose weight.

Fact: A grain product is any food made from wheat, rice, oats, cornmeal, barley, or another cereal grain. Grains are divided into two subgroups, whole grains and refined grains. Whole grains contain the entire grain kernel—the bran, germ, and endosperm. Examples include brown rice and whole-wheat bread, cereal, and pasta. Refined grains have been milled, a process that removes the bran and germ. This is done to give grains a finer texture and improve their shelf life, but it also removes dietary fiber, iron, and many B vitamins.

People who eat whole grains as part of a healthy diet may lower their chances of developing some chronic diseases. Government dietary guidelines advise making half your grains whole grains. For example, choose 100 percent whole-wheat bread instead of white bread, and brown rice instead of white rice.

TIP: To lose weight, reduce the number of calories you take in and increase the amount of physical activity you do each day. Create and follow a healthy eating plan that replaces less healthy options with a mix of fruits, veggies, whole grains, protein foods, and low-fat dairy:

- Eat a mix of fat-free or low-fat milk and milk products, fruits, veggies, and whole grains.

- Limit added sugars, cholesterol, salt (sodium), and saturated fat.

- Eat low-fat protein: beans, eggs, fish, lean meats, nuts, and poultry.

Physical Activity Myths

Myth: Lifting weights is not a good way to lose weight because it will make me "bulk up."

Fact: Lifting weights or doing activities like push-ups and crunches on a regular basis can help you build strong muscles, which can help you burn more calories. To strengthen muscles, you can lift weights, use large rubber bands (resistance bands), do push-ups or sit-ups, or do household or yard tasks that make you lift or dig. Doing strengthening activities 2 or 3 days a week will not "bulk you up." Only intense strength training, along with certain genetics, can build large muscles.

TIP: Government guidelines for physical activity recommend that adults should do activities at least two times a week to strengthen muscles. The guidelines also suggest that adults should get 150 to 300 minutes of moderately intense or vigorous aerobic activity each week—like brisk walking or biking. Aerobic activity makes you sweat and breathe faster.

For more on the benefits of physical activity and tips on how to be more active, check out the Government's guidelines for physical activity.

Myth: Physical activity only counts if I can do it for long periods of time.

Fact: You do not need to be active for long periods to achieve your 150 to 300 minutes of activity each week. Experts advise doing aerobic activity for periods of 10 minutes or longer at a time. You can spread these sessions out over the week.

TIP: Plan to do at least 10 minutes of physical activity three times a day on 5 or more days a week. This will help you meet the 150-minute goal. While at work, take a brief walking break. Use the stairs. Get off the bus one stop early. Go dancing with friends. Whether for a short or long period, bursts of activity may add up to the total amount of physical activity you need each week.

Don't Just Sit There!

Americans spend a lot of time sitting in front of computers, desks, hand-held devices, and TVs. Break up your day by moving around more and getting regular aerobic activity that makes you sweat and breathe faster.

- **Get 150 to 300 minutes of moderately intense or vigorous physical activity each week.** Basketball, brisk walks, hikes, hula hoops, runs, soccer, tennis—choose whatever you enjoy best! Even 10 minutes of activity at a time can add up over the week.

- **Strengthen your muscles at least twice a week.** Do push-ups or pull-ups, lift weights, do heavy gardening, or work with rubber resistance bands.

Chapter 44

Physical Fitness for People with Heart Conditions

Physical Activity: The Heart Connection[1]

Chances are, you already know that physical activity is good for you. "Sure," you may say, "When I get out and move around, I know it helps me to look and feel better." But you may not realize just how important regular physical activity is to your health. Inactive people are nearly twice as likely to develop heart disease as those who are active. Lack of physical activity also leads to more visits to the doctor, more hospitalizations, and more use of medicines for a variety of illnesses.

The good news is that physical activity can protect your heart in a number of important ways and keep you healthy overall.

Physical Activity Reduces Coronary Heart Disease Risk Factors[2]

When done regularly, moderate- and vigorous-intensity aerobic activity can lower your risk for CHD. CHD is a condition in which a

This chapter includes text excerpted from documents published by two public domain sources. Text under headings marked 1 are excerpted from "In Brief: Your Guide to Physical Activity and Your Heart," National Heart, Lung, and Blood Institute (NHLBI), January 2008. Reviewed September 2016; text under headings marked 2 are excerpted from "Benefits of Physical Activity," National Heart, Lung, and Blood Institute (NHLBI), June 22, 2016.

waxy substance called plaque builds up inside your coronary arteries. These arteries supply your heart muscle with oxygen-rich blood.

Plaque narrows the arteries and reduces blood flow to your heart muscle. Eventually, an area of plaque can rupture (break open). This causes a blood clot to form on the surface of the plaque.

If the clot becomes large enough, it can mostly or completely block blood flow through a coronary artery. Blocked blood flow to the heart muscle causes a heart attack.

Certain traits, conditions, or habits may raise your risk for CHD. Physical activity can help control some of these risk factors because it:

- Can lower blood pressure and triglyceride. Triglycerides are a type of fat in the blood.

- Can raise cholesterol levels. HDL sometimes is called "good" cholesterol.

- Helps your body manage blood sugar and insulin levels, which lowers your risk for type 2 diabetes.

- Reduces levels of C-reactive protein (CRP) in your body. This protein is a sign of inflammation. High levels of CRP may suggest an increased risk for CHD.

- Helps reduce overweight and obesity when combined with a reduced-calorie diet. Physical activity also helps you maintain a healthy weight over time once you have lost weight.

- May help you quit smoking. Smoking is a major risk factor for CHD.

Physical Activity Reduces Heart Attack Risk[2]

For people who have CHD, aerobic activity done regularly helps the heart work better. It also may reduce the risk of a second heart attack in people who already have had heart attacks.

Vigorous aerobic activity may not be safe for people who have CHD. Ask your doctor what types of activity are safe for you.

The Benefits Keep Coming[1]

In addition to protecting your heart, staying active has other effects:

- May help to prevent cancers of the breast, uterus, and colon

- Strengthens your lungs and helps them to work more efficiently

- Tones and strengthens your muscles
- Builds your stamina
- Keeps your joints in good condition
- Improves your balance
- May slow bone loss

Regular physical activity can also boost the way you feel in these ways:

- Give you more energy
- Help you to relax, cope better with stress, and beat the blues
- Build your confidence
- Allow you to fall asleep more quickly and sleep more soundly
- Provide you with an enjoyable way to share time with friends or family

Physical Activity: The Calorie Connection[1]

One way that regular physical activity protects against heart disease is by burning extra calories, which can help you to lose excess weight or stay at your healthy weight. To understand how physical activity affects calories, it's helpful to consider the concept of "energy balance." Energy balance is the amount of calories you take in relative to the amount of calories you burn. If you need to lose weight for your health, eating fewer calories and being more active is the best approach. You're more likely to be successful by combining a healthful, lower calorie diet with physical activity. For example, a 200-pound person who consumes 250 fewer calories per day and walks briskly each day for 1 1/2 miles will lose about 40 pounds in one year. Most of the energy you burn each day—about three-quarters of it—goes to activities that your body automatically engages in for survival, such as breathing, sleeping, and digesting food. The part of your energy output that you control is daily physical activity. Any activity you take part in beyond your body's automatic activities will burn extra calories.

Even seated activities, such as using the computer or watching TV, will burn calories—but only a very small number. That's why it's important to make time each day for moderate-to vigorous-intensity physical activity.

If you are just starting or significantly increasing your physical activity, take proper precautions and check with your doctor first.

Great Moves[1]

Given the numerous benefits of regular physical activity, you may be ready to get in motion! Three types of activity are important for a complete physical activity program: aerobic activity, resistance training, and flexibility exercises.

Aerobic activity is any physical activity that uses large muscle groups and causes your body to use more oxygen than it would while resting. Aerobic activity is the type of movement that most benefits the heart.

Examples of aerobic activity are brisk walking, jogging, and bicycling.

If you're just starting to be active, try brisk walking for short periods such as 5 or 10 minutes, and build up gradually to 30 to 60 minutes at least five days per week. Always start with a 5-minute, slower paced walk to warm up, and end with a 5-minute, slower paced walk to cool down.

Resistance training—also called strength training—can firm, strengthen, and tone your muscles, as well as improve bone strength, balance, and coordination. Examples of resistance training are pushups, lunges, and bicep curls using dumbbells.

Flexibility exercises stretch and lengthen your muscles. These activities help improve joint flexibility and keep muscles limber, thereby preventing injury. An example of a flexibility exercise is sitting crosslegged on the floor and gently pushing down on the tops of your legs to stretch the inner-thigh muscles.

Family Fitness[1]

When it comes to getting in shape, what's good for you is good for your whole family. Children and teenagers should be physically active for at least 60 minutes per day. A great way to pry kids off the couch—and help you to stay fit as well—is to do enjoyable activities together.

Some ideas include the following:

- Kick up your heels. Take turns picking out your favorite music, and dance up a storm in the living room.

- Explore the outdoors. Hit your local trail on weekends for some biking or hiking. Pack a healthy lunch, and let the kids choose the picnic spot.

- Get classy. Join family members in an active class, such as martial arts, yoga, or aerobics.

- Play pupil. Ask one of your children or grandchildren to teach you an active game or sport. Kids love to be the experts, and you'll get a work out learning a new activity!

- Use online resources. You'll find more family-friendly ideas for making smart food choices, increasing physical activity, and reducing "screen time" in front of the TV and other electronic attractions.

Creating Opportunities[1]

It's easier to stay physically active over time if you take advantage of everyday opportunities to move around.

- Use the stairs—both up and down—instead of the elevator.

- Start with one flight of stairs and gradually build up to more.

- Park a few blocks from the office or store and walk the rest of the way. If you take public transportation, get off a stop or two early and walk a few blocks.

- While working, take frequent activity breaks. Get up and stretch, walk around, and give your muscles and mind a chance to relax.

- Instead of eating that extra snack, take a brisk stroll around the neighborhood or your office building.

- Do housework, gardening, or yard work at a more vigorous pace.

- When you travel, walk around the train station, bus station, or airport rather than sitting and waiting.

Chapter 45

Physical Fitness for People with Bone Disorders

Chapter Contents

Section 45.1

Arthritis and Fitness

This section includes text excerpted from "Physical
Activity for Arthritis," Centers for Disease Control and
Prevention (CDC), April 11, 2016.

Physical Activity: The Arthritis Pain Reliever

Long gone are the days when healthcare providers told people with
arthritis to "rest their joints." In fact, physical activity can reduce
pain and improve function, mobility, mood, and quality of life for
most adults with many types of arthritis including osteoarthritis,
rheumatoid arthritis, fibromyalgia, and lupus. Physical activity can
also help people with arthritis manage other chronic conditions such
as diabetes, heart disease, and obesity. Most people with arthritis
can safely participate in a self-directed physical activity program or
join one of many proven programs available in communities across
the country. Some people may benefit from physical or occupational
therapy.

What Are the Benefits of Physical Activity for Adults with Arthritis?

Regular physical activity is just as important for people with arthritis or other rheumatic conditions as it is for all children and adults.
Scientific studies have shown that participation in moderate-intensity,
low-impact physical activity improves pain, function, mood, and quality of life without worsening symptoms or disease severity. Being physically active can also delay the onset of disability if you have arthritis.
But people with arthritis may have a difficult time being physically
active because of symptoms (e.g., pain, stiffness), their lack of confidence in knowing how much and what to do, and unclear expectations
of when they will see benefits. Both aerobic and muscle strengthening
activities are proven to work well, and both are recommended for
people with arthritis.

Physical Activity Guidelines for Americans

Adults with arthritis should follow guidelines that meets your personal health goals and matches your abilities. People with arthritis should also include daily flexibility exercises to maintain proper joint range of motion and do balance exercises if they are at risk of falling.

What Type of Activities Count?

Aerobic Activities

Aerobic activity is also called "cardio," endurance, or conditioning exercise. It is any activity that makes your heart beat faster and makes you breathe a little harder than when you are sitting, standing or lying. You want to do activity that is moderate or vigorous intensity and that does not twist or "pound" your joints too much. Some people with arthritis can do vigorous activities such as running and can even tolerate some activities that are harder on the joints like basketball or tennis. You should choose the activities that are right for you and that are enjoyable. Remember, each person is different, but there are a wide variety of activities that you can do to meet the Guidelines.

Table 45.1. Examples of Moderate and Vigorous Intensity Aerobic Activities

Moderate Intensity	Vigorous Intensity
• Brisk Walking. • Bicycling. • Swimming. • Mowing the grass, heavy yard work. • Doubles tennis. • Social dancing. • Conditioning Machines (e.g., stair climbers, elliptical, stationary bike). • Tai Chi, yoga. • Sports (e.g., softball, baseball, volleyball). • Skiing, roller and ice skating.	• Jogging/running. • Singles tennis. • Swimming. • Jumping rope. • Conditioning Machines (e.g., stair climbers, elliptical, stationary bike). • Sports (e.g., soccer, basketball, football, racquetball). • Aerobic dance or spinning classes.

Muscle Strengthening Activities

You should do activities that strengthen your muscles at least 2 days per week in addition to your aerobic activities. Muscle

439

strengthening activities are especially important for people with arthritis because having strong muscles takes some of the pressure off the joints.

You can do muscle strengthening exercises in your home, at a gym, or at a community center. You should do exercises that work all the major muscle groups of the body (e.g., legs, hips, back, abdomen, chest, shoulders, and arms). You should do at least 1 set of 8–12 repetitions for each muscle group. There are many ways you can do muscle strengthening activities:

- Lifting weights using machines, dumbbells, or weight cuffs.
- Working with resistance bands.
- Using your own bodyweight as resistance (e.g., push-ups, sit ups).
- Heavy gardening (e.g., digging, shoveling).
- Some group exercise classes.
- Muscle strengthening exercise videos.

Balance Activities

Many older adults and some adults with arthritis and other chronic diseases may be prone to falling. If you are worried about falling or are at risk of falling, you should include activities that improve balance at least 3 days per week as part of your activity plan. Balance activities can be part of your aerobic or your muscle strengthening activities. Examples of activities that improve balance include the following

- Tai Chi.
- Backward walking, side stepping, heel and toe walking.
- Standing on 1 foot.
- Some group exercise classes.

Additional Recommendations for People with Arthritis

Stay flexible. In addition to the activities recommended above, flexibility exercises are also important. Many people with arthritis have joint stiffness that makes daily tasks such as bathing and fixing meals difficult. Doing daily flexibility exercises for all upper (e.g., neck, shoulder, elbow, wrist, and finger) and lower (e.g., low back, hip, knee, ankle, and toes) joints of the body helps maintain essential range of motion.

More information for Older Adults

If you have arthritis, you should follow either the Active Adult or Active Older Adult recommendations, whichever meets your personal health goals and matches your abilities. You should do this activity in addition to your usual daily activity. You may notice that the recommended amount and type of activity are the same for the Active Adult and Active Older Adult except for the additional recommendation to include activities that promote balance. Read some additional details for the Active Older Adult below:

Prevent falls. Have you fallen in the past? Do you have trouble walking? If so, you may be at high risk of falling. Activities that improve or maintain balance should be included in your physical activity plan. Examples of activities that have been proven to help balance include walking backwards, standing on one leg, and Tai Chi. Some exercise classes offered in many local communities include exercises that are good for balance.

Stay active. Any physical activity is better than none. If you cannot do 150 minutes of moderate intensity activity every week, it is important to be as active as your health allows. People with arthritis often have symptoms that come and go. This may mean that one week you can do 150 minutes of moderate intensity activity and the next week you can't. You may have to change your activity level depending on your arthritis symptoms, but try to stay as active as your symptoms allow. Learn how to modify your activity with these tips for S.M.A.R.T. activity.

Adjust the level of effort. Some activities take more effort for older adults and those with low fitness or poor function. For example, walking at a brisk pace for a 23-year-old healthy male is moderate intensity, but the same activity may be vigorous activity for a 77-year-old male with diabetes. You should adjust the level of effort during activity so that it is comfortable for you. Find out how to measure your level of effort.

Talk to your doctor. If you have arthritis or another chronic health condition, you should already be under the care of a doctor or other healthcare provider. Healthcare providers and certified exercise professionals can answer your questions about how much and what types of activity are right for you.

How Hard Are You Working?

Moderate intensity activity makes your heart beat a little faster and you breathe a little harder. You can talk easily while doing moderate intensity activity, but you may not be able to sing comfortably.

Vigorous intensity activity makes your heart beat much faster and you may not be able to talk comfortably without stopping to catch your breath.

Relative intensity can be estimated using a scale of 0 to 10 where sitting is 0 and 10 is the highest level of effort possible. Moderate intensity activity is a 5 or 6 and vigorous intensity activity is a 7 or 8.

The **talk test** is a simple way to measure relative intensity. In general, if you're doing moderate-intensity activity you can talk, but not sing, during the activity. If you are doing vigorous-intensity activity, you will not be able to say more than a few words without pausing for a breath.

Tips for Starting and Maintaining a Physical Activity Program If You Have Arthritis

Safe, enjoyable physical activity is possible for most every adult with arthritis. The most important thing to remember is to find out what works best for you. At first glance, 150 minutes of activity per week sounds like a lot, but if you pay attention to the following tips you will be well on your way to getting the recommended amount of activity in no time!

Studies show that some increase in pain, stiffness, and swelling is normal when starting an activity program. If you have increased swelling or pain that does not get better with rest then talk to your healthcare provider. It may take 6–8 weeks for your joints to accommodate to your increased activity level, but sticking with your activity program will result in long-term pain relief.

Here is an easy way to remember these tips: Make **S.M.A.R.T** choices!

Start Low, and Go Slow

Many adults with arthritis are inactive, even though their doctor may have told them being active will help their arthritis. You may want to be more active but just don't know where to start or how much to do. You may be worried that using your joints and muscles may make your arthritis worse. The good news is that the opposite is true, physical activity will help your arthritis! The first key to starting activity safely is to start low. This may mean you can only walk 5 minutes at a time every other day. The second key is to go slow. People with arthritis may take more time for their body to adjust to a new level of activity. For example, healthy children can usually increase the amount of activity a little each week, while older adults and those with chronic conditions may take 3–4 weeks to adjust to a new activity level. You should add activity in small amounts, at least 10 minutes at a time, and allow enough time for your body to adjust to the new level before adding more activity.

Modify Activity as Needed

Remember, any activity is better than none. Your arthritis symptoms, such as pain, stiffness and fatigue, may come and go and you may have good days and bad days. You may want to stop activity completely when your arthritis symptoms increase. It is important that you first try to modify your activity to stay as active as possible without making your symptoms worse. Here are some ways you can do this:

If you currently do some activity or feel confident that you can safely plan your own activity program, you should look for safe places to be physically active. For example, if you walk in your neighborhood or a local park make sure the sidewalks or pathways are level and free of obstructions, are well-lighted, and are separated from heavy traffic.

Talk to a Health Professional

You should already be under the care of a healthcare professional for your arthritis, who is a good source of information about physical activity. Healthcare professionals and certified exercise professionals can answer your questions about how much and what types of activity match your abilities and health goals.

What Should I Do If I Have Pain When I Exercise?

Some soreness or aching in joints and surrounding muscles during and after exercise is normal for people with arthritis. This is especially true in the first 4 to 6 weeks of starting an exercise program. However, most people with arthritis find if they stick with exercise they will have significant long-term pain relief. Here are some tips to help you manage pain during and after exercise:

- Modify your exercise program by reducing the frequency (days per week) or duration (amount of time each session) until pain improves.

- Changing the type of exercise to reduce impact on the joints—for example switch from walking to water aerobics.

- Do proper warm-up and cool-down before and after exercise.

- Exercise at a comfortable pace—you should be able to carry on a conversation while exercising.

- Make sure you have good fitting, comfortable shoes.

Signs you should see your healthcare provider:

- Pain is sharp, stabbing, and constant.

- Pain that causes you to limp.

- Pain that lasts more than 2 hours after exercise or gets worse at night.

- Pain is not relieved by rest, medication, or hot/cold packs.

- Large increases in swelling or your joints feel "hot" or are red.

Section 45.2

Exercising Safely with Osteoporosis

This section contains text excerpted from the following sources: Text under the heading "Exercise and Osteoporosis" is excerpted from "Exercise and Osteoporosis," Go4Life, National Institute on Aging (NIA), March 27, 2015; Text beginning with the heading "Improve Your Strength" is excerpted from "Strength," Go4Life, National Institute on Aging (NIA), March 27, 2015.

Osteoporosis

Osteoporosis is a disease that weakens bones to the point where they break easily—most often in the hip, spine, and wrist. It is often called the "silent disease" because you may not notice any changes until a bone breaks.

Ten million Americans have osteoporosis. It is more common in women, but men also have this disease. The risk of osteoporosis grows as you get older. At the time of menopause, women may lose bone quickly for several years.

After that, the loss slows down but continues. In men, the loss of bone mass is slower, but by age 65 or 70, men and women lose bone at the same rate.

The good news is there are things you can do at any age to prevent weakened bones:

- Eat foods rich in calcium and vitamin D.

- Include regular weight-bearing exercise in your lifestyle.

- Stop smoking.

- Limit how much alcohol you drink.

These are the best ways to keep your bones strong and healthy.

Your bones and muscles will be stronger if you are physically active. Weight-bearing exercises, done three to four times a week, are best for preventing osteoporosis. Walking, jogging, playing tennis, and dancing are examples of weight-bearing exercises. Try some strengthening and balance exercises too. They may help you avoid falls, which could cause a broken bone.

Improve Your Strength

To strengthen your muscles, you need to lift or push weight. Even very small changes in muscle strength can make a real difference in function. Stronger muscles can make it easier to do everyday things like get up from a chair, climb stairs, carry groceries, open jars, and even play with your grandchildren. Lower-body strength exercises also will improve your balance.

Be sure to try all four types of exercise—Endurance, Strength, Balance, and Flexibility.

Safety Tips

- Talk with your doctor if you are unsure about doing a particular exercise, especially if you've had hip or back surgery.

- Don't hold your breath during strength exercises. Holding your breath while straining can cause changes in blood pressure.

Breathe in slowly through your nose and breathe out slowly through your mouth.

• Breathe out as you lift or push, and breathe in as you relax.

• For some exercises, you may want to start alternating arms and work your way up to using both arms at the same time.

• To prevent injury, don't jerk or thrust weights. Use smooth, steady movements.

• Muscle soreness lasting a few days and slight fatigue are normal after muscle-building exercises, at least at first. After doing these exercises for a few weeks, you will probably not be sore after your workout.

How Much, How Often

Try to do strength exercises for all of your major muscle groups on 2 or more days per week for 30-minute sessions each, but don't exercise the same muscle group on any 2 days in a row.

• Depending on your condition, you might need to start out using 1- or 2-pound weights or no weight at all.

• Use a light weight the first week and then gradually add more weight. You need to challenge your muscles to get the most benefit from strength exercises.

• It should feel somewhere between hard and very hard for you to lift or push the weight. If you can't lift or push a weight 8 times in a row, it's too heavy.

• Take 3 seconds to lift or push a weight into place, hold the position for 1 second, and take another 3 seconds to return to your starting position. Return the weight slowly; don't let it drop.

Progressing

Gradually increase the amount of weight you use to build strength. Start out with a weight you can lift only 8 times. Use that weight until you can lift it easily 10 to 15 times. When you can do 2 sets of 10 to 15 repetitions easily, add more weight so that, again, you can lift it only 8 times. Repeat until you reach your goal.

Section 45.3

Managing Osteogenesis Imperfecta with Exercise and Activity

This section includes text excerpted from "Exercise and Activity: Key Elements in the Management of OI," National Institute of Arthritis and Musculoskeletal and Skin Diseases (NIAMS), May 2015.

What Is Osteogenesis Imperfecta (OI)?

Osteogenesis imperfecta (OI) is a connective tissue disorder characterized by fragile bones, weak muscles, and loose ligaments. Bone problems can include bowing of the long bones, scoliosis (curvature of the spine), a barrel chest, and joint problems. Varying degrees of short stature and decreased muscle mass and strength also may be present.

Not so long ago, parents were advised to "protect" their children with this disorder by carrying them on pillows and avoiding recreational activities. But this well-intentioned approach did not protect children from fractures (broken bones) and may have hindered their development and achievement of independent functioning.

Bone growth depends on muscle pull as well as loading (weight bearing) through standing, walking, and lifting. Immobilization may result in loss of muscle and skeletal mass. It can take as long as a year to restore this bone mass following a relatively short period of immobilization. Over the years, it has become clear that physical activity is an important part of managing OI in both children and adults.

Research indicates that physical activity is important because it promotes:

- general health through
  - cardiovascular fitness
  - mental alertness
  - weight control
  - improved sleep quality

- improved ability to handle infection

- reduced risk for some cancers

- maximum bone density

- optimal physical function to support independence in daily activities

- optimal psychological and social well-being by improving self-confidence and the ability to interact socially with peers.

Children and adults with OI will benefit from a regular program of physical activity to promote optimal function through muscle strengthening, aerobic exercise, and recreational pursuits. Specifics of the exercise program vary depending on the person's age, level of function, severity of OI, and needs and desires. A well-designed program can combine activities to prevent problems as well as to restore function.

Activity programs may include specific exercises recommended by rehabilitation professionals (physiatrists, physical therapists, occupational therapists, and recreation therapists) as well as sports and other recreational activities. Having fun and feeling a sense of accomplishment are legitimate goals for an exercise program. In addition, diet, weight control, and commitment to a healthy lifestyle are essential to longevity and an improved quality of life.

The optimal long-term goal for children with OI is good health and independence in all areas of function (social, educational, self-care, locomotion, and recreation), using adaptive devices as needed. Goals for adults with OI include maintaining independence, preserving bone density, and supporting cardiovascular function. To achieve these goals, it is often necessary to improve muscle strength and body alignment.

When to Begin

The first year of life includes many motor skill transitions and is a critical window of opportunity for babies who are born with muscle weakness, alignment problems, and fragility. Physical therapy should begin as soon as the infant exhibits weakness or motor skill delays when compared with other infants of the same age. This might be first noticed because the baby cannot hold up his or her head independently or sit without support until later than most other children.

Treatments for such problems are often aimed at proper positioning and placing children in positions that encourage their use of certain muscle groups. Proper positioning elicits specific anti gravity muscular effort, which is the basis for learning to sit and later on stand. Babies with large heads will face additional challenges and limitations in developing the ability to move against gravity.

An infant or child with weakness or motor skill delays should be working for brief periods daily or at least 5 days a week to improve muscle strength and motor skills. In the process, the child gains endurance and independence in self-care activities. Treatment should not be confined to "therapy hours" only. Very short exercise efforts during the day, as short as 5 minutes, will often result in improvement more quickly than an hour-long session once or twice a week.

Depending on the child's age, the interventions can take several forms, including positioning, specific exercises, and developmental activities (such as standing in a standing device). Ideally, family members and care providers would integrate the activities naturally into the child's day. Playtime can be purposeful, but it should still be fun for both the parent and the child.

Children with OI can excel in the water, particularly if the activity is presented as an opportunity for recreation and independent exploration, rather than a demand to exercise. Water exercise can begin during infancy, with the child lying on his or back in 2 to 3 inches of warm water to promote independent kicking. Over time, the child can progress to independent activity in the water, first in a swim vest or other support, then swimming without support. Walking in the water may be possible for individuals who are unable to walk outside the pool. Water activities in childhood can be the foundation for a lifelong, enjoyable fitness activity.

Adults with OI can benefit from water activity as well. It is an excellent form of aerobic conditioning and may have some benefit with respect to strengthening. Because water activities do little to promote bone health, however, adults also should try to add walking or other weight-bearing exercise to their physical activity program.

Safety

People of any age who have OI can safely exercise. Obstacles to consider when evaluating an activity include prior fracture history, degree of bending of long bones, degree of muscle weakness, joint stiffness or laxity (looseness), joint alignment, poor exercise tolerance, and lack of stamina. Inability to accomplish daily activities without specialized equipment also can affect which activities can be done safely. For example, long-term sitting in a wheelchair may be associated with hip flexion contractures and compensatory back curvatures, which often are associated with back pain, joint stiffness, osteoporosis, and obesity. A safe physical activity program would include getting out of the chair and changing body positions at least every 2 hours when possible.

People who have OI should avoid some activities. These include jumping, diving, and contact sports as well as activities that promote falls, abrupt joint compressions, or high rotary (twisting) forces on bones.

Steps for Developing a Successful Exercise Program at Any Age

1. Determine the person's capabilities by asking: "What can the child or adult do?"

2. Determine the goal you want to pursue by asking: "What is the child or adult trying to achieve?"

3. Determine the constraints or limitations to achieving the goal by asking: "Is limited range of motion, strength, alignment, or joint instability preventing successful performance?" These limitations may have to be addressed before the goal can be accomplished, perhaps by modifying the exercise program.

4. Determine which equipment or treatments are available to help accomplish the goal. A wide range of devices can support improved function. Examples include bathroom safety equipment, walking aids, and devices for reaching objects in high or low places. A consultation with an occupational therapist may be necessary to help choose the best devices to accomplish a specific goal.

It's Never Too Late to Begin

Adults and older children who do not exercise are encouraged to make a new commitment to a healthy lifestyle and become more physically active. They should include enjoyable exercises that will improve strength, balance, and endurance and, if possible, promote socialization. Rehabilitation specialists or exercise specialists who are familiar with OI or osteoporosis can help design an appropriate program. Enjoyment plus improved function can be found through physical activity at every age.

Chapter 46

Physical Fitness for People with Asthma

Chapter Contents

Section 46.1

Exercise for People with Asthma

This section includes text excerpted from "Meeting the Challenge,"
Centers for Disease Control and Prevention (CDC), May 9, 2015.

Who Has Asthma?

Asthma—which makes it hard to breathe, and causes coughing and
wheezing—affects about five million American kids and teens?

That's almost 1 in 10!

Famous people like rapper Coolio have asthma, although he's better
known for his hit songs like "Gangsta's Paradise" than for his fight
against the illness.

Physical Activity and Asthma?

Things like cold or dry air, dust, pollen, pollution, cigarette smoke,
or stress can "trigger" asthma. This can make your body pump out
chemicals that close off your airways, making it hard for air to get into
to your lungs, and causing an asthma attack.

Physical activity can trigger asthma attacks too. Experts don't
know for sure why physical activity sometimes brings one on, but they
suspect that fast breathing through the mouth (like what happens
when you get winded) can irritate the airways. In addition, when air
pollution levels are high, physical activity in the afternoon is harder
on the lungs than morning activity—pollution levels rise later in the
day.

Get Fit

So, should you get a doctor's note and skip gym class? Sorry, no.
Doctors want their asthma patients to get active, especially in asth-
ma-friendly activities like these: Swimming, bicycling, golf, inline
skating, and weightlifting.

Why Are These Good Choices If You Want to Be Physically Active?

- They let you control how hard and fast you breathe
- They let you breathe through your nose at all times
- They don't dry out your airways
- They mix short, intense activities with long endurance workouts
- You can do them in a controlled environment (for example, a gym with air that's not too cold or dry)
- Usually you do them with other people, who can help you if an attack comes on

Getting regular physical activity can improve your breathing, and lead to fewer asthma attacks. Just remember to follow these tips. (In fact, this is good advice for everyone, not just those with asthma.)

- Ease into it.

  Start your workout with a warm-up, and don't overdo it by running five miles on your first day if you get winded walking around the block! Finish up with a cool-down.

- Take a buddy.

  It's more fun and a friend can help if you get into trouble.

- Respect your body.

  Stay away from the things that trigger your asthma. Help out your airways by breathing through your nose instead of your mouth. Take it easy on days when your asthma symptoms are really bugging you. And stick to the medicine routine that your doctor has set up.

- Take breaks.

  Treat yourself to rest and drink plenty of water.

- Mix it up.

  For example, try going inline skating one day and taking a long walk the next.

Feel Good

To feel your best, do the right stuff to control your asthma. And listen to your doctors—they're on your team!

Dr. Asthma says that people with asthma "should expect to live a life that really isn't affected by asthma, except for having to follow the directions." He also says to speak up if you are having symptoms, and remember to "keep a good attitude and keep working to control the disease."

So, get out there and get moving! With good habits and today's medicines, you can go for the gold—or just join your friends on the basketball court, in the pool, on the dance floor.

Section 46.2

Exercise-Induced Asthma

This section contains text excerpted from the following sources: Text in this section begins with excerpts from "Asthma and Physical Activity in the School," National Heart, Lung, and Blood Institute (NHLBI), April 2012. Reviewed September 2016; text beginning with the heading "Definition and Overview" is excerpted from "Exercise-Induced Bronchoconstriction (EIB) with or without Chronic Asthma," Agency for Healthcare Research and Quality (AHRQ), U.S. Department of Health and Human Services (HHS), July 31, 2012. Reviewed September 2016.

Exercise and other physical activity can bring on symptoms in most people who have asthma. Symptoms may occur either during or right after being active. This is called **exercise-induced asthma** (or exercise-induced bronchospasm).

But regular physical activity is good for all of us. In fact, doctors recommend that most people, including those who have asthma, get at least 2 hours and 30 minutes of aerobic physical activity that requires moderate effort every week (at least 1 hour a day for children 6–17 years of age). This activity should be for at least 10 minutes at a time.

The good news is that if your asthma is well controlled, physical activity should not be a problem. In fact, most people who have asthma should be able to participate in any physical activity they like without having asthma symptoms. Here are some things you can do to prevent or reduce exercise-induced asthma:

- Ask your doctor about using your quick-relief medicine 5 minutes before exercise. This usually can prevent and control exercise-induced asthma. You can also use this medicine to relieve symptoms during and after exercise. But remember to let your doctor know if you have to use it often during or after exercise. It may be a sign that you need to start taking daily long term control medicine or to increase the dose of your long-term control medicine.

- Try warming up before you exercise or do physical activity. This may help you handle continuous exercise without having to stop repeatedly to take more medicine. Good ways to warm up include walking, doing flexibility exercises, or doing other low-intensity activities.

- Try to avoid your other asthma triggers while exercising or doing other physical activity. For example, if cold, dry air makes your asthma worse, wear a scarf or cold air mask when exercising outdoors in winter.

- If you have been having mild asthma symptoms, consider reducing the intensity or length of the activity you do.

- Try exercising indoors when outside temperatures are extreme, or the ozone level is high. The same is true if you are allergic, and the grass has recently been mowed, or pollen counts are high.

- When first starting to be active, try increasing your level of activity gradually over time.

Remember, asthma should not limit your participation or success in physical activities—even more intense and sustained activities like running or playing basketball or soccer.

Exercise-induced asthma (also called exercise-induced bronchospasm) is asthma that is triggered by physical activity. Vigorous exercise will cause symptoms for most students who have asthma if their asthma is not well-controlled. Some students experience asthma symptoms only when they exercise. Asthma varies from student to student and often from season to season or even hour by hour. At times, programs for students who have asthma may need to be temporarily modified, such as by varying the type, intensity, duration, and/or frequency of activity. At all times, students who have asthma should be included in activities as much as possible. Remaining behind in the gym or library or frequently sitting on the bench can set the stage for teasing, loss of self-esteem, unnecessary restriction of activity, and low levels of physical fitness.

Definition and Overview

- Exercise-induced bronchospasm (EIB) is defined as the transient narrowing of the lower airways that occurs after vigorous exercise. It may appear with or without asthma. The term exercise-induced asthma (EIA) should not be used because exercise does not induce asthma but rather is a trigger of bronchoconstriction.

- EIB occurs in response to heating and humidifying large volumes of air during a short period. The most important determinants of expression of EIB response and severity are the water content of the inspired air and/or the level of ventilation achieved and sustained during exercise.

- Respiratory water loss at high ventilation is associated with airway cooling and dehydration and an increase in osmolarity of the airway surface. The predominant theory of EIB is the osmotic theory, although the thermal theory may also play a role.

- Exercise itself is not necessary to cause airways to narrow; voluntary hyperpnea of dry air may induce bronchoconstriction similar to exercise. Eucapnic voluntary hyperpnea is used as a surrogate for exercise in the diagnosis of EIB, particularly in athletes.

- People who have EIB without asthma associated with airway inflammation and the presence of eosinophils are likely to be responsive to corticosteroids.

- EIB is accompanied by release of mediators such as prostaglandins (PGs), leukotrienes (LTs), and histamine.

- In approximately half of patients who have EIB, there is an interval of refractoriness lasting approximately 2 to 3 hours immediately after an episode of EIB during which additional exercise produces little or no bronchoconstriction.

Genetics and Environment

- Gene expression and environmental interaction may be relevant to the EIB phenotype.

- Oxidative stress caused by environmental pollutants that are inhaled during exercise may play an important role in the development and exaggeration of EIB.

- The pathogenesis of EIB in elite athletes may relate to effects on the airways arising from humidifying large volumes of dry air over months of training with or without exposure to environmental irritants, allergens, and viral agents.

Prevalence

- EIB is reported in most asthmatic patients.

- Patients with more severe or less well-controlled asthma are more likely to manifest EIB than patients with less severe or better controlled disease.

- The true prevalence of EIB in the general population is poorly defined because epidemiologic studies of EIB have not differentiated asthmatic vs. nonasthmatic populations. In addition, there is no consensus for the end point indicative of a positive response, and the conditions under which exercise is performed frequently differ.

- The prevalence of EIB in elite athletes appears to be higher than in the general population and depends on the type of sport, the maximum exercise level, and environmental conditions.

- The prevalence of EIB varies with history, type of challenge, and conditions under which the challenge is performed.

- The prevalence of EIB with and without asthma may be influenced by age, sex, and ethnicity.

Diagnosis

- Self-reported symptoms alone are not reliable for diagnosis of EIB.

- Optimal EIB management may require confirmation of the diagnosis using objective methods.

- Self-reported symptom-based diagnosis of EIB in the elite athlete lacks sensitivity and specificity and establishes the necessity for standardized, objective challenges using spirometry.

- The indirect challenge (e.g., exercise or surrogate such as eucapnic voluntary hyperpnea (EVH)) is preferred over a direct challenge (e.g., methacholine) for assessing EIB in the elite athlete.

- EVH is the preferred surrogate challenge for the elite athlete participating in competitive sports.

- The intensity of the exercise challenge for the elite athlete should be 95% or greater than actual or estimated maximal heart rate (HR max), and dry medical-grade air should be used in performing the challenge.

- Hyperosmolar aerosols may also be used as surrogates to exercise.

Differential Diagnosis

- Exercise-induced laryngeal dysfunction (EILD), primarily VCD and other glottic abnormalities, may be elicited by exercise and mimic EIB. Inspiratory stridor is a differentiating hallmark sign with EILD and not with EIB alone. Flattening of the inspiratory curve on spirometric maneuver may be seen concomitant with symptoms. EILD may occur alone or with EIB. Failure to respond to asthma management is a key historical feature suggesting EILD.

- Exercise-induced dyspnea and hyperventilation can masquerade as asthma, especially in children and adolescents.

- Shortness of breath with exercise may be associated with underlying conditions due to obstructive lung disease, such as chronic obstructive pulmonary disease (COPD), or restrictive lung physiology, such as obesity, skeletal defects (e.g., pectus excavatum), diaphragmatic paralysis, and interstitial fibrosis.

- Shortness of breath accompanied by pruritus and urticaria, with varying other systemic symptoms, suggests exercise-induced anaphylaxis (EIAna) rather than EIB.

- In the absence of objective evidence of EIB, breathlessness with exercise, with or without chest pain, may be caused by cardiovascular, pulmonary, or gastroenterologic mechanisms other than asthma. Appropriate cardiopulmonary testing and/or referral to a cardiologist, pulmonologist, or gastroenterologist may be necessary.

- Exercise-induced dyspnea is seen as a physiologic limitation in otherwise healthy active individuals without bronchospasm.

- The association between EIB and gastroesophageal reflux disease (GERD) is controversial, and probably there is no relationship.

- Psychological factors need to be considered in the differential diagnosis of EIB.

- Dyspnea on exertion, which is prevalent in otherwise healthy, obese individuals, is not associated with EIB.

- Mitochondrial enzyme deficiency with myopathy is a rare cause of exercise limitation.

Chapter 47

Physical Fitness for People with Diabetes

How Can Physical Activity Help Me Take Care of My Diabetes?

Physical activity and keeping a healthy weight can help you take care of your diabetes and prevent diabetes problems. Physical activity helps your blood glucose, also called blood sugar, stay in your target range.

Physical activity also helps the hormone insulin absorb glucose into all your body's cells, including your muscles, for energy. Muscles use glucose better than fat does. Building and using muscle through physical activity can help prevent high blood glucose. If your body doesn't make enough insulin, or if the insulin doesn't work the way it should, the body's cells don't use glucose. Your blood glucose levels then get too high, causing diabetes.

Starting a physical activity program can help you lose weight or keep a healthy weight and keep your blood glucose levels on target. Even without reaching a healthy weight, just a 10 or 15 pound weight loss makes a difference in reducing the risk of diabetes problems.

This chapter includes text excerpted from "Diabetes and Physical Activity," National Institute of Diabetes and Digestive and Kidney Diseases (NIDDK), August 2014.

What Should I Do before I Start a Physical Activity Program?

Before you start a physical activity program, you should:

- talk with your healthcare team
- plan ahead
- find an exercise buddy
- decide how you'll track your physical activity
- decide how you'll reward yourself

Talk with your healthcare team. Your healthcare team may include a doctor, nurse, dietitian, diabetes educator, and others. Always talk with your healthcare team before you start a new physical activity program. Your healthcare team will tell you a target range for your blood glucose levels.

People with diabetes who take insulin or certain diabetes medicines are more likely to have low blood glucose, also called hypoglycemia. If your blood glucose levels drop too low, you could pass out, have a seizure, or go into a coma. Physical activity can make hypoglycemia more likely or worse in people who take insulin or certain diabetes medicines, so planning ahead is key. It's important to stay active. Ask your healthcare team how to stay active safely.

Physical activity works together with healthy eating and diabetes medicines to prevent diabetes problems. Studies show that people with type 2 diabetes who lose weight with physical activity and make healthy changes to their eating plan are less likely to need diabetes and heart medicines. Ask your healthcare team about your healthy eating plan and all your medicines. Ask if you need to change the amount of medicine you take or the food you eat before any physical activity.

Plan ahead. Decide in advance what type of physical activity you'll do. Before you start, also choose:

- the days and times you'll be physically active
- the length of each physical activity session
- your plan for warming up, stretching, and cooling down for each physical activity session
- a backup plan, such as where you'll walk if the weather is bad
- how you will measure your progress

To make sure you stay active, find activities you like to do. If you keep finding excuses not to be physically active, think about why:

- Are your goals realistic?
- Do you need a change in activity?
- Would another time be more convenient?

Find an exercise buddy. Many people find they are more likely to be physically active if someone joins them. Ask a friend or family member to be your exercise buddy. When you do physical activities with a buddy you may find that you:

- enjoy the company
- stick to the physical activity plan
- are more eager to do physical activities

Being active with your family may help everyone stay at a healthy weight. Keeping a healthy weight may prevent them from developing diabetes or prediabetes. Prediabetes is when the amount of glucose in your blood is above normal yet not high enough to be called diabetes.

Decide how you'll track your physical activity. Write down your blood glucose levels and when and how long you are physically active in a record book. You'll be able to track your progress and see how physical activity affects your blood glucose. You can find tools to help track your daily activities at www.ndep.nih.gov.

Decide how you'll reward yourself. Reward yourself with a nonfood item or activity when you reach your goals. For example, treat yourself to a movie or buy a new plant for the garden.

What Kinds of Physical Activity Can Help Me?

Many kinds of physical activity can help you take care of your diabetes. Even small amounts of physical activity can help. You can measure your physical activity level by how much effort you use.

Doctors suggest that you aim for 30 to 60 minutes of moderate to vigorous physical activity most days of the week. Children and adolescents with type 2 diabetes who are 10 to 17 years old should aim for 60 minutes of moderate to vigorous activity every day.

Your healthcare team can tell you more about what kind of physical activity is best for you. They can also tell you when and how much you can increase your physical activity level.

Light physical activity. Light activity is easy. Your physical activity level is light if you:

- are breathing normally
- are not sweating
- can talk normally or even sing

Moderate physical activity. Moderate activity feels somewhat hard. Your physical activity level is moderate if you:

- are breathing quickly, yet you're not out of breath
- are lightly sweating after about 10 minutes of activity
- can talk normally, yet you can't sing

Vigorous physical activity. Vigorous, or intense, activity feels hard. Your physical activity level is vigorous if you:

- are breathing deeply and quickly
- are sweating after a few minutes of activity
- can't talk normally without stopping for a breath

Not all physical activity has to take place at the same time. You might take a walk for 20 minutes, lift hand weights for 10 minutes, and walk up and down the stairs for 5 minutes.

Breaking the physical activity into different groups can help. You can:

- do aerobic exercise
- do strength training to build muscle
- do stretching exercises
- add extra activity to your daily routine

Do Aerobic Exercise

Aerobic exercise is activity that uses large muscles, makes your heart beat faster, and makes you breathe harder. Doing moderate to vigorous aerobic exercise for 30 to 60 minutes a day most days of the week provides many benefits. You can even split up these minutes into several parts.

Talk with your healthcare team about how to warm up and cool down before and after you exercise. Start slowly, with 5 to 10 minutes a day, and add a little more time each week. Try:

- walking briskly

- hiking

- climbing stairs

- swimming or taking a water-aerobics class

- dancing

- riding a bicycle outdoors or a stationary bicycle indoors

- taking an exercise class

- playing basketball, tennis, or other sports

- in-line skating, ice skating, or skateboarding

Do Strength Training to Build Muscle

Strength training is a light to moderate physical activity that builds muscle and keeps your bones healthy. When you have more muscle and less fat, you'll burn more calories because muscle burns more calories than fat, even between exercise sessions. Burning more calories can help you lose and keep off weight.

Whether you're a man or a woman, you can do strength training with hand weights, elastic bands, or weight machines two to three times a week. You can do strength training at home, at a fitness center, or in a class. Start with a light weight and slowly increase the size of your weights as your muscles become stronger.

Do Stretching Exercises

Stretching exercises are a light to moderate physical activity that both men and women can do. For example, yoga is a type of stretching that focuses on your breathing and helps you relax. Your healthcare team can suggest whether yoga is right for you.

Even if you have problems moving or balancing, certain types of yoga can help. For example, chair yoga has stretches you can do when sitting in a chair. When you stretch, you increase your flexibility, lower your stress, and help prevent sore muscles.

Add Extra Activity to Your Daily Routine

Increase daily activity by spending less time watching TV or at the computer. Try these simple ways to add light, moderate, or vigorous physical activities in your life every day:

- Walk around while you talk on the phone.

- If you have kids or grandkids, visit a zoo or a park with them.

- Take a walk through your neighborhood.

- When you watch TV, get up and walk around the room during commercials.

- Do chores, such as work in the garden or rake leaves, clean the house, or wash the car.

- Stretch out your chores. For example, make two trips to take the laundry downstairs instead of one.

- Park at the far end of the shopping center parking lot and walk to the store.

- Take the stairs instead of the elevator.

- Stretch or walk around instead of taking a coffee break and eating.

- ketones in your blood or urine. Ketones are chemicals your body might make when your blood glucose levels are too high and your insulin level is too low. If you are physically active when you have ketones in your blood or urine, your blood glucose levels may go even higher.

Light or moderate physical activity can help lower blood glucose if you have type 2 diabetes and you don't have ketones. Ketones are rare in people with type 2 diabetes. Ask your healthcare team whether you should be physically active when your blood glucose levels are high.

Points to Remember

- Starting a physical activity program can help you lose weight or keep a healthy weight and keep your blood glucose levels on target.

- Always talk with your healthcare team before you start a new physical activity program.

- Ask your healthcare team if you need to change the amount of medicine you take or the food you eat before any physical activity.

- Talk with your healthcare team about what types of physical activity are safe for you, such as walking, weight lifting, or housework.

- To make sure you stay active, find activities you like to do. Ask a friend or family member to be your exercise buddy.

- Write down your blood glucose levels and when and how long you are physically active in a record book.

- Doctors suggest that you aim for 30 to 60 minutes of moderate to vigorous physical activity most days of the week.

- Children and adolescents with type 2 diabetes who are 10 to 17 years old should aim for 60 minutes of moderate to vigorous activity every day.

- Not all physical activity has to take place at the same time. For example, you might take a walk for 20 minutes, lift hand weights for 10 minutes, and walk up and down the stairs for 5 minutes.

- Doing moderate to vigorous aerobic exercise for 30 to 60 minutes a day most days of the week provides many benefits. You can even split up these minutes into several parts.

- Start exercising slowly, with 5 to 10 minutes a day, and add a little more time each week. Try walking briskly, hiking, or climbing stairs.

- Whether you're a man or a woman, you can do strength training with hand weights, elastic bands, or weight machines two to three times a week.

- Stretching exercises are a light to moderate physical activity that both men and women can do. When you stretch, you increase your flexibility, lower your stress, and help prevent sore muscles.

- Increase daily activity by spending less time watching TV or at the computer.

- Try these simple ways to add light, moderate, or vigorous physical activities in your life every day:

  - Walk around while you talk on the phone.

467

- Take a walk through your neighborhood.

- Do chores, such as work in the garden or rake leaves, clean the house, or wash the car.

- If you have type 1 diabetes, try not to do vigorous physical activity when you have ketones in your blood or urine.

Chapter 48

Physical Fitness and Cancer

Chapter Contents

469

Section 48.1

Physical Fitness and Cancer Prevention

This section includes text excerpted from "Increased Physical Activity
Associated with Lower Risk of 13 Types of Cancer," National Cancer
Institute (NCI), May 16, 2016.

A study of the relationship between physical activity and cancer
has shown that greater levels of leisure-time physical activity were
associated with a lower risk of developing 13 different types of cancer.
The risk of developing seven cancer types was 20 percent (or more)
lower among the most active participants (90th percentile of activity)
as compared with the least active participants (10th percentile of activity). These findings, from researchers at the National Cancer Institute
(NCI), part of the National Institutes of Health, and the American
Cancer Society, confirm and extend the evidence for a benefit of physical activity on cancer risk and support its role as a key component of
population-wide cancer prevention and control efforts. The study, by
Steven C. Moore, Ph.D., NCI, and colleagues, appeared May 16, 2016,
in *JAMA Internal Medicine.*

Hundreds of previous studies have examined associations between
physical activity and cancer risk and shown reduced risks for colon,
breast, and endometrial cancers; however, results have been inconclusive for most cancer types due to small numbers of participants in
the studies. This study pooled data on 1.44 million people, ages 19 to
98, from the United States and Europe, and was able to examine a
broad range of cancers, including rare malignancies. Participants were
followed for a median of 11 years during which 187,000 new cases of
cancer occurred.

The investigators confirmed that leisure-time physical activity, as
assessed by self-reported surveys, was associated with a lower risk
of colon, breast, and endometrial cancers. They also determined that
leisure-time physical activity was associated with a lower risk of 10
additional cancers, with the greatest risk reductions for esophageal
adenocarcinoma, liver cancer, cancer of the gastric cardia, kidney cancer, and myeloid leukemia. Myeloma and cancers of the head and neck,
rectum, and bladder also showed reduced risks that were significant,

but not as strong. Risk was reduced for lung cancer, but only for current and former smokers; the reasons for this are still being studied.

"Leisure-time physical activity is known to reduce risks of heart disease and risk of death from all causes, and our study demonstrates that it is also associated with lower risks of many types of cancer," said Moore. "Furthermore, our results support that these associations are broadly generalizable to different populations, including people who are overweight or obese, or those with a history of smoking. Healthcare professionals counseling inactive adults should promote physical activity as a component of a healthy lifestyle and cancer prevention."

Leisure-time physical activity is defined as exercise done at one's own discretion, often to improve or maintain fitness or health. Examples include walking, running, swimming, and other moderate to vigorous intensity activities. The median level of activity in the study was about 150 minutes of moderate-intensity activity per week, which is comparable to the current recommended minimum level of physical activity for the U.S. population.

There are a number of mechanisms through which physical activity could affect cancer risk. It has been hypothesized that cancer growth could be initiated or abetted by three metabolic pathways that are also affected by exercise: sex steroids (estrogens and androgens); insulin and insulin-like growth factors; and proteins involved with both insulin metabolism and inflammation. Additionally, several non-hormonal mechanisms have been hypothesized to link physical activity to cancer risk, including inflammation, immune function, oxidative stress, and for colon cancer, a reduction in time that it takes for waste to pass through the gastrointestinal tract.

Most associations between physical activity and lower cancer risk changed little when adjusted for body mass index, suggesting that physical activity acts through mechanisms other than lowering body weight to reduce cancer risk. Associations between physical activity and cancer were also similar in subgroups of normal weight and overweight participants, and in current smokers or people who never smoked.

The study was a large-scale effort of the Physical Activity Collaboration of NCI's Cohort Consortium, which was formed to estimate physical activity and disease associations using pooled prospective data and a standardized analytical approach.

"For years, we've had substantial evidence supporting a role for physical activity in three leading cancers: colon, breast, and endometrial cancers, which together account for nearly one in four cancers in the United States," said Alpa V. Patel, Ph.D., a co-author from the

American Cancer Society. "This study linking physical activity to 10 additional cancers shows its impact may be even more relevant, and that physical activity has far reaching value for cancer prevention."

The National Cancer Institute leads the National Cancer Program and the NIH's efforts to dramatically reduce the prevalence of cancer and improve the lives of cancer patients and their families, through research into prevention and cancer biology, the development of new interventions, and the training and mentoring of new researchers.

About the National Institutes of Health (NIH): NIH, the nation's medical research agency, includes 27 Institutes and Centers and is a component of the U.S. Department of Health and Human Services. NIH is the primary federal agency conducting and supporting basic, clinical, and translational medical research, and is investigating the causes, treatments, and cures for both common and rare diseases.

The American Cancer Society saves lives and creates a world with less cancer and more birthdays by helping you stay well, helping you get well, by finding cures and fighting back. As the nation's largest non-governmental investor in cancer research, contributing about $3.4 billion, we turn what we know about cancer into what we do.

Section 48.2

Exercise during and after Cancer Treatment

This section includes text excerpted from "Nutrition and Physical Activity Guidelines for Cancer Survivors," Agency for Healthcare Research and Quality (AHRQ), U.S. Department of Health and Human Services (HHS), July 2012. Reviewed August 2016.

Exercise and Cancer Treatment

Existing evidence strongly suggests that exercise is not only safe and feasible during cancer treatment, but that it can also improve physical functioning, fatigue, and multiple aspects of quality of life.

The decision regarding when to initiate and how to maintain physical activity should be individualized to the patient's condition and personal preferences. Exercise during cancer treatment improves multiple posttreatment adverse effects on bone health, muscle strength, and other quality-of-life measures. Persons receiving chemotherapy and/or radiation therapy who are already on an exercise program may need to exercise at a lower intensity and/or for a shorter duration during their treatment, but the principal goal should be to maintain activity as much as possible. Some clinicians advise certain survivors to wait to determine their extent of side effects with chemotherapy before beginning an exercise program. For those who were sedentary before diagnosis, low-intensity activities such as stretching and brief, slow walks should be adopted and slowly advanced.

For older individuals and those with bone metastases or osteoporosis, or significant impairments such as arthritis or peripheral neuropathy, careful attention should be given to balance and safety to reduce the risk of falls and injuries. The presence of a caregiver or exercise professional during exercise sessions can be helpful. If the disease or treatment necessitates periods of bed rest, then reduced fitness and strength, as well as loss of lean body mass, can be expected. Physical therapy during bed rest is therefore advisable to maintain strength and range of motion and can help to counteract fatigue and depression.

Recovery Immediately after Treatment

After cancer therapy has been completed, the next phase of cancer survivorship is recovery. In this phase, many symptoms and side effects of treatment that have affected nutritional and physical well-being begin to resolve. Survivors may require ongoing nutritional assessment and guidance in this phase of survival. For those who emerge from treatment underweight or with compromised nutritional status, continued supportive care, including nutritional counseling and pharmacotherapy to relieve symptoms and stimulate appetite, is helpful in the recovery process. After treatment, a program of regular physical activity is essential to aid in the process of recovery and improve fitness.

Long-Term Disease-Free Living or Stable Disease

During this phase, setting and achieving lifelong goals for an appropriate weight, a physically active lifestyle, and a healthy diet are important to promote overall health, quality of life, and longevity. While cancer survivorship is a relatively new area of study and much needs to be learned regarding the optimal diet and physical activity practices for cancer survivors, current evidence supports recommendations in three basic areas: weight management, physical activity, and dietary patterns. The guidelines are as follows:

Achieve and maintain a healthy weight.

- If overweight or obese, limit consumption of high-calorie foods and beverages and increase physical activity to promote weight loss.

Engage in regular physical activity.

- Avoid inactivity and return to normal daily activities as soon as possible following diagnosis.

- Aim to exercise at least 150 minutes per week.

- Include strength training exercises at least 2 days per week.

Achieve a dietary pattern that is high in vegetables, fruits, and whole grains.

- Follow the *American Cancer Society Guidelines* on nutrition and physical activity for cancer prevention.

Because individuals who have been diagnosed with cancer are at a significantly higher risk of developing second primary cancers, and may also be at an increased risk of chronic diseases such as cardiovascular disease, diabetes, and osteoporosis, the guidelines established to prevent those diseases are especially important for cancer survivors. Because family members of cancer survivors may also be at a higher risk of developing cancer, they should also be encouraged to follow the American Cancer Society (ACS) nutrition and physical activity guidelines for cancer prevention.

Achieving and maintaining a healthy weight, as well as consuming a nutrient-rich diet and maintaining a physically active lifestyle, are important to improve long-term health and well-being.

Exercise has been shown to improve cardiovascular fitness, muscle strength, body composition, fatigue, anxiety, depression, self-esteem, happiness, and several components of quality of life (physical, functional, and emotional) in cancer survivors. In addition, exercise studies have targeted certain symptoms particular to specific cancers and the adverse effects of specific therapies (e.g., lymphedema in survivors of breast cancer) and shown beneficial effects that are more cancer-specific.

At least 20 prospective observational studies have shown that physically active cancer survivors have a lower risk of cancer recurrences and improved survival compared with those who are inactive, although studies remain limited to breast, colorectal, prostate, and ovarian cancer, and randomized clinical trials are still needed to better define the impact of exercise on such outcomes.

Living with Advanced Cancer

For individuals living with advanced cancer, a healthy diet and some physical activity may be important factors in establishing and maintaining a sense of well-being and enhancing their quality of life. Although advanced cancer is sometimes accompanied by substantial weight loss, it is not inevitable that individuals with cancer lose weight or experience malnutrition. Many patients with advanced cancer need to adapt their food choices and meal patterns to meet nutritional needs and to manage cancer symptoms or treatment side effects such as fatigue, bowel changes, and a diminished sense of taste or appetite. For persons experiencing anorexia, negative changes in weight, or difficulty in gaining weight, convincing evidence exists that some medications (e.g., megestrol acetate) can help to enhance appetite.

Additional nutritional supplementation such as nutrient-dense beverages and foods can be consumed by those who cannot eat or drink enough to maintain sufficient energy intake. The use of enteral nutrition and parenteral nutrition support should be individualized with recognition of overall treatment goals (control or palliation) and the associated risks of medical complications and/or ethical dilemmas. Both the American Society for Parenteral and Enteral Nutrition and the Academy of Nutrition and Dietetics position papers recommend that nutrition support be used selectively and with clear purpose.

The evidence of a benefit from exercise for survivors of advanced cancer is insufficient to make general recommendations. Recommendations for nutrition and physical activity in those who are living with advanced cancer are best based on individual nutrition needs and physical abilities.

Body Weight Issues in Nutrition and Physical Activity for Cancer Survivors

Increasing evidence indicates that being overweight increases the risk of recurrence and reduces the likelihood of disease-free and overall survival among those diagnosed with cancer. Such data suggest that the avoidance of weight gain and weight maintenance throughout treatment may be important for survivors who are normal weight, overweight, or obese at the time of diagnosis, and that intentional weight loss following treatment recovery among those who are overweight and obese may be associated with health-related benefits.

It is hypothesized that improvements in cancer-related outcomes are possible, and likely probable, through intentional weight reduction. Evidence exists that weight loss that results from intentional exercise and caloric restriction can improve the hormonal milieu and quality of life and physical functioning among survivors who are obese or overweight. It may be difficult for individuals to pursue a host of new dietary, exercise, and behavioral strategies to reduce body weight through reduced energy intake and increased energy expenditure while at the same time balancing the demands of daily life during initial treatments. Thus, for many, active efforts toward intentional weight loss may be postponed until surgery, chemotherapy, and/or radiation treatment is complete.

However, for cancer survivors who are overweight or obese and who choose to pursue weight loss, there appears to be no contraindication to modest weight loss (i.e., a maximum of 2 pounds per week) during treatment, as long as the treating oncologists approve, weight loss is monitored closely, and it does not interfere with treatment. Safe weight loss should be achieved through a nutritious diet that is reduced in energy density and increased physical activity tailored to the specific needs of the patient.

After cancer treatment, weight gain or loss should be managed with a combination of dietary, physical activity, and behavioral strategies. For some who need to gain weight, this means increasing energy intake to exceed energy expended and for others who need to lose weight, reducing caloric intake and increasing energy expenditure via increased physical activity to exceed energy intake. Reducing the energy density of the diet by emphasizing low-energy dense foods (e.g., water- and fiber-rich vegetables and fruits) and limiting the intake of foods and beverages high in fat and added sugar promotes healthy weight control. Limiting portion sizes of energy-dense foods is an important accompanying strategy. Increased physical activity is also an important element to prevent weight gain, retain or regain muscle mass, promote weight loss, and promote the maintenance of weight loss in patients who are overweight or obese.

For survivors who are severely obese and have more pressing health issues, more structured weight loss programs or pharmacologic or surgical means may be indicated. It should be noted that among those who need to lose weight, even if ideal weight is not achieved, it is likely that any weight loss achieved by physical activity and healthful eating is beneficial, with weight losses of 5% to 10% still likely to have significant health benefits. Although most evidence related to these weight management strategies does not come from studies of cancer survivors per se, it is likely that these approaches can apply in the special circumstances of the cancer survivor.

Throughout the cancer continuum, therefore, individuals should strive to achieve and maintain a healthy weight, as defined by a body mass index (BMI) between 18.5 kg/m2 and 25 kg/m2. Some cancer survivors can be malnourished and underweight at diagnosis or as a result of aggressive cancer treatments. For these individuals, further weight loss can impair their quality of life, interfere with the completion of treatment, delay healing, and increase the risk of complications. In survivors with these difficulties, dietary intake and factors affecting energy expenditure should be carefully assessed.

For those at risk of unintentional weight loss, multifaceted interventions should focus on increasing food intake to achieve a positive energy balance and therefore increase weight. Physical activity may be useful to the underweight survivor when tailored to provide stress reduction and to increase strength and lean body mass, but exceptionally high levels of physical activity make weight gain more difficult.

Physical Activity in Cancer Survivors

Despite the many benefits of exercise for cancer survivors, particular issues may affect the ability of survivors to exercise. Effects of treatment may also increase the risk of exercise-related injuries and adverse effects, and therefore specific precautions may be advisable, including:

- Survivors with severe anemia should delay exercise, other than activities of daily living, until the anemia is improved.

- Survivors with compromised immune function should avoid public gyms and public pools until their white blood cell counts return to safe levels. Survivors who have completed a bone marrow transplant are usually advised to avoid such exposures for one year after transplantation.

- Survivors experiencing severe fatigue from their therapy may not feel up to an exercise program, and therefore they may be encouraged to do 10 minutes of light exercises daily.

- Survivors undergoing radiation should avoid chlorine exposure to irradiated skin (e.g., from swimming pools).

- Survivors with indwelling catheters or feeding tubes should be cautious or avoid pool, lake, or ocean water or other microbial exposures that may result in infections, as well as resistance training of muscles in the area of the catheter to avoid dislodgment.

- Survivors with multiple or uncontrolled comorbidities need to consider modifications to their exercise program in consultation with their physicians.

- Survivors with significant peripheral neuropathies or ataxia may have a reduced ability to use the affected limbs because of weakness or loss of balance. They may do better with a stationary reclining bicycle, for example, than walking on a treadmill.

After consideration of these and other specific precautions, it is recommended that cancer survivors follow the survivor-specific guidelines written by an expert panel convened by the American College of Sports Medicine (ACSM). The ACSM panel recommended that individuals avoid inactivity and return to normal activity as soon as possible after diagnosis or treatment. For aerobic physical activity, the ACSM panel recommended that survivors follow the *U.S. Department of Health and Human Services 2008 Physical Activity Guidelines for Americans.* According to those guidelines, adults aged 18 to 64 years should

Table 48.1. Examples of Moderate and Vigorous Activities

Moderate Activities (I Can Talk While I Do Them, But I Can't Sing)	Vigorous Activity (I Can Only Say a Few Words without Stopping to Catch My Breath)
• Ballroom and line dancing • Biking on level ground or with few hills • Canoeing • General gardening (raking, trimming shrubs) • Sports where you catch and throw (baseball, softball, volleyball) • Tennis (doubles) • Using your manual wheelchair • Using hand cyclers (also called ergometers) • Walking briskly • Water aerobics	• Aerobic dance • Biking faster than 10 miles per hour • Fast dancing • Heavy gardening (digging, hoeing) • Hiking uphill • Jumping rope • Martial arts (such as karate) • Race walking, jogging, or running • Sports with a lot of running (basketball, hockey, soccer) • Swimming fast or swimming laps • Tennis (singles)

engage in at least 150 minutes per week of moderate intensity or 75 minutes per week of vigorous intensity aerobic physical activity, or an equivalent combination of moderate and vigorous intensity aerobic physical activity (see the Table below). Some activity is better than none and exceeding the guidelines is likely to provide additional health benefits. Activity should be done in episodes of at least 10 minutes per session and preferably spread throughout the week. Furthermore, adults should do muscle-strengthening activities involving all major muscle groups at least two days per week. Adults aged older than 65 years should also follow these recommendations if possible, but if chronic conditions limit activity, older adults should be as physically active as their abilities allow and avoid long periods of physical inactivity. Cancer type-specific recommendations will be discussed in the individual cancer sections below.

Supporting Exercise Behavior Change

Unless behavioral support interventions are provided, the majority of cancer survivors will not benefit fully from regular physical activity. Behavioral support interventions to assist cancer survivors in adopting and maintaining a physically active lifestyle have been reviewed elsewhere. Some successful strategies include short-term supervised exercise (e.g., 12 weeks), support groups, telephone counseling, motivational interviewing, and cancer survivor-specific print materials. The key point for cancer care professionals is that cancer survivors have unique motives, barriers, and preferences for physical activity.

Part Seven

Health and Wellness Trends

Chapter 49

Fitness and Exercise Trends

Physical fitness and exercise are two areas of modern life that are particularly subject to fluctuations in consumer interest. New fitness equipment and exercise programs catch the attention of those looking for the greatest results, replacing older approaches that have fallen out of favor. Some popular exercise programs quickly become fads, fading away after a brief period of widespread success in the fitness industry. Other fitness practices develop into trends, resulting in a more lasting change in the way people approach physical fitness. Some of the more popular current trends in fitness and exercise are described below.

Newer Trends

Wearable fitness trackers have become extremely popular among those with an interest in overall health and well-being. These portable devices use sensors and other technology to records various biometric data such as heart rate, and physical activities such as walking, running, stair climbing, and so on. Wearable fitness trackers often work in conjunction with smart phone apps or other web-enabled technology.

Functional fitness is a relatively new trend among fitness enthusiasts. Functional fitness refers to exercise that is performed to enhance one's ability to carry out tasks of daily living. Those who practice functional fitness generally seek to increase their strength, balance, coordination, and endurance in order to increase overall quality of life.

"Latest Trends in Fitness and Exercise," © 2017 Omnigraphics. Reviewed September 2016.

As the population of the U.S. ages, the popularity of fitness programs tailored specifically for older adults continues to grow. With the increase among senior citizens and retirees who are interested in continuing an active lifestyle, demand is increasing for fitness programs to serve this demographic.

High-intensity interval training (HIIT) is another popular fitness trend. This style of workout involves short periods of intense activity followed by short periods of rest. A high-intensity interval workout generally lasts about 30 minutes, although some sessions can run longer.

The use of special flexibility/mobility roller equipment is rising, particularly among those who experience issues with full range of motion. These rollers can be used during warm-up or cool-down periods, to work on areas of the body that are trigger points, or muscles that need focused attention or deep tissue work.

Weight Training

Strength training, also known as weightlifting or bodybuilding, is another somewhat timeless fitness trend that has never fallen out of favor. Strength training involves lifting weights, either free weights or through the use of weight-lifting machines, in a manner that targets specific muscles or groups of muscles. In strength training, various weights are lifted in repetitions known as sets, with periods of rest between sets. Strength training can be performed at a gym or at home, using traditional weights and/or weightlifting machines.

Bodyweight training, also known as calisthenics, is a minimalist form of exercise that requires no special equipment. Bodyweight training uses a person's own body mass as resistance, for example, exercises such as push-ups, sit-ups, and jumping jacks. This type of exercise was once the most popular form of physical training in the United States. Although it never completely fell out of favor, bodyweight training has at various times been eclipsed by newer activities and workouts based around gym equipment. Bodyweight training is experiencing a resurgence in popularity among those looking for a "back to basics" approach to fitness.

Personal Trainers, Fitness Coaches, and Wellness

Personal training continues to be a popular trend in fitness. Modern fitness enthusiasts are demanding fitness training services provided by educated, certified, experienced fitness professionals. Consumers of personal training services have become more aware of the benefits of working with a certified trainer, and many consumers look for trainers that have certain credentials or qualifications. Group personal training has gained popularity among those looking for a more cost-effective way to access the services of a personal trainer. In group personal training, a small group of people share the cost of personal training sessions. Under this arrangement, the personal trainer divides his or her time in the training session among all the group members. Online fitness training is another option that is growing in popularity among those who wish to access the services of a personal trainer at a time or place that is most convenient for them.

Wellness coaching is a form of personal fitness training that uses a more integrative approach to behavior modification. Wellness coaching often focuses on disease prevention, rehabilitation, and health maintenance. Sessions can occur in person, by phone or video, or other format, including individual one-on-one sessions or group meetings.

Wellness tourism is a relatively new trend among fitness enthusiasts. The term "wellness" encompasses the total state of a person's health, including physical, mental, and social aspects, with particular focus on proactive measures that promote, maintain, and improve one's overall healthiness. Wellness tourism, also known as fitness tourism, is any form of recreational travel that supports the goals of total personal wellness. Wellness tourism focuses on disease prevention and enhancement of healthy lifestyles through visits to spas, hot springs, and other therapeutic retreat centers.

Continuing Trends

Programs that combine exercise and weight loss continue to be popular choices for many fitness enthusiasts. These programs combine physical fitness coaching with nutrition and dietary instruction to promote a more rounded approach to health and well-being.

Circuit training is another form of workout that has remained popular among fitness enthusiasts. Circuit training involves a selection of exercises that are done in sequence, normally to promote strength and endurance. One circuit is the completion of all the exercises in the program. Circuit training can include virtually any form of exercise, such as weightlifting, aerobics, and so on.

Yoga remains one of the most popular and enduring fitness trends in recent years. Sometimes practiced for stress reduction and relaxation, yoga can also be a form of exercise centered on stretching the body and assuming specific poses for specific amounts of time.

References

1. Brown, Jill S. "Top Fitness Trends for 2016: Does Your Favorite Make the List?" Huffington Post, November 23, 2015.

2. Roberts. Amy. "Forecast: The Top 10 Fitness Trends in 2016," Men's Fitness, 2016.

3. Thompson, Walter R. "Worldwide Survey of Fitness Trends for 2016: 10th Anniversary Edition," ACSM's Health and Fitness Journal, November/December 2015.

Chapter 50

Wellness or Fitness Tourism

What Is Wellness Tourism?

The term "wellness" encompasses the total state of a person's health, including physical, mental, and social aspects, with particular focus on proactive measures that promote, maintain, and improve one's overall healthiness. Wellness tourism, also known as fitness tourism, is any form of recreational travel that supports the goals of total personal wellness. Wellness tourism focuses on disease prevention and enhancement of healthy lifestyles through visits to spas, hot springs, and other therapeutic retreat centers. In contrast, medical tourism addresses existing health problems through treatment at hospitals or other medical centers.

Types of Wellness Tourism

There are many different types of wellness tourism opportunities that offer experiences and services addressing a broad spectrum of healthy living. Some wellness tourism destinations combine more than one area of focus, while others concentrate on a single aspect of overall health.

- **Eco Adventure:** Experiential destinations that typically emphasize time spent in nature, with activities such as hiking, biking, kayaking, paddle boarding, etc., and usually include guided tours. Some eco adventures include activities that are designed to be personally challenging, such as high ropes courses, extreme sports, or outdoor survival experiences.

- **Fitness:** Fitness retreats typically provide coaching and direction that emphasizes physical health, including gym workouts and other exercise programs such as pilates, stretching, cross-training, and so on. Some fitness retreats offer extreme sports activities or intensive boot-camp style physical programs.

- **Health:** These wellness tourism destinations typically focus on integrative health, often incorporating alternative medicine treatments, and therapies. Some health retreats focus on a specific issue such as stress management or relaxation techniques, while others promote overall health and well-being.

- **Healthy Eating:** Wellness centers that focus on healthy eating often provide instruction and guidance on nutrition, body cleansing and detoxification, organic eating, whole food diets, vegan or vegetarian living, weight management, and so on. Immersive weight-loss retreat centers typically combine nutrition and diet programs with fitness and exercise in a relaxed environment that fosters camaraderie among attendees.

- **Mind-Body:** These retreat centers often focus on wellness practices such as yoga, martial arts, meditation, tai chi, qigong, biofeedback, and so on.

- **Personal Growth and Development:** These lifestyle retreats often include activities intended to provide deep experiences of reflection and/or introspection through music, arts, writing, reading, life coaching, and so on.

- **Spa and Beauty:** Health resorts and specialty cruises provide a range of spa services including massage, therapeutic baths, hot springs, body treatments, facials, and other salon services.

- **Spiritual Connection:** Wellness centers that emphasize spiritual connection practices often include activities such as yoga, prayer, volunteering, time alone, time in silence, meditation, and so on.

Wellness Tourism Trends in the United States

Interest in wellness tourism is increasing in the United States, with billions of dollars being spent at these types of destinations each year.

Wellness tourism is popular among people who strive for a healthy lifestyle and want to incorporate those habits and interests into their travel experiences. In general, wellness tourists seek out experiences and destinations that help them maintain healthy lifestyles, often through activities that promote rejuvenation and relaxation, meaning and connection to self or others, authentic experiences as opposed to traditional tourist activities, and opportunities to learn about disease prevention and maintenance of overall good health. Wellness tourists are generally categorized in two groups: primary purpose and secondary purpose.

Primary-purpose wellness tourists are those who travel to wellness tourism destinations such as those listed above. Primary-purpose wellness tourists choose a vacation destination specifically for the wellness programs, services, or experiences that are offered.

Secondary-purpose wellness tourists are those who partake of wellness-related activities as part of their travel, for example visiting a gym, spa, or wellness center while on vacation or a business trip. Secondary-purpose wellness tourists strive to maintain healthy lifestyles and general wellness while travelling for other purposes.

References

1. "The Global Wellness Tourism Economy Executive Summary," Global Wellness Institute, October 2013.

2. "Wellness Tourism, a US$500 Billion Travel Industry," The Yucatan Times, July 31, 2015.

3. "Wellness tourism: An emerging trend in travel," Ontario Blue Cross, January 27, 2016.

Chapter 51

Online Fitness Training

What Is Online Fitness Training?

Online fitness training refers to the practice of working with a personal trainer or fitness coach via the Internet instead of in person. In most online fitness training programs, people subscribe to receive access to exercise programs and/or additional information and services from a personal trainer. Exercise programs are typically provided via video and are sometimes supplemented with written materials provided by email, web site, online chat, or other format.

General online fitness training usually consists of access to videos only. These videos contain recorded exercise routines to provide a virtual workout or exercise class experience, with no interaction between the instructor and the subscriber. Subscribers follow along with the video, performing the same moves shown on screen. In this format, the same videos are provided to all subscribers.

Personalized online fitness training often includes exercise programs and routines designed especially for the individual subscriber. This form of online fitness training generally includes some level of interactivity with the fitness trainer, which allows the consumer to ask questions and receive additional guidance.

Personalized online fitness training is sometimes offered in varying levels or packages. The most basic package might include a small monthly fee for access to online videos and web site materials related to fitness, exercise, nutrition, or an online discussion area where

"Online Fitness Training," © 2017 Omnigraphics. Reviewed September 2016.

subscribers share tips, personal experiences, and motivate each other. Another package might include more personalized information for a higher monthly fee. In this level, each subscriber typically has access to an individual trainer who provides exercise and nutrition plans and feedback tailored to individual goals. Interaction between the trainer and the subscriber can be by phone, email, and/or webcam. At the highest service level, subscribers can often gain unlimited access to a personal trainer who works with them at every level, including assessment, goal setting, accountability, progression, and so on.

Are Online Training Programs Effective?

Online fitness training programs can be effective for subscribers who are self-motivated and able to commit to following a program on their own, without a trainer by their side during workouts. Advantages to online fitness training include:

- **Accessibility of personal trainers:** For those who travel often or live in an area without access to an experienced personal trainer.

- **Access to well-known trainers:** Online fitness training allows subscribers to benefit from working with a highly experienced trainer no matter where they are located.

- **Access to specialized trainers:** For those who want specialized training, online fitness training can be a way to work with established experts who are located in distant areas.

- **Reference checking:** Online fitness trainers often gain their reputation through client reviews, social media activity, and other online forums. Subscribers can thoroughly research an online trainer before engaging in a potentially costly relationship.

- **Lower cost of training:** An expert personal trainer has limited time to work with clients in person, and high demand can influence the cost of training sessions. In some cases, monthly subscription fees may be the same as a one-hour session of in-person training.

- **Flexibility:** Subscribers can access workouts at any convenient time and place.

- **Support:** Online trainers often provide more support options than in-person trainers through the use of email or other forms of communication.

Disadvantages of Online Training Programs

There are also disadvantages to online fitness training programs. Some of these include:

- **Lack of personalization:** Some fitness programs are not personalized for an individual's goals, but intended to serve as many people as possible.

- **Lack of motivation:** Subscribers need to be able to motivate themselves without the trainer at their side during workouts.

- **Cost:** Even the lowest monthly fee can be a burden for some potential subscribers.

- **Lack of guidance on technique:** Without the trainer present during workouts, there is no immediate feedback or correction on exercise form, method, or performance.

- **Difficult to assess progress:** Online trainers sometimes have difficulty accurately measuring the progress of clients because the trainer is not present during workouts.

Is Online Training Right for You?

As with in-person fitness training, consumers should carefully evaluate the offerings, skills, and experience of any potential online fitness trainers. Some points to keep in mind include:

- Can an individual trainer help you meet your goals? Do their programs address your areas of concern? Look for a trainer who provides workouts that work for you.

- Is an individual trainer knowledgeable of current practices in health and fitness? What are their qualifications and experience?

- Can an individual trainer provide references from former or current clients? Can you verify that their programs produce results?

- Is an individual trainer reviewed or discussed online? Web searches can often provide insight on an individual trainer's reputation.

- Does an individual trainer offer something that you can't get on your own or through one or two sessions with an in-person trainer?

References

1. Laidler, Scott. "Does online personal training work?" The Telegraph, April 24, 2014.

2. "The Next Frontier of Fitness: An Introduction to Online Personal Training," Bodybuilding.com, May 29, 2013.

3. Smith, Dave. "The 50 Best Free Workout Resources You Can Find Online," Huffington Post, June 7, 2016.

Chapter 52

Fitness Wearables and Wearable Technology

The broad scope of digital health includes categories such as mobile health (mHealth), health information technology (IT), wearable devices, telehealth and telemedicine, and personalized medicine.

Providers and other stakeholders are using digital health in their efforts to:

- Reduce inefficiencies
- Improve access
- Reduce costs
- Increase quality
- Make medicine more personalized for patients

Patients and consumers can use digital health to better manage and track their health and wellness related activities. The use of technologies such as smart phones, social networks and internet applications is not only changing the way we communicate, but is also providing innovative ways for us to monitor our health and well-being and giving us greater access to information. Together these advancements are leading to a convergence of people, information, technology, and connectivity to improve healthcare and health outcomes.

Why Is the FDA Focusing on Digital Health?

Many medical devices now have the ability to connect to and communicate with other devices or systems. Devices that are already U.S. Food and Drug Administration (FDA) approved or cleared are being updated to add digital features. New types of devices that already have these capabilities are being explored.

Many stakeholders are involved in digital health activities, including patients, healthcare practitioners, researchers, traditional medical device industry firms, and firms new to FDA regulatory requirements, such as mobile application developers.

FDA's Center for Devices and Radiological Health (CDRH) is excited about these advances and the convergence of medical devices with connectivity and consumer technology.

The following are topics in the digital health field on which the FDA has been working to provide clarity using practical approaches that balance benefits and risks:

- Wireless Medical Devices

- Mobile medical apps

- Health IT

- Telemedicine

- Medical Device Data Systems

- Medical device Interoperability

- Software as a Medical Device (SaMD)

- General Wellness

- Cybersecurity

How Is the FDA Advancing Digital Health?

CDRH has established the Digital Health Program which seeks to better protect and promote public health and provide continued regulatory clarity by:

- Fostering collaborations and enhancing outreach to digital health customers

- Developing and implementing regulatory strategies and policies for digital health technologies

Wearable Trackers

Wearable trackers can help motivate you during workouts and provide information about your daily routine or fitness in combination with your smartphone without requiring potentially disruptive manual calculations or records. This paper summarizes and compares wearable fitness devices, also called "fitness trackers" or "activity trackers."

These devices are becoming increasingly popular in personal health-care, motivating people to exercise more throughout the day without the need for lifestyle changes. The various choices in the market for wearable devices are also increasing, with customers searching for products that best suit their personal needs. Further, using a wearable device or fitness tracker can help people reach a fitness goal or finish line. Generally, companies display advertising for these kinds of products and depict them as beneficial, user friendly, and accurate. However, there are no objective research results to prove the veracity of their words. This research features subjective and objective experimental results, which reveal that some devices perform better than others.

Ingestibles, Wearables and Embeddables

Routine tests can be anything but. Appointment times are often inconvenient. You may be at the mercy of walk-in labs and testing facilities, where waiting could be uncertain and often longer than many people can accommodate. Personal health – which should be a top priority – can suffer when important diagnostic tests fall off our to-do lists.

Recent advances in broadband-enabled sensor technology offer the potential for the emergence of more convenient, ultimately less-costly – and less-invasive – solutions. For example, we may soon see widespread use of smart clothing (or smart "tattoo" applications) that use skin-based sensors to measure things like heart rate, respiration and blood pressure. These new types of technologies are generically called "ingestibles," "wearables" and "embeddables."

Ingestibles are broadband-enabled digital tools that we actually "eat." For example, there are "smart" pills that use wireless technology to help monitor internal reactions to medications. Or imagine a smart pill that tracks blood levels of medications in a patient's body throughout the day to help physicians find optimum dosage levels, avoid overmedicating, and truly individualize treatment. Also, miniature pill-shaped video cameras may one day soon replace colonoscopies or endoscopies. Patients would simply swallow a "pill," which would collect and transmit images as it makes its way through the digestive system.

Wearables are digital tools you can "wear," such as wristwatch-like devices that have sensors to monitor your heart rate and other vital signs. Beyond medical monitoring, such wearables may also help improve athletic performance, track fitness goals or help prevent dangerous falls in the elderly. In fact, designers are now able to put sensors in T-shirts and other clothing to monitor perspiration as a stress indicator. And, "tattoo-like" sensor that could be peeled off after use or that might be absorbed by the body are another similar advance. These sensors gather data through skin contact and transmit information wirelessly to smartphones and remote diagnostic facilities.

Embeddables are miniature devices that are actually inserted under the skin or deeper into the body. A heart pacemaker is one kind of embeddable device. In the future, embeddables may use nanotechnology and be so tiny that doctors would simply "inject" them into our bodies. Some promising applications in this area could help diabetes patients monitor their blood sugar levels reliably and automatically, without the need to prick their fingers or otherwise draw blood.

Part Eight

Additional Help and Information

Chapter 53

Glossary of Terms Related to Fitness and Exercise

absolute intensity: The amount of energy used by the body per minute of activity.

aerobic exercise: Any continuous activity of large muscle groups that forces your heart and lungs to work harder. Aerobic means your heart and lungs are using oxygen.

aerobic physical activity: Aerobic (or endurance) physical activities use large muscle groups (back, chest, and legs) to increase heart rate and breathing for an extended period of time.

balance training: Static and dynamic exercises that are designed to improve individuals' ability to withstand challenges from postural sway or destabilizing stimuli caused by self-motion, the environment, or other objects.

balance: A performance-related component of physical fitness that involves the maintenance of the body's equilibrium while stationary or moving.

baseline activity: The light-intensity activities of daily life, such as standing, walking slowly, and lifting lightweight objects. People who do only baseline activity are considered to be inactive.

This glossary contains terms excerpted from documents produced by several sources deemed reliable.

body composition: A health-related component of physical fitness that applies to body weight and the relative amounts of muscle, fat, bone, and other vital tissues of the body. Most often, the components are limited to fat and lean body mass (or fat-free mass).

body mass index (BMI): A measure of body weight relative to height. BMI is a tool that is often used to determine if a person is at a healthy weight, overweight, or obese, and whether a person's health is at risk due to his or her weight.

bone-strengthening activity: Physical activity primarily designed to increase the strength of specific sites in bones that make up the skeletal system.

calisthenics: Physical exercises done without equipment to build muscular strength, endurance, and flexibility.

calorie: A unit of energy in food. Foods have carbohydrates, proteins, and/or fats. Some beverages have alcohol. Carbohydrates and proteins have four calories per gram. Fat has nine calories per gram. Alcohol has seven calories per gram.

carbohydrate: A major source of energy in the diet. There are two kinds of carbohydrates—simple carbohydrates and complex carbohydrates: simple carbohydrates are sugars and complex carbohydrates include both starches and fiber.

cholesterol: A fatty substance present in all parts of the body. It is a component of cell membranes and is used to make vitamin D and some hormones. Some cholesterol in the body is produced by the liver and some is derived from food, particularly animal products.

cool down: A gradual reduction of the intensity of physical activity to allow physiological processes to return to normal.

dehydration: Excessive loss of body water that the body needs to carry on normal functions at an optimal level.

diabetes: A disease in which blood glucose (blood sugar) levels are above normal. There are two main types of diabetes. Type 1 diabetes is caused by a problem with the body's defense system, called the immune system. This form of diabetes usually starts in childhood or adolescence. Type 2 diabetes is the most common form of diabetes. It starts most often in adulthood.

diet: What a person eats and drinks. Any type of eating plan.

duration: The length of time in which an activity or exercise is performed. Duration is generally expressed in minutes.

energy expenditure: The amount of energy that you use measured in calories. You use calories to breathe, send blood through your blood vessels, digest food, maintain posture, and be physically active.

exercise: A subcategory of physical activity that is planned, structured, repetitive, and purposive in the sense that the improvement or maintenance of one or more components of physical fitness is the objective.

fat: A major source of energy in the diet. All food fats have nine calories per gram. Fat helps the body absorb fat-soluble vitamins, such as vitamins A, D, E, and K, and carotenoids. Some kinds of fats, especially saturated fats and trans fats, may raise blood cholesterol and increase the risk for heart disease. Other fats, such as unsaturated fats, do not raise blood cholesterol.

flexibility: A health- and performance-related component of physical fitness that is the range of motion possible at a joint. Flexibility is specific to each joint and depends on a number of specific variables, including but not limited to the tightness of specific ligaments and tendons.

frequency: The number of times an exercise or activity is performed. Frequency is generally expressed in sessions, episodes, or bouts per week.

glucose: Glucose is a major source of energy for our bodies and a building block for many carbohydrates. The food digestion process breaks down carbohydrates in foods and drinks into glucose. After digestion, glucose is carried in the blood and goes to body cells where it is used for energy or stored.

health: A human condition with physical, social and psychological dimensions, each characterized on a continuum with positive and negative poles. Positive health is associated with a capacity to enjoy life and to withstand challenges; it is not merely the absence of disease. Negative health is associated with illness, and in the extreme, with premature death.

healthy weight: Compared to overweight or obese, a body weight that is less likely to be linked with any weight-related health problems, such as type 2 diabetes, heart disease, high blood pressure, and high blood cholesterol. A body mass index (BMI) of 18.5 to 24.9 is considered a healthy weight, though not all individuals with a BMI in this range may be at a healthy level of body fat; they may have more body fat tissue and less muscle. A person with a BMI of 25 to 29.9 is considered overweight, and a person with a BMI of 30 or more is considered obese.

heart disease: A number of abnormal conditions affecting the heart and the blood vessels in the heart. The most common type of heart disease is coronary artery disease, which is the gradual buildup of plaques in the coronary arteries, the blood vessels that bring blood to the heart. This disease develops slowly and silently, over decades. It can go virtually unnoticed until it produces a heart attack.

heart rate: Reserve is the difference between the resting heart rate and the maximal heart rate.

high blood pressure: Your blood pressure rises and falls throughout the day. An optimal blood pressure is less than 120/80 mmHg. When blood pressure stays high—greater than or equal to 140/90 mmHg—you have high blood pressure, also called "hypertension." With high blood pressure, the heart works harder, your arteries take a beating, and your chances of a stroke, heart attack, and kidney problems are greater.

high-density lipoprotein (HDL): HDL is a compound made up of fat and protein that carries cholesterol in the blood to the liver, where it is broken down and excreted. Commonly called "good" cholesterol, high levels of HDL cholesterol are linked to a lower risk of heart disease.

hydration: The amount of fluid in your body. It is important to replace any fluid your body loses during physical activity.

hypertension: Also called high blood pressure, it is having blood pressure greater than 140 over 90 mmHg (millimeters of mercury). Long-term high blood pressure can damage blood vessels and organs, including the heart, kidneys, eyes, and brain.

insulin: A hormone made by the pancreas, insulin helps move glucose (sugar) from the blood to muscles and other tissues. Insulin controls blood sugar levels.

intensity: Intensity refers to how much work is being performed or the magnitude of the effort required to perform an activity or exercise.

interval training: An exercise session in which the intensity and duration of exercise are consciously alternated between harder and easier work. Often used to improve aerobic capacity and/or anaerobic endurance in people who exercise regularly or who are physically well trained.

leisure-time physical activity: A recreational activity generally associated with pleasure and/or health and fitness. Such activities are varied as to type and intensity. Some leisure-time activities are of light intensity such as sitting in a boat fishing; others are of moderate activity, such as low impact aerobics. Those that are classified as vigorous intensity are more strenuous, such as high impact aerobics or running.

low-density lipoprotein (LDL): LDL is a compound made up of fat and protein that carries cholesterol in the blood from the liver to other parts of the body. High levels of LDL cholesterol, commonly called "bad" cholesterol, cause a buildup of cholesterol in the arteries and increase the risk of heart disease. An LDL level of less than 100 mg/dL is considered optimal, 100 to 129 mg/dL is considered near or above optimal, 130 to 159 mg/dL is considered borderline high, 160 to 189 mg/dL is considered high, and 190 mg/dL or greater is considered very high.

metabolic syndrome: A person with metabolic syndrome has a group of medical problems that, when they occur together, may increase the risk of heart disease and diabetes. These problems are a large waist size, high blood pressure, high blood sugar levels, high levels of triglycerides, and low levels of high-density lipoprotein (HDL).

metabolism: All of the processes in the body that make and use energy, such as digesting food and nutrients and removing waste through urine and feces.

moderate-intensity physical activity: On an absolute scale, physical activity that is done at 3.0 to 5.9 times the intensity of rest. On a scale relative to an individual's personal capacity, moderate-intensity physical activity is usually a 5 or 6 on a scale of 0 to 10.

muscle-strengthening activity: Physical activity, including exercise that increases skeletal muscle strength, power, endurance, and mass.

nutrition: The process of the body using food to sustain life.

obesity: Excess body fat. Because body fat is usually not measured, a ratio of body weight to height is often used instead. It is defined as BMI. An adult who has a BMI of 30 or higher is considered obese.

oils: Fats that are liquid at room temperature, oils come from many different plants and from seafood. Some common oils include canola, corn, olive, peanut, safflower, soybean, and sunflower oils. A number of foods are naturally high in oils, such as avocados, olives, nuts, and some fish.

osteoarthritis: A joint disease that mostly affects cartilage, the slippery tissue that covers the ends of bones in a joint. The top layer of cartilage breaks down and wears away. This allows bones under the cartilage to rub together, which causes pain, swelling, and loss of motion of the joint.

osteoporosis: A bone disease that is characterized by progressive loss of bone density and thinning of bone tissue, causing bones to break easily.

overload: The amount of new activity added to a person's usual level of activity. The risk of injury to bones, muscles, and joints is directly related to the size of the gap between these two levels. This gap is called the amount of overload.

overweight: A body mass index (BMI) of 25 to 29.9. Body weight comes from fat, muscle, bone, and body water. It is important to remember that although BMI correlates with the amount of body fat, BMI does not directly measure body fat. As a result, some people, such as athletes, may have a BMI that identifies them as overweight even though they do not have excess body fat.

pancreas: A gland and an organ that makes enzymes to help the body break down and use nutrients in food. The pancreas also produces the hormone insulin and releases it into the bloodstream to help the body control blood sugar levels.

pedometer: A step counter that is worn at the waist or on a person's waistband. It tallies the number of steps a person takes each day. Walking 2,000 steps is equal to about one mile and roughly 100 calories are burned over and above calories for resting metabolism.

physical activity: Any bodily movement produced by the contraction of skeletal muscle that increases energy expenditure above a basal level. In these Guidelines, physical activity generally refers to the subset of physical activity that enhances health.

physical fitness: The ability to carry out daily tasks with vigor and alertness, without undue fatigue, and with ample energy to enjoy leisure-time pursuits and respond to emergencies.

progression: The process of increasing the intensity, duration, frequency, or amount of activity or exercise as the body adapts to a given activity pattern.

protein: One of the nutrients that provide calories to the body. Protein is an essential nutrient that helps build many parts of the body, including blood, bone, muscle, and skin. Protein provides 4 calories per gram.

relative intensity: The level of effort required by a person to do an activity. When using relative intensity, people pay attention to how physical activity affects their heart rate and breathing.

repetitions: The number of times a person lifts a weight in muscle-strengthening activities. Repetitions are analogous to duration in aerobic activity.

saturated fat: This type of fat is solid at room temperature. Saturated fat is found in full-fat dairy products (like butter, cheese, cream, regular ice cream, and whole milk), coconut oil, lard, palm oil, ready-to-eat meats, and the skin and fat of chicken and turkey, among other foods. Saturated fats have the same number of calories as other types of fat, and may contribute to weight gain if eaten in excess. Eating a diet high in saturated fat also raises blood cholesterol and risk of heart disease.

serving size: A standard amount of a food, such as a cup or an ounce.

strength: A health and performance component of physical fitness that is the ability of a muscle or muscle group to exert force.

stretching: Stretching includes movements that lengthen muscles to their maximum extension and move joints to the limits of their extension.

stroke: A stroke occurs when blood flow to your brain stops. Within minutes, brain cells begin to die. There are two kinds of stroke. The more common kind, called ischemic stroke, is caused by a blood clot that blocks or plugs a blood vessel in the brain. The other kind, called hemorrhagic stroke, is caused by a blood vessel that breaks and bleeds into the brain. "Mini-strokes," or transient ischemic attacks (TIAs), occur when the blood supply to the brain is stopped for a short time.

sugar-sweetened beverages: Drinks that are sweetened with added sugars often add a large number of calories. These beverages include, but are not limited to, energy and sports drinks, fruit drinks, soda, and fruit juices.

target heart rate: A safe heart rate recommended for fitness workouts; it depends on age and gender. It is the rate you want the heart to work (beats per minute) during a certain activity. You can use it to help determine the intensity of an activity.

vigorous-intensity physical activity: On an absolute scale, physical activity that is done at 6.0 or more times the intensity of rest. On a scale relative to an individual's personal capacity, vigorous-intensity physical activity is usually a 7 or 8 on a scale of 0 to 10.

warm-up: A gradual increase in the intensity of exercise to allow physiological processes to prepare for greater energy outputs. Changes include a rise in body temperature, cardiorespiratory changes (i.e., increased heart and ventilation rate), and increase in muscle elasticity and contractility.

weight control: This refers to achieving and maintaining a healthy weight with healthy eating and physical activity.

Chapter 54

Directory of Fitness Resources

Government Agencies That Provide Information about Fitness and Exercise

Americans with Disabilities Act (ADA)

U.S. Department of Justice
950 Pennsylvania Ave. NW
Civil Rights Division, Disability
Rights Section-NYA
Washington, DC 20530
Toll-Free: 800-514-0301
Phone: 202-307-0663
Toll-Free TTY: 800-514-0383
Fax: 202-307-1197
Website: www.ada.gov
E-mail: FTA.ADAassistance@
dot.gov

Centers for Disease Control and Prevention (CDC)

Division of Nutrition, Physical
Activity, and Obesity (DNPAO)
1600 Clifton Rd.
Atlanta, GA 30329-4027
Toll-Free: 800-CDC-INFO
(800-232-4636)
Toll-Free TTY: 888-232-6348
Website: http://www.cdc.gov/
nccdphp/dnpao
E-mail: cdcinfo@cdc.gov

Resources in this chapter were compiled from several sources deemed reliable; all contact information was verified and updated in September 2016.

National Cancer Institute (NCI)
NCI Public Inquiries Office
9609 Medical Center Dr.
Bldg. 9609 MSC 9760
Bethesda, MD 20892-9760
Toll-Free: 800-4-CANCER
(800-422-6237)
Website: www.cancer.gov

National Center for Complementary and Integrative Health (NCCIH)
NCCIH Clearinghouse
9000 Rockville Pike
Bethesda, MD 20892
Toll-Free: 888-644-6226
TTY: 866-464-3615
Website: www.nccih.nih.gov
E-mail: info@nccih.nih.gov

National Diabetes Information Clearinghouse (NDIC)
1 Information Way
Bethesda, MD 20892-3560
Toll-Free: 800-860-8747
Toll-Free TTY: 866-569-1162
Fax: 703-738-4929
Website: www.niddk.nih.gov
E-mail: healthinfo@niddk.nih.gov

National Heart, Lung, and Blood Institute (NHLBI)
NHLBI Health Information Center
P.O. Box 30105
Bethesda, MD 20824-0105
Phone: 301-592-8573
TTY: 240-629-3255
Fax: 301-592-8563
Website: www.nhlbi.nih.gov
E-mail: nhlbiinfo@nhlbi.nih.gov

National Institute of Arthritis and Musculoskeletal and Skin Diseases (NIAMS)
Information Clearinghouse
National Institutes of Health
1 AMS Cir.
Bethesda, MD 20892-3675
Toll-Free: 877-22-NIAMS
(877-226-4267)
Phone: 301-495-4484
TTY: 301-565-2966
Fax: 301-718-6366
Website: www.niams.nih.gov
E-mail: NIAMSinfo@mail.nih.gov

National Institute of Diabetes and Digestive and Kidney Diseases (NIDDK)
Office of Communications and Public Liaison
9000 Rockville Pike
Bethesda, MD 20892
Phone: 301-496-3583
Website: www.niddk.nih.gov

National Institute of Mental Health (NIMH)
6001 Executive Blvd.
Rockville, MD 20852
Toll-Free: 866-615-NIMH
(866-615-6464)
Phone: 301-443-4513
Toll-Free TTY: 866-415-8051
TTY: 301-443-8431
Fax: 301-443-4279
Website: www.nimh.nih.gov
E-mail: nimhinfo@nih.gov

National Institute on Aging (NIA)
31 Center Dr. MSC 2292
Bethesda, MD 20892
Phone: 301-496-1752
Toll-Free TTY: 800-222-4225
Fax: 301-496-1072
Website: www.nia.nih.gov
E-mail: niaic@nia.nih.gov

National Institutes of Health (NIH)
9000 Rockville Pike
Bethesda, MD 20892
Phone: 301-496-4000
TTY: 301-402-9612
Website: www.nih.gov
E-mail: NIHinfo@od.nih.gov

National Library of Medicine (NLM)
Reference and Web Services
8600 Rockville Pike
Bethesda, MD 20894
Toll-Free: 888-FIND-NLM
(888-346-3656)
Phone: 301-594-5983
Toll-Free TDD: 800-735-2258
Fax: 301-402-1384
Website: www.nlm.nih.gov
E-mail: custserv@nlm.nih.gov

National Women's Health Information Center
U.S. Department of Health and Human Services (HHS)
200 Independence Ave. S.W.
Rm. 712E
Washington, DC 20201
Toll-Free: 800-994-9662
Phone: 202-690-7650
Toll-Free TDD: 888-220-5446
Website: www.womenshealth.gov

President's Council on Physical Fitness and Sports (PCPFS)
1101 Wootton Pkwy
Ste. 560
Rockville, MD 20852
Phone: 240-276-9567
Fax: 240-276-9860
Website: www.fitness.gov
E-mail: fitness@hhs.gov

U.S. Consumer Product Safety Commission (CPSC)
4330 E.W. Hwy
Bethesda, MD 20814
Toll-Free: 800-638-2772
(Hotline)
Phone: 301-504-7923
Toll-Free TTY: 800-638-8270
Fax: 301-504-0124; 301-504-0025
Website: www.cpsc.gov

U.S. Department of Health and Human Services (HHS)
200 Independence Ave. S.W.
Washington, DC 20201
Toll-Free: 877-696-6775
(Hotline)
Website: www.hhs.gov

Weight-Control Information Network (WIN)
National Institute of Diabetes and Digestive and Kidney Diseases (NIDDK)
1 WIN Way
Bethesda, MD 20892-3665
Toll-Free: 877-946-4627
Fax: 202-828-1028
Website: www.win.niddk.nih.gov
E-mail: win@info.niddk.nih.gov

Private Organizations That Provide Information about Fitness and Exercise

Action for Healthy Kids
600 W. Van Buren St.
Ste. #720
Chicago, IL 60607
Toll-Free: 800-416-5136
Fax: 312-212-0098
Website: www.
actionforhealthykids.org

Aerobics and Fitness Association of America (AFAA)
1750 E. Northrop Blvd.
Ste. 200
Chandler, AZ 85286-1744
Toll-Free: 800-446-2322
Website: www.afaa.com

American Academy of Orthopaedic Surgeons (AAOS)
9400 W. Higgins Rd.
Rosemont, IL 60018
Phone: 847-823-7186
Fax: 847-823-8125
Website: www.aaos.org
E-mail: custserv@aaos.org

Physical Education and Health Education-Shape America
1900 Association Dr.
Reston, VA 20191
Toll-Free: 800-213-7193
Phone: 703-476-3400
Fax: 703-476-9527
Website: www.shapeamerica.org

American College of Sports Medicine (ACSM)
401 W. Michigan St.
Indianapolis, IN 46202-3233
Phone: 317-637-9200
Fax: 317-634-7817
Website: www.acsm.org

American Council on Exercise (ACE)
4851 Paramount Dr.
San Diego, CA 92123
Toll-Free: 888-825-3636
Phone: 858-279-8227
Fax: 858-576-6564
Website: www.acefitness .org
E-mail: support@acefitness.org

American Diabetes Association (ADA)
1701 N. Beauregard St.
Alexandria, VA 22311
Phone: 800-DIABETES
(800-342-2383)
Website: www.diabetes.org

American Heart Association (AHA)
7272 Greenville Ave.
Dallas, TX 75231
Toll-Free: 800-AHA-USA1
(800-242-8721)
Website: www.heart.org

American Stroke Association
7272 Greenville Ave.
Dallas, TX 75231
Toll-Free: 888-4-STROKE
(888-478-7653)
Website: www.strokeassociation.
org

American Lung Association
55 W. Wacker Dr.
Ste. 1150
Chicago, IL 60601
Toll-Free: 800-LUNGUSA (800-586-4872) (Helpline)
Phone: 202-785-3355
Fax: 202-452-1805
Website: www.lung.org
E-mail: info@lung.org

American Orthopaedic Society for Sports Medicine (AOSSM)
9400 W. Higgins Rd.
Ste. 300
Rosemont, IL 60018
Toll-Free: 877-321-3500
Phone: 847-292-4900
Fax: 847-292-4905
Website: www.sportsmed.org
E-mail: aossm@aossm.org

American Physical Therapy Association (APTA)
1111 N. Fairfax St.
Alexandria, VA 22314-1488
Toll-Free: 800-999-2782
Phone: 703-684-APTA
(800-684-2782)
TDD: 703-683-6748
Fax: 703-684-7343
Website: www.apta.org
E-mail: memberservices@apta.org

American Physiological Society (APS)
9650 Rockville Pike
Bethesda, MD 20814-3991
Phone: 301-634-7164
Fax: 301-634-7241
Website: www.the-aps.org

American Running Association (ARA)
4405 E.W. Hwy
Ste. 405
Bethesda, MD 20814
Phone: 800-776-2732 ext. 13 or ext. 12
Fax: 301-913-9520
Website: www.americanrunning.
org

Arthritis Foundation (AF)
1355 Peachtree St. N.E.
6th Fl.
Atlanta, GA 30309
Toll-Free: 800-283-7800
Website: www.arthritis.org

Asthma and Allergy Foundation of America (AAFA)
8201 Corporate Dr.
Ste. 1000
Landover, MD 20785
Toll-Free: 800-7-ASTHMA
(800-727-8462)
Website: www.aafa.org
E-mail: info@aafa.org

Aquatic Exercise Association (AEA)
P.O. Box 1609
Nokomis, FL 34274-1609
Toll-Free: 888-232-9283
Phone: 941-486-8600
Website: www.aeawave.com

Cleveland Clinic
9500 Euclid Ave.
Cleveland, OH 44195
Toll-Free: 800-223-2273
Phone: 216-444-2200
TTY: 216-444-0261
Website: my.clevelandclinic.org
E-mail: myconsult@ccf.org

Disabled Sports USA (DS / USA)
451 Hungerford Dr.
Ste. 100
Rockville, MD 20850
Phone: 301-217-0960
Fax: 301-217-0968
Website: www.
disabledsportsusa.org
E-mail: information@dsusa.org

HealthyWomen (HW)
P.O. Box 430
Red Bank, NJ 07701
Toll-Free: 877-986-9472
Phone: 732-530-3425
Fax: 732-865-7225
Website: www.healthywomen.
org
E-mail: info@healthywomen.org

IDEA Health and Fitness Association
10190 Telesis Ct.
San Diego, CA 92121
Toll-Free: 800-999-4332 ext. 7
Phone: 858-535-8979 ext. 7
Fax: 619-344-0380
Website: www.ideafit.com
E-mail: contact@ideafit.com

International Fitness Association (IFA)
12472 Lake Underhill Rd.
Ste. 341
Orlando, FL 32828-7144
Toll-Free: 800-227-1976
Phone: 407-579-8610
Website: www.ifafitness.com

National Alliance for Youth Sports (NAYS)
2050 Vista Pkwy
West Palm Beach, FL 33411
Toll-Free: 800-688-KIDS
(800-688-5437)
Phone: 800-688-5437
Fax: 561-684-2546
Website: www.nays.org
E-mail: nays@nays.org

National Association for Health and Fitness (NAHF)
c/o Be Active New York State
10 Kings Mill Ct.
Albany, NY 12205-3632
Phone: 716-583-0521
Fax: 716-851-4309
Website: www.physicalfitness.org
E-mail: wellness@city-buffalo.org

National Center on Physical Activity and Disability (NCPAD)
University of Illinois at Chicago
Department of Disability and
Human Development
4000 Ridgeway Dr.
Birmingham, AL 35209
Toll-Free: 800-900-8086
Fax: 205-313-7475
Website: www.ncpad.org
E-mail: email@nchpad.org

National Coalition for Promoting Physical Activity (NCPPA)
1150 Connecticut Ave. N.W.
Ste. 300
Washington, DC 20036
Phone: 202-454-7521
Fax: 202-454-7598
Website: www.ncppa.org
E-mail: NCPPA@heart.org

National Osteoporosis Foundation (NOF)
251 18th St. S.
Ste. 630
Arlington, VA 22202
Toll-Free: 800-231-4222
Phone: 202-223-2226
Website: www.nof.org
E-mail: info@nof.org

National Recreation and Park Association (NRPA)
22377 Belmont Ridge Rd.
Ashburn, VA 20148
Toll-Free: 800-626-NRPA
(800-626-6772)
Website: www.nrpa.org

National Strength and Conditioning Association (NSCA)
1885 Bob Johnson Dr.
Colorado Springs, CO 80906
Toll-Free: 800-815-6826
Phone: 719-632-6722
Fax: 719-632-6367
Website: www.nsca.com
E-mail: nsca@nsca-lift.org

The Nemours Foundation
10140 Centurion Pkwy N.
Jacksonville, FL 32256
Phone: 904-697-4100
Website: www.nemours.org

PE Central
2516 Blossom Trail W.
Blacksburg, VA 24060
Phone: 540-953-1043
Fax: 866-776-9170
Website: www.pecentral.org
E-mail: pec@pecentral.org

Women's Sports Foundation
Eisenhower Park 1899
Hempstead Tpke
Ste. 400
East Meadow, NY 11554
Toll-Free: 800-227-3988
Phone: 516-542-4700
Fax: 516-542-0095
Website: www.
womenssportsfoundation.org
E-mail: Info@
WomensSportsFoundation.org

Index

Index

Page numbers followed by 'n' indicate a footnote. Page numbers in *italics* indicate a table or illustration.

536